Ocular Surface Disease

OCULAR SURFACE DISEASE

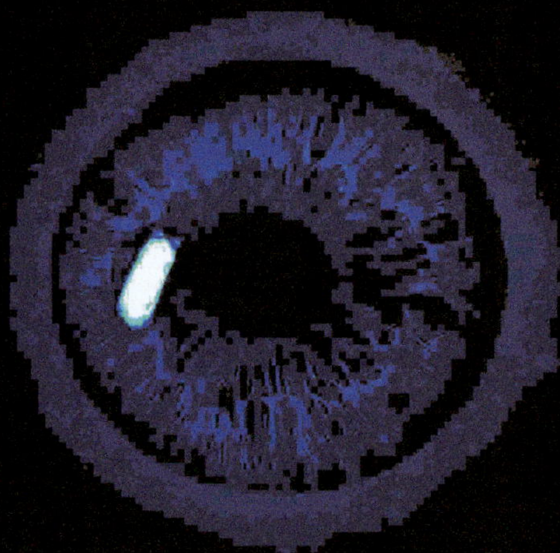

A Case-Based Update

Editor: Ali R. Djalilian, M.D.

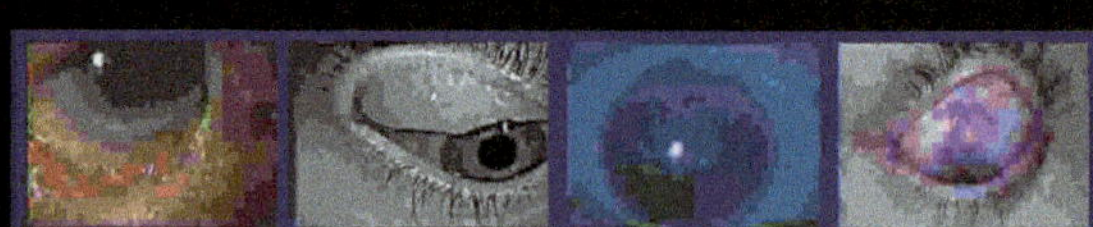

Ali R. Djalilian
Editor

Ocular Surface Disease

A Case-Based Guide

Springer

Editor
Ali R. Djalilian
Cornea Service
Illinois Eye and Ear Infirmary
Chicago, IL
USA

Additional material to this book can be downloaded from https://link.springer.com/book/10.1007/978-3-319-15823-5.

ISBN 978-3-319-15822-8 ISBN 978-3-319-15823-5 (eBook)
DOI 10.1007/978-3-319-15823-5

Library of Congress Control Number: 2017955574

Printed on acid-free paper

This Springer imprint is published by Springer Nature
The registered company is Springer International Publishing AG
The registered company address is: Gewerbestrasse 11, 6330 Cham, Switzerland

Preface

It is well known that some of the best clinical diagnosis and management pearls cannot be found in regular textbooks or journal papers. Inspired by the great teachers and colleagues who have taught me most of what I know today, I decided to put this book together using a case-based format to help disseminate some of that hard to find information in ocular surface disease. I was fortunate that the best and the brightest in this field offered to graciously share with the readers their clinical experiences in this rapidly evolving field.

Each chapter is built around three actual patient cases with varying degrees of complexity. Detailed aspects of the care are described throughout the entire patient course in order to provide practical information and illustrate real-world challenges—in the end it is all about patients. The book covers the most common ocular surface diseases ranging from tear film insufficiency to the more severe cicatricial diseases such as pemphigoid and Stevens-Johnson syndrome. The contributors have chosen fantastic cases that should make this book useful for clinicians with a wide range of experiences. The more medical chapters are in the first half, while the more surgically oriented chapters are in the latter half, but the chapters/cases can be read in any order.

In addition to all the outstanding contributors without whom this book would have never been possible, I want to thank the publisher, Springer, who first proposed this book and who waited patiently for the final product. I have to acknowledge Dr. Robert Swan who came up with the question and answer format while writing the chapter on cicatricial conjunctival disease with Dr. Foster—I adopted this format for all the chapters.

I also want to take this opportunity to express my sincere gratitude to all the mentors and close colleagues who have supported me throughout my career. I want to specifically acknowledge Dr. Ed Holland who inspired me to pursue ophthalmology and focus on ocular surface disease and the late Dr. Bob Nussenblatt, the quintessential clinician-scientist and role model who attracted me to the National Institutes of Health—my gateway to the world of biomedical research.

Last but not least, I want to thank my immediate family, my wife and kids, and my siblings and parents, whose unconditional love and support have enabled me to pursue all my dreams.

Chicago, IL Ali R. Djalilian, MD

Contents

Contributors

Vinay K. Aakalu, MD, MPH Department of Ophthalmology and Visual Sciences, University of Illinois at Chicago, Chicago, IL, USA

Alessandro Abbouda, MD Cornea Service, New England Eye Center, Boston, MA, USA

Department of Ophthalmology, Center for Translational Ocular Immunology, Tufts Medical Center, Tufts University School of Medicine, Boston, MA, USA

Ahmad A. Aref, MD Department of Ophthalmology and Visual Sciences, Illinois Eye and Ear Infirmary, University of Illinois at Chicago College of Medicine, Chicago, IL, USA

Sarah Avila, BS Miami Veterans Administration Medical Center, Miami, FL, USA

Bascom Palmer Eye Institute, University of Miami, Miami, FL, USA

Priti Batta, MD New York Eye and Ear Infirmary, New York, NY, USA

Benjamin Botsford, BS Tufts University School of Medicine, Boston, MA, USA

Charles S. Bouchard, MD, MA Loyola University Medical Center, Maywood, IL, USA

Vatinee Y. Bunya, MD Department of Ophthalmology, Scheie Eye Institute, University of Pennsylvania, Philadelphia, PA, USA

Victoria Butcko, OD The Jesse Brown VA Medical Center, Chicago, IL, USA

Jennifer Cao, MD Massachusetts Eye Research and Surgery Institution (MERSI), Waltham, MA, USA

Ocular Immunology and Uveitis Foundation, Waltham, MA, USA

Anny MS Cheng, MD Ocular Surface Center and Ocular Surface Research and Education Foundation, Miami, FL, USA

Florida International University, Herbert Wertheim College of Medicine, Miami, FL, USA

Jessica B. Ciralsky, MD Weill Cornell Medical College, New York, NY, USA

Ali R. Djalilian, MD Department of Ophthalmology and Visual Sciences, Illinois Eye and Ear Infirmary, University of Illinois at Chicago, Chicago, IL, USA

Nisreen Ezuddin, BS Miami Veterans Administration Medical Center, Miami, FL, USA

Bascom Palmer Eye Institute, University of Miami, Miami, FL, USA

Marjan Farid, MD Gavin Herbert Eye Institute, UC-Irvine, Irvine, CA, USA

Asim V. Farooq, MD Department of Ophthalmology, University of Chicago, Chicago, IL, USA

Department of Ophthalmology and Visual Sciences, Washington University in St. Louis, St. Louis, MO, USA

Nicole M. Fuerst, MD Department of Ophthalmology, Scheie Eye Institute, University of Pennsylvania, Philadelphia, PA, USA

Anat Galor, MD, MSPH Miami Veterans Administration Medical Center, Miami, FL, USA

Bascom Palmer Eye Institute, University of Miami, Miami, FL, USA

Giancarlo A. Garcia, MS Gavin Herbert Eye Institute, UC-Irvine, Irvine, CA, USA

Elham Ghahari, MD Department of Ophthalmology and Visual Sciences, Illinois Eye and Ear Infirmary, University of Illinois at Chicago, Chicago, IL, USA

Hamed Ghassemi, MD Farabi Eye Hospital, Tehran University, Tehran, Iran

Sunali Goyal, MD Department of Ophthalmology, University of Arkansas for Medical Sciences, Little Rock, AR, USA

Darren G. Gregory, MD University of Colorado School of Medicine, Aurora, CO, USA

Pedram Hamrah, MD, FRCS Cornea Service, New England Eye Center, Boston, MA, USA

Department of Ophthalmology, Center for Translational Ocular Immunology, Tufts Medical Center, Tufts University School of Medicine, Boston, MA, USA

Edward J. Holland, MD Cincinnati Eye Institute, University of Cincinnati, Cincinnati, OH, USA

Kimberly M. Hsu, MD Illinois Eye and Ear Infirmary, University of Illinois Chicago, Chicago, IL, USA

Andrew J.W. Huang, MD, MPH Department of Ophthalmology and Visual Sciences, Washington University in St. Louis, St. Louis, MO, USA

Tsutomu Inatomi, MD, PhD Department of Ophthalmology, Kyoto Prefectural University of Medicine, Kyoto, Japan

Sandeep Jain, MD Department of Ophthalmology and Visual Sciences, Illinois Eye and Ear Infirmary, University of Illinois at Chicago, Chicago, IL, USA

Bennie H. Jeng, MD Department of Ophthalmology and Visual Sciences, University of Maryland School of Medicine, Baltimore, MD, USA

Shigeru Kinoshita, MD, PhD Department of Frontier Medical Science and Technology for Ophthalmology, Kyoto Prefectural University of Medicine, Kyoto, Japan

Noriko Koizumi, MD, PhD Department of Biomedical Engineering, Faculty of Life and Medical Sciences, Doshisha University, Kyoto, Japan

Department of Ophthalmology, Kyoto Prefectural University of Medicine, Kyoto, Japan

Jordan Margo, MD Department of Ophthalmology and Visual Sciences, University of Maryland School of Medicine, Baltimore, MD, USA

Mina Massaro-Giordano, MD Department of Ophthalmology, Scheie Eye Institute, University of Pennsylvania, Philadelphia, PA, USA

Farhan I. Merali, MD, MBA Wilmer Ophthalmological Institute, Johns Hopkins University School of Medicine, Baltimore, MD, USA

Takahiro Nakamura, MD, PhD Department of Ophthalmology, Kyoto Prefectural University of Medicine, Kyoto, Japan

Stephen E. Orlin, MD Department of Ophthalmology, Scheie Eye Institute, University of Pennsylvania, Philadelphia, PA, USA

Jeanie Paik, MD New York Eye and Ear Infirmary, New York, NY, USA

Chau Pham, MD Department of Ophthalmology, Washington University, St. Louis, MO, USA

Angelique Pillar, MD Department of Ophthalmology and Visual Sciences, University of Maryland School of Medicine, Baltimore, MD, USA

Nicholas Pondelis, BA Department of Ophthalmology, Center for Translational Ocular Immunology, Tufts Medical Center, Tufts University School of Medicine, Boston, MA, USA

Pete Setabutr, MD Department of Ophthalmology and Visual Sciences, University of Illinois at Chicago, Chicago, IL, USA

Duaa Sharfi, MD Department of Ophthalmology and Visual Sciences, Illinois Eye and Ear Infirmary, University of Illinois at Chicago, Chicago, IL, USA

Joanne Shen, MD Mayo Clinic, Scottsdale, AZ, USA

Ellen Shorter, OD University of Illinois at Chicago, Chicago, IL, USA

Kimberly C. Sippel, MD Weill Cornell Medical College, New York, NY, USA

Ketki Soin, MD Department of Ophthalmology and Visual Sciences, Illinois Eye and Ear Infirmary, University of Illinois at Chicago, Chicago, IL, USA

M. Soledad Cortina, MD Illinois Eye and Ear Infirmary, University of Illinois Chicago, Chicago, IL, USA

Nishant G. Soni, MD Department of Ophthalmology and Visual Sciences, University of Maryland School of Medicine, Baltimore, MD, USA

Chie Sotozono, MD, PhD Department of Ophthalmology, Kyoto Prefectural University of Medicine, Kyoto, Japan

C. Stephen Foster, MD, FACS Massachusetts Eye Research and Surgery Institution (MERSI), Waltham, MA, USA

Ocular Immunology and Uveitis Foundation, Waltham, MA, USA

Harvard Medical School, Boston, MA, USA

Michael E. Sulewski, MD Department of Ophthalmology, Scheie Eye Institute, University of Pennsylvania, Philadelphia, PA, USA

Robert T. Swan, MD Massachusetts Eye Research and Surgery Institution (MERSI), Waltham, MA, USA

Ocular Immunology and Uveitis Foundation, Waltham, MA, USA

Aisha Traish, MD University of Illinois Hospital, Chicago, IL, USA

Scheffer C.G. Tseng, MD, PhD Ocular Surface Center and Ocular Surface Research and Education Foundation, Miami, FL, USA

Frederick B. Vivino, MD, MS Department of Rheumatology, University of Pennsylvania, Philadelphia, PA, USA

Samuel C. Yiu, MD, PhD Wilmer Ophthalmological Institute, Johns Hopkins University School of Medicine, Baltimore, MD, USA

Tufts University School of Medicine, Boston, MA, USA

Mehran Zarei-Ghanavati, MD Farabi Eye Hospital, Tehran University, Tehran, Iran

Chapter 1
Aqueous-Deficient Dry Eye Disease: Evaluation and Management

Benjamin Botsford, Farhan I. Merali, and Samuel C. Yiu

Case 1

BJ is a 52-year-old female who complains of tearing, burning, and a gritty feeling in both eyes for the last year but with progressive worsening of severity. The patient notes that it has become increasingly difficult for her to read books, as she develops increased burning. She also notices that her eyes feel worse on windy days. She has a past medical history of hypertension and takes hydrochlorothiazide. She has no prior ocular history besides being myopic and sees an optometrist for examination and refraction every 2 years. She has not yet tried anything to relieve her current symptoms (Table 1.1).

B. Botsford, BS
Tufts University School of Medicine, Boston, MA, USA

F.I. Merali, MD, MBA
Wilmer Ophthalmological Institute, Johns Hopkins University School of Medicine, 400 N Broadway, Smith Building, 6041 Baltimore, MD 21231, USA

S.C. Yiu, MD, PhD (✉)
Tufts University School of Medicine, Boston, MA, USA

Wilmer Ophthalmological Institute, Johns Hopkins University School of Medicine, 400 N Broadway, Smith Building, 6041 Baltimore, MD 21231, USA
e-mail: syiu2@jhmi.edu

A.R. Djalilian (ed.), *Ocular Surface Disease*,
https://doi.org/10.1007/978-3-319-15823-5_1

Table 1.1 The DEWS dry eye diagnosis and management grid[a]

Dry eye severity level	1	2	3	4
Discomfort, severity, and frequency	Mild/episodic/environmental stress	Moderate/episodic or chronic/ environmental stress or no stress	Severe/frequent or constant without stress	Severe and disabling, constant
Visual symptoms	None or episodic mild fatigue	Annoying and/or activity-limiting episodic	Annoying, chronic, and/or constant limiting activity	Constant and/or possibly disabling
Lid/meibomian glands	MGD variably present		Frequent	Trichiasis, keratinization, symblepharon
TFBUT (s)	Variable	≤10	≤5	Immediate
Corneal staining (NEI Scale 0–15)	None to mild	Variable	Central	Severe punctate erosions
Conjunctival staining (NEI Scale 0–18)	None to mild	Variable	Moderate to marked	Marked
Schirmer test (no anesthesia) (mm/5 min)	Variable	≤10	≤5	≤2
Recommended management	1. Patient education 2. Diet modification 3. Lid therapy 4. Artificial tear/gel supplements 5. Environmental control	Add: 1. Anti-inflammatories 2. Tetracycline 3. Punctal plugs 4. Moisture chamber spectacles	Add: 1. Autologous serum 2. Bandage or large-diameter rigid contact lenses 3. Permanent punctal occlusion	Add: 1. Systemic anti-inflammatory agents 2. Surgical intervention

[a]Modified with permission from 2007 DEWS report [38]

What Additional Questions Do You Want to Ask This Patient to Further Understand the Possible Etiology of Her Complaints?

The patient's initial complaints are very suggestive of dry eye disease. The symptoms of dry eye disease vary among patients, but may include tearing, burning, the sensation of dryness, sensitivity to light, transiently blurred vision, and foreign body or gritty sensations. Exacerbation with activities like reading or watching TV that cause reduction in blink frequency or by environmental factors such as heating, air conditioning, and wind can be suggestive of dry eye disease. Symptoms are often worse toward the end of the day, with the exception being nocturnal lagophthalmos in which case morning is usually worse. The initial evaluation for a patient with these symptoms may be difficult as symptoms may be heterogeneous or vague. A full and comprehensive history should be taken, including identification of potential exacerbating factors, such as medications or environments, and patient behaviors, as discussed below.

Questions about the patient's work environment should be conducted, as well as inquiring about activities that require visual concentration, such as reading or working on a computer. Computer use is associated with a decrease blink frequency through suppression of blinking, causing prolonged exposure of the ocular surface and disruption of the tear film [1]. Identifying the number of hours the patient may read or look at a computer monitor is useful for recognizing exposure as a risk factor and for elucidating potential behavioral modifications that may benefit the patient. Additional environmental factors such as direct exposure to ventilation can worsen symptoms, and desiccating environments involving heat or air conditioning may precipitate or worsen dry eye disease.

Other risk factors may include female gender and old age. Postmenopausal patients presenting with dry eye symptoms should be queried about possible hormonal replacement therapy, as replacement with either estrogen or estrogen and progestin has been shown to increase the risk for developing dry eye [2].

Any medications that the patient takes should be carefully evaluated. Ocular medications, especially glaucoma medications containing the preservative benzalkonium chloride [3, 4] have been shown to precipitate dry eye disease by causing tear film instability, loss of goblet cells, conjunctival squamous apoptosis, and disruption of the corneal epithelial barrier [5]. Systemic medications such as antihistamines, systemic retinoids, antidepressants or antianxiety medications with anticholinergic side effects, as well as diuretics may cause or contribute to a patient's symptoms. Asking a patient if they have recently started any new medications and determining temporal relation in regard to their symptoms may be useful in identifying problem medications that should be discontinued or substituted.

While allergic conjunctivitis is not typically a component of dry eye disease, symptoms of the two entities may overlap. It is therefore important to inquire about environmental allergens and a history of seasonal allergies. It is also useful to elicit the presence of symptoms of allergic conjunctivitis, such as itching and eye rubbing. Avoidance of allergens or other irritants may be a useful intervention for relieving symptoms that may be attributable to those causes.

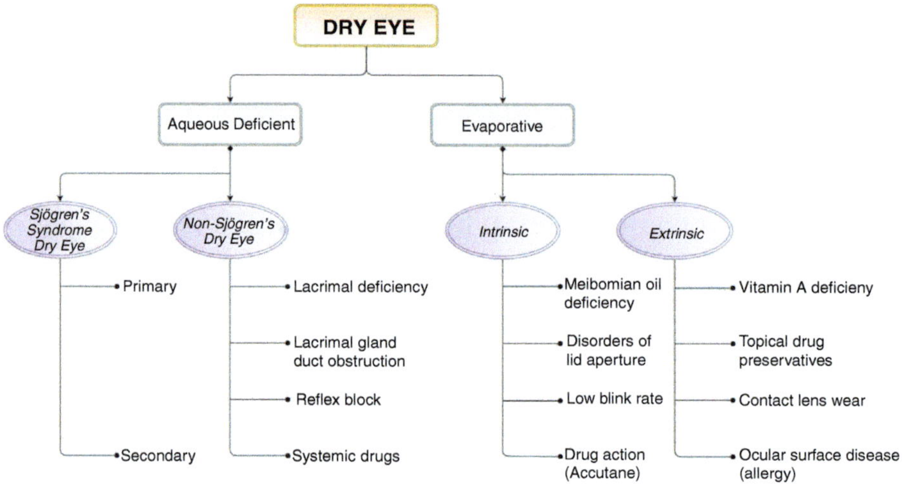

Fig. 1.1 Etiopathogenic classification of dry eye disease

Contact lens wear should be assessed, as use can be a significant contributor to for dry eye disease. The patient should also be asked about any prior history of refractive surgery. Postoperative corneal hypoesthesia caused by the resection of corneal nerves during surgery can lead to dry eye through a decrease in reflex tear secretion. Usually, corneal nerves will regenerate postoperatively but may leave the patient with dry eye symptoms for multiple months before healing occurs [6].

For any patient presenting with symptoms of dry eye disease, it is important to rule out systemic causes as the underlying etiology (Fig. 1.1). Any history of chemotherapy or radiation should be elicited as these treatment modalities can damage the lacrimal and meibomian glands and cause hypofunction, leading to aqueous-deficient dry eye disease (AD-DED) as well as evaporative dry eye. A thorough review of systems should be conducted with the following disease processes in mind, as they can cause ocular surface dryness: diabetes, rheumatoid arthritis, hepatitis C, HIV, sarcoidosis, thyroid disease, lupus, Sjogren's syndrome (SS), graft-versus-host disease, and cicatricial pemphigoid. It is prudent to question about fatigue, joint problems, dry mouth, vaginal dryness, skin lesions or rashes, shortness of breath, hearing loss, urinary difficulties, headaches, fever, peripheral edema, and peripheral neuropathy to work up these systemic conditions, as treatment will need to address the underlying condition. History of snoring and daytime sleepiness should likewise raise the suspicion for sleep apnea (often in patient with lax eyelids). The ophthalmologist may very well be the first provider to diagnose a systemic condition associated with dry eye. SS is a particularly important consideration in the initial assessment of a patient as prevalence of primary SS may be as high as 10–11% in patients presenting with clinically significant AD-DED [7]. Questions about family history of autoimmune diseases can also provide further clues. Positive review of systems concerning for systemic illness necessitates further investigation and/or referral.

The patient works as a secretary at an elementary school and uses her computer frequently throughout the day. Additionally, she sits close to a heating vent. She often uses over-the-counter Benadryl to help her sleep. She does not wear contact lenses and denies any other medications. She denies any arthritis, rashes, dry mouth, vaginal dryness, peripheral neuropathy, or fatigue. Family history is negative for any autoimmune diseases. She smokes half a pack of cigarettes per day.

What Should You Look for on Physical Exam to Aid in Diagnosis of the Patient?

As typical of any patient, best corrected visual acuity (BCVA) should be assessed. BCVA may be diminished or may transiently fluctuate in patients with dry eye as due to tear film instability [8]. The tear film contributes to the refractive power of the cornea, and disruptions may produce higher-order aberrations that interfere with visual acuity. Dry eye patients often complain of a reduction in visual acuity with driving, reading a computer, and maintaining gaze as the ocular surface may dry out from suppression of the blink reflex. Assessment of functional visual acuity (FVA), or the measure of visual acuity during sustained eye opening without blinking, may therefore be a good tool for assessment of dry eye patients [9]. FVA has been shown to be diminished in both SS and non-SS dry eye disease [10].

An external examination of the patient should be conducted to evaluate for any evidence of rosacea, enlarged lacrimal glands, or Bell's palsy. Eyelids and lid margins should be investigated as for evidence of blepharitis, meibomian gland dysfunction, infrequent or incomplete blink, and lagophthalmos as these conditions may be addressed individually. Careful evaluation of the conjunctiva should also be conducted, and chemosis, chalasis, injection, scarring, forniceal foreshortening, subepithelial scarring, and the presence of papillae or follicles should be noted. Lid eversion should be performed. Meticulous examination may demonstrate other causes of the patient's symptoms unrelated to dry eye disease.

The tear film should be evaluated, including the size of the tear meniscus and the tear breakup time (TBUT). TBUT is conducted by instilling a small amount of fluorescein in the inferior cul-de-sac, followed by evaluating the stability of the tear film after the patient blinks. Blinking distributes the tear film across the ocular surface, and a broad beam of cobalt blue light at the slit lamp can be used to assess the time it takes from the last blink until the first dark patch appears, which represents tear film dissolution. Patients with AD-DED have significantly faster tear breakup times, with times of less than 10 s considered to be abnormal.

Ocular surface staining is another important tool used to assess dry eye severity. Staining can be used to identify abnormalities of the corneal surface and of the bulbar conjunctiva. Punctate staining of the inferior cornea and inferior bulbar conjunctiva are the most typical pattern seen in dry eye. Multiple stains can be used. Fluorescein is the most common and will stain areas of the conjunctiva and cornea where tight junctions have been disrupted, though corneal staining will be much more prominent. Peak staining occurs approximately 2 min after instillation. If conjunctivalization of the cornea has occurred, however, fluorescein staining will have limited utility.

Lissamine green and rose bengal dyes can be used to stain devitalized cells and allow for more prominent staining of the bulbar conjunctiva. These dyes may pick up more subtle changes and are useful for detecting milder forms of dry eye disease. Inferior staining may suggest MGD or exposure, while superior staining suggests superior limbic keratoconjunctivitis. Lissamine green possesses advantages over rose bengal as it is less toxic to the ocular surface [11].

On examination, visual acuity is 20/25 in both eyes with correction. Pupils are equal, round, and reactive without afferent pupillary defect bilaterally. Intraocular pressure (IOP) is 15 mm Hg on the right and 16 mm Hg on the left. Her lids and lashes appear normal with no evidence of meibomian gland dysfunction, lagophthalmos, or other findings. Her conjunctivas are normal. The patient's tear meniscus appears reduced, and her tear breakup time is 10 s. Corneal staining with fluorescein reveals no punctate epithelial erosions, while lissamine green reveals minimal punctate staining of the bulbar conjunctiva in the exposure zone bilaterally.

What Additional Ancillary Testing Would Be Appropriate?

The Schirmer test is the classic test for diagnosis of decreased lacrimal secretion of the aqueous portion of the tear film. The Schirmer test is performed by placing a strip of paper in the inferior cul-de-sac and allowing the strip be wetted by produced tears over a period of 5 min. A positive Schirmer test is <5 mm of wetting with anesthetic and <10 mm without anesthetic [12], as anesthetic will reduce reflex tear secretion. Performing the Schirmer test with anesthetic has been shown to have more variable results than without [13]. The relatively low cutoff of the Schirmer test produces greater specificity at the cost of decreased sensitivity. The results of the Schirmer test may be variable between visits and should not be used as the sole criterion for diagnosis of AD-DED. However, serially abnormal results over time are highly suggestive.

Considering the importance of tear hyperosmolarity in the pathogenesis of dry eye disease, directly measuring tear osmolarity has been implemented in clinical practices since FDA approval of the osmolarity measuring device (TearLab, San Diego, CA) in 2009. It has reported to be another test to consider as part of an overall diagnostic picture [14]. Elevated tear osmolarity is suggestive of dry eye disease, and hyperosmolar tears stress the ocular surface leading to inflammation and perpetuation of the condition. Values >312 mOsm/L were found to be 73% sensitive and 92% specific for dry eye disease in one study; [15] however, tear osmolarity values may not be correlated with symptoms [16], and some studies also suggested variability in measurements [17]. However, the variability of the measurements may actually be diagnostic of an unstable tear film and hence dry eye disease. Overall, the role of tear osmolarity in the diagnosis and monitoring of dry eyes is evolving and with further studies will likely play a role in the management of the disease.

Overall, no perfect test or examination finding exists to confirm the diagnosis of dry eye disease. Heterogeneity of patient symptoms, poor correlation of symptoms with exam findings [18] and test results, and variability of exam findings and tests between visits [19, 20] can provide substantial challenges for the ophthalmologist. The overall picture generated from the patient's symptoms, exam findings, and ancillary testing must be synthesized to provide increased sensitivity and specificity in diagnosis.

The patient's Schirmer test without anesthesia is >20 mm. You check her tear osmolarity and find it to be 310 mOsm/L.

What Treatment Should Be Initiated?

Due to the poor correlation between symptoms and signs/test findings in dry eye disease, particularly in mild dry eye disease, the patient's ancillary testing findings should not prevent any interventions. Patients with suggestive symptoms should be placed on trial treatments if other potential etiologies for their symptoms have been ruled out. Our patient should be informed that though the symptoms may improve with lifestyle changes and treatment, the condition is not typically cured but managed.

The initial approach should involve identification of environmental and behavioral risk factors and suggestion of appropriate modifications, as well as initiation of artificial tear supplementation. Scheduling a follow-up visit to assess success of these interventions is prudent, and remaining patient and optimistic is important as disease management can be challenging and punctuated by signs or symptoms that are refractory to treatment.

For aid with desiccating environments, the use of humidifiers may alleviate symptoms caused by excessive heat or air conditioning. Additional care should be taken to improve the dynamics of air movement in an office environment, and work stations may be moved out of the direct line of ducts and vents. Long hours of work on computers should be interrupted by regular breaks. Additionally, placing the monitor below eye level can decrease the interpalpebral aperture, limiting the surface area of the exposed ocular surface, thereby aiding in reduction of tear film evaporation [21].

Smoking cessation counseling should be provided as cigarette use has been found to have adverse effects to the precorneal tear film [22, 23], including the lipid layer [24]. Identifying any offending drugs such as diuretics and anticholinergic medication as discussed above and having patients stop or consider alternatives is important. Discontinuing the Benadryl and following up with her PCP to find other sleep aids that do not have anticholinergic effects will likely be beneficial. Finally, we encourage patients to drink ample amounts of fluids.

Over-the-counter artificial tear supplementation may also be initiated. There are no significant differences between different brands and formulations of artificial tears, and patients can take whichever brand they prefer. While artificial tears without preservatives are preferred, their cost makes them prohibitive unless they become necessary. Artificial tears are generally safe in patients who use them up to four times a day. Ideally, ocular surface lubrication should be done before the patient starts to have symptoms related to ocular surface damage. Instructing the patient to use them three times a day before meals may provide a good aid to remember to use them regularly. Additionally, instructing to instill drops before reading or visual display terminal use may also help prevent exacerbations of symptoms.

You recommend behavioral modifications, asking her to take more frequent breaks from the computer, quit smoking, and move her desk away from the heating vent. She expresses desire to purchase a humidifier for her office, and you advise her to take artificial tears as needed up to four times a day to help with her symptoms. You schedule her for a 4-month follow-up visit and advise her to contact you sooner if further problems arise.

Four months later, she notes improvement with her symptoms at work. She is much more comfortable in her office and takes artificial tears before starting computer work and a couple of times after lunch, as her symptoms are worse in the afternoon. She notes that taking them before her eyes feel dry seems to provide additional benefit in prevention of her symptoms. While she has struggled to quit smoking, she has been able to cut down on the number of cigarettes she smokes a day and has discussed cessation options with her primary care doctor to assist her.

Her exam is unremarkable with no PEEs and a TBUT of 13 s. You schedule her for a yearly follow-up visit and wish her well and advise her to continue with her current regimen.

Case 2

RR is a 70-year-old male with past medical history of diabetes mellitus type 2, glaucoma, and dry eye disease here for a follow-up appointment for further management of his dry eye disease. He reports feeling a sensation of dryness and sensitivity to light and has been unable to watch television for extended periods of time due to burning and blurring of vision. For the last 6 months, he has been using over-the-counter artificial tears without any relief. He reports that he is requiring them up to six times per day. He placed a humidifier in his room and has attempted to take frequent breaks but has not noticed any difference. He also notices that he has eye irritation first thing in the morning when he wakes up. His current medications include metformin, glyburide, latanoprost, and artificial tears with preservatives. His last hemoglobin A1C was 8.6.

On examination, his visual acuity is 20/40 bilaterally with spectacle correction. His IOP is 20 mm Hg bilaterally. External exam and lids and lashes are

normal. He has mild conjunctival injection bilaterally and no evidence of lid margin disease. TBUT is 8 s and he has 2+ PEEs on his inferior cornea on fluorescein staining. Schirmer test performed without anesthesia is 6 mm and his tear osmolarity is 318 mOsm/L.

What Are the Patient's Risk Factors for Dry Eye Disease, and How Can These Be Addressed?

The patient's diabetes mellitus may be contributing to his dry eye disease. Dry eye is more prevalent in diabetics, especially those with poor glycemic control [25]. Diabetes can cause corneal hypoesthesia that is correlated with decreased tear secretion [26]. Corneal sensation can be tested to identify a potential source of decreased reflex tear secretion. Better management of his diabetic care by his primary care physician is necessary and may prevent additional sequelae of the disease, and a careful retinal examination should also be conducted.

His glaucoma medications may also be a contributing factor. Benzalkonium chloride in the drops combined with the preservatives in the artificial tears may contribute to dry eye disease [3, 4]. Switching to preservative-free glaucoma drops may assist in reduction of his symptoms. Additionally, switching to preservative-free artificial tears may be necessary, as he is requiring artificial tears more than four times a day. A nighttime lubrication ointment should also be started to provide ocular surface lubrication at night, as the patient is experiencing symptoms upon awakening.

What Additional Treatments May Be Initiated?

In patients with moderate dry eyes, a key question is what role inflammation is playing. While some patients may display signs of inflammation on exam, this may not always be the case. A useful test to determine the role of inflammation is to measure MMP9 levels in the tears (InflammaDry). A positive test helps to guide the therapy more toward controlling inflammation, although patients with a negative test should also be considered for anti-inflammatory therapy.

An easy first choice for targeting inflammation is omega-3 fatty acid. A recent meta-analysis concluded that omega-3 supplements improve the TBUT and Schirmer test without significant change in ocular surface disease index assessment of patient symptomatology [27]. The inconsistency of the results may be in part related to the difference in the formulations and dosages used in various studies. A very recent multicenter placebo-controlled study found significant improvement in the signs and symptoms of dry eyes using a re-esterified formulation which presumably improves absorption [28]. Patients should be advised to look for fish oil formulations that provide at least 500 mg of EPA (eicosapentaenoic acid) and DHA (docosahexaenoic acid) per day. As an alternative, we recommend at least three servings of fish high in omega-3 (salmon, tuna, and halibut) per week. Flax seed, chia seed, and walnuts also contain omega-3, but this is in the form of alpha-linoleic acid which must be converted to EPA/DHA in the body—a process that is not very efficient. Therefore, these plant sources may not be as efficient and we recommend primarily fish sources.

Corticosteroids can provide immense relief of dry eye symptoms due to their immunomodulatory actions. However, side effects limit their use to short-term courses. Repetitive short-term pulsatile administration of topical corticosteroids is a promising method of harnessing their beneficial effects, while minimizing the risk of adverse events [9]. Loteprednol (or fluorometholone) is our first choice, as it provides higher potency with a lower side effect profile. A 2-week course of loteprednol or FML TID can help suppress inflammation followed by a slow taper off or down to 1–2 drops per week. If available, a preservative-free steroid (e.g., compounded methylprednisolone) may be used instead as it minimizes the detrimental effects of the preservatives. Either way, a positive clinical response to steroids confirms that inflammation is contributing to the signs/symptoms of that patients, and therefore they may be a good candidate for Restasis (and/or Xiidra) as the steroids are tapered off.

Restasis (topical cyclosporine A 0.05%) exerts immunosuppressive and anti-inflammatory actions through various pathways, but primarily by suppressing T cells. Restasis is a great option for a number of patients, though it often requires a long-term commitment and presents high costs. As such, it should be initiated with some discretion. Restasis may be initiated in patients who have persistent dry eye symptoms despite behavioral modifications, ample artificial tear supplementation, use of nighttime ointments, or dietary modifications. Additionally, these patients should display evidence of decreased tear production, as shown by elevated tear osmolarity or decreased Schirmer test values. As noted above, one strategy may be to first try a course of topical steroids and, if the patient responds, then consider Restasis for long-term anti-inflammatory therapy. Kick-starting anti-inflammatory therapy with steroids seems prudent given that Restasis is less efficient at suppressing active inflammation.

Our experience with Restasis suggests that patients may sometimes take up to 6 months to reach its full benefit. The dose can be increased to three to four times a day to achieve further benefit, though this can precipitate worsening side effects of burning [29, 30]. Recently, another medication lifitegrast (Xiidra) has been approved as an anti-inflammatory therapy for dry eye disease. The experience at this time is limited, although the results from the clinical trials are very promising for moderate dry eye patients.

Another useful measure in this patient, or any patient on BAK-preserved glaucoma drops, is to switch to preservative-free options. We have had a number of patients who have noted improvement in their signs and symptoms from this change.

Punctal occlusion may also be a consideration in a patient whose signs and/or symptoms are not adequately controlled with anti-inflammatory therapy [31]. Prior to this step, it is best to treat acute inflammation as inflammatory mediators present in the tear film will linger longer if tear drainage is blocked, potentially exacerbating symptoms and causing further damage to the ocular surface. Initiation of Restasis and a short course of topical corticosteroids before insertion of the plug can help alleviate these concerns. It is important to inform the patient that punctal plugs will frequently dislodge but can be reinserted. Absorbable and nonabsorbable plugs made of silicone or thermal labile polymer are available. Silicone plugs provide added utility as they are removable if the patient develops epiphora or irritation. Insertion of the largest plug that fits into the duct helps prevent plug dislodgement. As benefit from punctal occlusion has been shown to not peak until approximately 8 weeks after placement, a period of follow-up of at least this length is recommended to assess the patient's maximal response to therapy [32].

For patients with moderate disease (level 2), typically occluding only one of the puncta in each eye is considered since occluding both upper and lower will quite likely lead to epiphora. We prefer to use lower punctal silicone plugs for most patients, although collagen or other dissolvable plugs can be used for a "trial" period. Silicone plugs may be left in if the patient expresses benefit or removed if no improvement is seen. In patients who experience epiphora, perforated plugs (flow through) are an attractive option. The choice of plug remains the practitioner's preference. Permanent cauterization is reserved for patients who express benefit from punctual plugs but require frequent replacement, often due to plugs dislodging and sometimes irritating the ocular surface.

You suggest that he should begin artificial tear supplementation with preservative-free artificial tears. Since he also has symptoms upon awakening, you prescribe him a nighttime lubricant eye ointment. Additionally, you inform him that the preservatives in his latanoprost may also be contributing to his condition. You recommend he discuss with his glaucoma doctor switching to a preservative-free formulation. You also advise him that he may benefit from omega-3 supplementation.

Lastly, you inform him that his diabetes can also contribute to his condition. You recommend he follow up with his primary care physician to help determine how he can optimize his glycemic control. You schedule him for a 3-month follow-up and advise him to come sooner if any issues arise.

Three months later, he returns. He reports mild improvement with the changes in his medications and dietary changes. He states he began taking a fish oil supplement that he found online, has been using PFATs six to seven times per day, has been using a nighttime lubricant gel, and has made further dietary modifications with slightly better glycemic control. However, he notes the symptoms are still highly bothersome and that the PFATs only seem to provide brief benefit. On examination, his TBUT is now 9 s and he has 2+ PEEs on his inferior cornea on fluorescein staining. Schirmer testing performed without anesthesia is 5 mm and his tear osmolarity is 315 mOsm/L.

You advise the patient that he would likely benefit from Restasis. You start him a bi-daily administration and advise him that the most common side effect is a burning sensation. You tell him he may consider refrigeration of the drops and repeated use of a vial over the course of 1 day to save costs. You make note that the medication may often take a long time before he experiences

benefit and that some patients may take 6 months to even a year. You avoid prescribing him a short course of steroids due to his history of glaucoma. He is scheduled for another 3-month follow-up to assess his response to the medication.

Upon follow-up, he reports improvement in his symptoms. He feels he is using his PFATs less frequently, now four to five times a day. On examination, his TBUT is 11 s and he has trace PEEs on exam on the inferior cornea. Schirmer testing performed without anesthesia is 9 mm and his tear osmolarity is 312 mOsm/L. You advise him he is likely benefitting from the medication and schedule a 6-month follow-up appointment. In the future, you may consider punctal plugs (inferior only) if his symptoms are not completely controlled.

Case 3

MC is a 62-year-old female with past medical history of Sjogren's syndrome who is referred to your office for further management of her dry eye disease. She notes an almost constant feeling of burning, dryness, and foreign body sensation. She reports that she has been on Restasis twice a day bilaterally for the past year. Her rheumatologist started her on Plaquenil which she has taken for the last year and a half. She has had lower punctal plugs placed 3 months ago and believes they are still in place. She takes preservative-free artificial tears ten times per day but says the relief provided only lasts for a few, brief seconds when she uses them. She has missed multiple days of work this year due to her symptoms and is frustrated that nothing has helped her so far. She states that she is miserable and the problems are severely affecting her quality of life.

On examination, her best corrected visual acuity is 20/40 bilaterally with spectacle correction. Her intraocular pressures are 16 mm Hg in both eyes. External exam and lids and lashes are unremarkable. Conjunctivas appear mildly injected. TBUT is 3 s. She has mucous standing in the inferior fornix. She has 3+ PEE on inferior cornea. Schirmer testing without anesthesia is 4 mm, and her tear osmolarity is 320 mOsm/L.

What Additional Treatment Options Might You Offer to This Patient?

Patients with Sjogren's syndrome clearly have inflammatory disease. In the presence of active inflammation, a short course of topical steroids, particularly if available in a preservative-free preparation, may be useful for reducing inflammation on the surface. In patients with more significant inflammation, a short course of oral steroids may also be highly effective. In general, the patient should be questioned about their systemic disease and whether it is active, in which case, a recommendation is made for the rheumatologist to increase the patient's systemic therapy.

The use of punctal occlusion in patients with severe disease is different from that in patients with more moderate disease (e.g., Case 2). In particular, in patient with severe disease, occluding a single punctum in each eye is unlikely to have any measurable effect, and instead total occlusion must be considered. This is best done as a trial of using plugs (dissolvable or permanent) in both upper and lower puncta and evaluating the patient response. If there is a positive clinical response, then cautery punctal occlusion of the puncta is offered as a more permanent solution (given the likelihood of plugs falling out with time).

Secretagogues like oral pilocarpine and cevimeline that mimic parasympathetic activity can be used in the treatment of dry eye disease, especially in patients with coexisting dry mouth such as SS. These agents are discussed in more detail in the chapter on SS.

Another good option for patients with level 3 disease is autologous serum tears. Autologous serum eye drops—produced by separating the liquid from the cellular components of a patient's own blood—are an important tool in dry eye disease, as the serum contains substances that support proliferation, differentiation, and maturation of the ocular surface epithelium. Additionally the serum contains immunomodulatory mediators. Availability of serum eye drops may vary depending on the availability of pharmacies that can compound them. Studies have shown improvement in symptoms and TBUT despite no changes in other objective measures [33]. In patients with AD-DED, we typically start with 20% serum (diluted in BSS). Patients are instructed to use the drops at least four to six times a day (or more) and to maintain the unopened bottles in the freezer and opened bottle in the fridge up to 1 week. While there has been some concern with the use of serum from patients with active systemic diseases, we have not experienced any complications in patients with Sjogren's syndrome, and the only group where caution may need to be exercised are allergic diseases.

Recently, sutureless amniotic membranes, such as the ProKera and AmbioDisk, have been approved by the FDA for use in dry eye disease. Amniotic membranes have long been used in ophthalmology to promote healing of the ocular surface and to curb inflammation through downregulation of inflammatory cytokines. Patients with severe dry eye disease may benefit from a trial with an amniotic membrane. However, this treatment may represent only a temporizing measure, and it is unclear the duration of the benefit or how often the procedure would need to be repeated. Further studies are required to appraise its efficacy [34].

Scleral contact lenses such as PROSE lenses have been a revolutionary treatment for patients with severe dry eye disease and many other ocular conditions. Many patients endorse the comfort and the ability for the lenses to alleviate symptoms by recapitulating the ocular surface and housing medication and lubrication. However, the cost of the lenses may be prohibitive, and insurance coverage of lenses remains uncertain and inconsistent. Despite these barriers, the customizability of the lenses provides tremendous opportunity for improvement of patient quality of life, with improvements in symptoms, objective measures, and visual acuity in dry eye disease [35, 36]. PROSE lenses can also be utilized for debilitating diseases of the ocular surface such as graft-versus-host disease with substantial success [37]. These are discussed in more detail elsewhere in this book.

You discuss her options and she decides to be fitted for scleral lenses. You arrange her an appointment to be fitted and advise her that the cost may be rather expensive and her insurance company may not pay for all of it. She explains that she is aware of the potential cost to her and proceeds with a scleral contact lens trial.

At a follow-up appointment later, she reports significant relief from wearing the lenses. Her symptoms during the day have dramatically improved. Her visual acuity is 20/20 OU with the lenses in place, and she has 1+ PEE on the inferior cornea. TBUT, Schirmer testing, and tear osmolarity are unchanged. She expresses gratitude and is happy with her decision to try the lenses.

Acknowledgments *Financial Disclosures*: None of the authors have any financial disclosures regarding the contents discussed in this manuscript. *Conflict of Interest*: None of the authors have any conflicts of interest with the contents discussed in this manuscript.

References

1. Blehm C, Vishnu S, Khattak A, Mitra S, Yee RW. Computer vision syndrome: a review. Surv Ophthalmol. 2005;50(3):253–62.
2. Schaumberg DA, Buring JE, Sullivan DA, Dana MR. Hormone replacement therapy and dry eye syndrome. JAMA. 2001;286(17):2114–9.
3. Leung EW, Medeiros FA, Weinreb RN. Prevalence of ocular surface disease in glaucoma patients. J Glaucoma. 2008;17(5):350–5.
4. Saade CE, Lari HB, Berezina TL, Fechtner RD, Khouri AS. Topical glaucoma therapy and ocular surface disease: a prospective, controlled cohort study. Can J Ophthalmol. 2015;50(2):132–6.
5. Baudouin C, Labbe A, Liang H, Pauly A, Brignole-Baudouin F. Preservatives in eyedrops: the good, the bad and the ugly. Prog Retin Eye Res. 2010;29(4):312–34.
6. Murakami Y, Manche EE. Prospective, randomized comparison of self-reported postoperative dry eye and visual fluctuation in LASIK and photorefractive keratectomy. Ophthalmology. 2012;119(11):2220–4.
7. Liew MS, Zhang M, Kim E, Akpek EK. Prevalence and predictors of Sjogren's syndrome in a prospective cohort of patients with aqueous-deficient dry eye. Br J Ophthalmol. 2012;96(12):1498–503.
8. Ibrahim OM, Dogru M, Kaido M, Kojima T, Fujishima H, Tsubota K. Functional visual acuity assessment of severe atopic keratoconjunctivitis. Cornea. 2014;33(Suppl 11):S13–8.
9. Lin H, Yiu SC. Dry eye disease: a review of diagnostic approaches and treatments. Saudi J Ophthalmol. 2014;28(3):173–81.
10. Goto E, Yagi Y, Matsumoto Y, Tsubota K. Impaired functional visual acuity of dry eye patients. Am J Ophthalmol. 2002;133(2):181–6.
11. Machado LM, Castro RS, Fontes BM. Staining patterns in dry eye syndrome: rose bengal versus lissamine green. Cornea. 2009;28(7):732–4.

12. Pflugfelder SC, Tseng SC, Sanabria O, Kell H, Garcia CG, Felix C, et al. Evaluation of subjective assessments and objective diagnostic tests for diagnosing tear-film disorders known to cause ocular irritation. Cornea. 1998;17(1):38–56.
13. Clinch TE, Benedetto DA, Felberg NT, Laibson PR. Schirmer's test. A closer look. Arch Ophthalmol. 1983;101(9):1383–6.
14. Sullivan BD, Whitmer D, Nichols KK, Tomlinson A, Foulks GN, Geerling G, et al. An objective approach to dry eye disease severity. Invest Ophthalmol Vis Sci. 2010;51(12):6125–30.
15. Lemp MA, Bron AJ, Baudouin C, Benitez Del Castillo JM, Geffen D, Tauber J et al. Tear osmolarity in the diagnosis and management of dry eye disease. Am J Ophthalmol. 2011; 151(5): 792–798, e791.
16. Yeh TN, Graham AD, Lin MC. Relationships among tear film stability, osmolarity, and dryness symptoms. Optom Vis Sci. 2015.
17. Bunya VY, Fuerst NM, Pistilli M, McCabe BE, Salvo R, Macchi I, et al. Variability of tear osmolarity in patients with dry eye. JAMA Ophthalmol. 2015;133(6):662–7.
18. Schein OD, Tielsch JM, Munoz B, Bandeen-Roche K, West S. Relation between signs and symptoms of dry eye in the elderly. A population-based perspective. Ophthalmology. 1997;104(9):1395–401.
19. Goren MB, Goren SB. Diagnostic tests in patients with symptoms of keratoconjunctivitis sicca. Am J Ophthalmol. 1988;106(5):570–4.
20. Sullivan BD, Crews LA, Sonmez B, de la Paz MF, Comert E, Charoenrook V, et al. Clinical utility of objective tests for dry eye disease: variability over time and implications for clinical trials and disease management. Cornea. 2012;31(9):1000–8.
21. Tsubota K, Nakamori K. Effects of ocular surface area and blink rate on tear dynamics. Arch Ophthalmol. 1995;113(2):155–8.
22. Thomas J, Jacob GP, Abraham L, Noushad B. The effect of smoking on the ocular surface and the precorneal tear film. Australas Med J. 2012;5(4):221–6.
23. Matsumoto Y, Dogru M, Goto E, Sasaki Y, Inoue H, Saito I, et al. Alterations of the tear film and ocular surface health in chronic smokers. Eye (Lond). 2008;22(7):961–8.
24. Altinors DD, Akca S, Akova YA, Bilezikci B, Goto E, Dogru M, et al. Smoking associated with damage to the lipid layer of the ocular surface. Am J Ophthalmol. 2006;141(6):1016–21.
25. Kaiserman I, Kaiserman N, Nakar S, Vinker S. Dry eye in diabetic patients. Am J Ophthalmol. 2005;139(3):498–503.
26. Lv H, Li A, Zhang X, Xu M, Qiao Y, Zhang J, et al. Meta-analysis and review on the changes of tear function and corneal sensitivity in diabetic patients. Acta Ophthalmol. 2014;92(2):e96–104.
27. Liu A, Ji J. Omega-3 essential fatty acids therapy for dry eye syndrome: a meta-analysis of randomized controlled studies. Med Sci Monit. 2014;20:1583–9.
28. Holland EJ, Bucci FA, Epitropoulos AT, et al. Effect of oral re-esterified omega-3 nutritional supplementation on dry-eye disease: double-masked randomized placebo-controlled study. American Society of Cataract and Refractive Surgery Paper Session 2-B, April 19, 2015, San Diego, CA.
29. Dastjerdi MH, Hamrah P, Dana R. High-frequency topical cyclosporine 0.05% in the treatment of severe dry eye refractory to twice-daily regimen. Cornea. 2009;28(10):1091–6.
30. Su MY, Perry HD, Barsam A, Perry AR, Donnenfeld ED, Wittpenn JR, et al. The effect of decreasing the dosage of cyclosporine A 0.05% on dry eye disease after 1 year of twice-daily therapy. Cornea. 2011;30(10):1098–104.
31. Ervin AM, Wojciechowski R, Schein O. Punctal occlusion for dry eye syndrome. Cochrane Database Syst Rev. 2010;9:Cd006775.
32. Nava-Castaneda A, Tovilla-Canales JL, Rodriguez L, Tovilla YPJL, Jones CE. Effects of lacrimal occlusion with collagen and silicone plugs on patients with conjunctivitis associated with dry eye. Cornea. 2003;22(1):10–4.
33. Celebi AR, Ulusoy C, Mirza GE. The efficacy of autologous serum eye drops for severe dry eye syndrome: a randomized double-blind crossover study. Graefes Arch Clin Exp Ophthalmol. 2014;252(4):619–26.

34. Suri K, Kosker M, Raber IM, Hammersmith KM, Nagra PK, Ayres BD, et al. Sutureless amniotic membrane ProKera for ocular surface disorders: short-term results. Eye Contact Lens. 2013;39(5):341–7.
35. Bavinger JC, DeLoss K, Mian SI. Scleral lens use in dry eye syndrome. Curr Opin Ophthalmol. 2015;26(4):319–24.
36. Dimit R, Gire A, Pflugfelder SC, Bergmanson JP. Patient ocular conditions and clinical outcomes using a PROSE scleral device. Cont Lens Anterior Eye. 2013;36(4):159–63.
37. Jacobs DS, Rosenthal P. Boston scleral lens prosthetic device for treatment of severe dry eye in chronic graft-versus-host disease. Cornea. 2007;26(10):1195–9.
38. The definition and classification of dry eye disease: report of the Definition and Classification Subcommittee of the International Dry Eye WorkShop (2007). Ocul Surf. 2007;5(2):75–92.

Chapter 2
Update in the Diagnosis and Management of Meibomian Gland Dysfunction

Joanne Shen

Case 1

The patient is a 48-year-old dentist referred for dry eye symptoms. His past medical history is significant for gastroesophageal reflux treated with Zantac. Otherwise, he is healthy and takes no other systemic medications. He denies seasonal allergies. He has no family history of eye disease.

His past ocular history is significant for 20 years of soft contact lens wear and then PRK for myopia 3 years prior to his visit. For the past 18 months, he has dry, gritty feeling in his eyes, awakens with Velcro feeling under his eyelids, and occasional tearing when he is preforming dental procedures. He is using preservative-free tears four times a day without sustained relief. He was diagnosed by his optometrist with dry eye disease and treated with 6 months of Restasis which did not improve his symptoms. He heard about LipiFlow and wanted to see if this would help him.

On examination, his distance vision is 20/20 in each eye and near vision is 20/30 in each eye, both measured without correction. His pupils are reactive without an afferent pupillary defect. His intraocular pressure by Icare tonometry is 16 in each eye. Evaluation of the periocular skin shows no evidence of rash or other lesions. All four puncta are patent. There is no trichiasis or *Demodex* sleeving of lashes. There is no significant eyelid laxity or lagophthalmos. The meibomian glands show plugging and inspissation bilaterally. Meibomian gland evaluation (MGE) shows three glands on the right lower lid and one gland on the left lower lid yielding liquid turbid secretions.

J. Shen, MD
Mayo Clinic, 13400 East Shea Boulevard, Scottsdale, AZ 85259, USA
e-mail: shen.joanne@mayo.edu

A.R. Djalilian (ed.), *Ocular Surface Disease*,
https://doi.org/10.1007/978-3-319-15823-5_2

The eyelid margin appears normal in architecture. His conjunctivae are mildly injected bilaterally. On upper and lower eyelid eversion, there is trace papillary reaction but no follicles, subepithelial fibrosis, or foreign bodies. The right bulbar conjunctiva does not stain with lissamine green but stains 1+ medially in the left eye. No superior limbic keratoconjunctivitis is seen. Sclerae appear normal. Corneas have no punctate epithelial erosions and TBUT is 2 s bilaterally. His anterior chambers are deep and quiet, and irides are normal. His crystalline lenses are clear bilaterally. His optic nerve cup-to-disk ratio is 0.3 bilaterally. The remainder of his dilated fundus exam is normal.

What Diagnosis Do These Findings Suggest?

This patient appears to have meibomian gland dysfunction with low TBUT. Having tonometry performed by the technician with a noncontact system like Icare can allow evaluation of the ocular surface without artifactual worsening of the ocular surface signs after instillation of topical anesthetic.

How Do You Approach Symptoms of Dry Eye?

The history is obviously very important. Patients with MGD-related dry eyes typically report having irritation upon awakening, but other conditions such as lagophthalmus may also lead to similar symptoms. A common question I like to ask: "How do your eyes feel first thing upon awakening?" Patients may need nocturnal lagophthalmos addressed with night mask or Saran Wrap occlusion if the answer is: "Dry."

The patient is examined carefully looking for tear component deficiencies and mechanical eyelid and blink issues that would limit the ability to keep a stable tear film. A detailed exam supplemented by special testing can give more confidence in determining what deficiencies exist.

Lastly, a dry eye questionnaire can help quantitate the severity of symptoms and detect modest levels of improvement to reassure patients at subsequent visits.

The patient's OSDI score is 45, indicating moderately severe dry eye symptoms.

What Other Testing Should Be Performed?

Schirmer's test can be helpful in evaluating for aqueous tear deficiency. Also, a high Schirmer's test would be a reassuring sign that the patient has intact reflex tearing which can be protective against corneal epithelial breakdown.

Patient's Schirmer's test without anesthesia after 10 min is normal, yielding 20 mm in the right eye and 24 mm in the left eye. He denies a history of dry mouth and does not appear to have aqueous deficiency.

What Newer Technologies Can Be Helpful in Evaluating and Quantifying Meibomian Gland Dysfunction?

Imaging systems can now provide a detailed view of the meibomian glands in the upper and lower lid as well as tear film interferometry which can be used to evaluate the tear film thickness and quality of the lipid layer (Fig. 2.1).

The patient underwent a LipiView scan which demonstrated the average interferometry color units (ICU) to be low at 45 in both eyes (normal is >50).

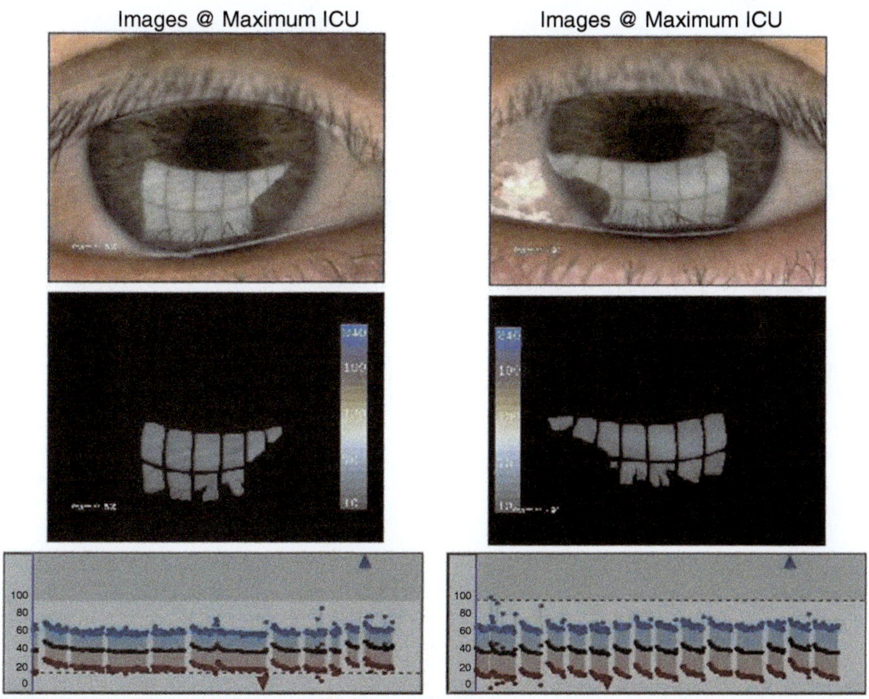

Video Length	19.1 sec	Avg ICU	45
Max ICU	55 @ 523	Min ICU	42 @ 366
Std. Dev.	3	CF: 1.00	PB: 9/10

Video Length	19.1 sec	Avg ICU	45
Max ICU	57 @ 491	Min ICU	40 @ 208
Std. Dev.	3	CF: 1.00	PB: 14/10

Fig. 2.1 LipiView scan of the both eyes of a patient with MGD-related dry eyes

The patient has 15 blinks in a 19 s testing interval which is a very high rate with concern for blepharospasm (Fig. 2.1). There are also very flat waveforms, unlike the example shown of a normal tear interferometry testing (Fig. 2.2).

Video imaging also captures the blink mechanism. Incomplete blinking can be observed and this dysfunction will exacerbate evaporation, contributing to symptoms especially in arid climates/conditions. Past contact lens wearers and eyelid surgery patients are at risk for incomplete blink due to loss of feedback with the cornea sensation masked by contact lenses or mechanical inability for the eyelids to meet.

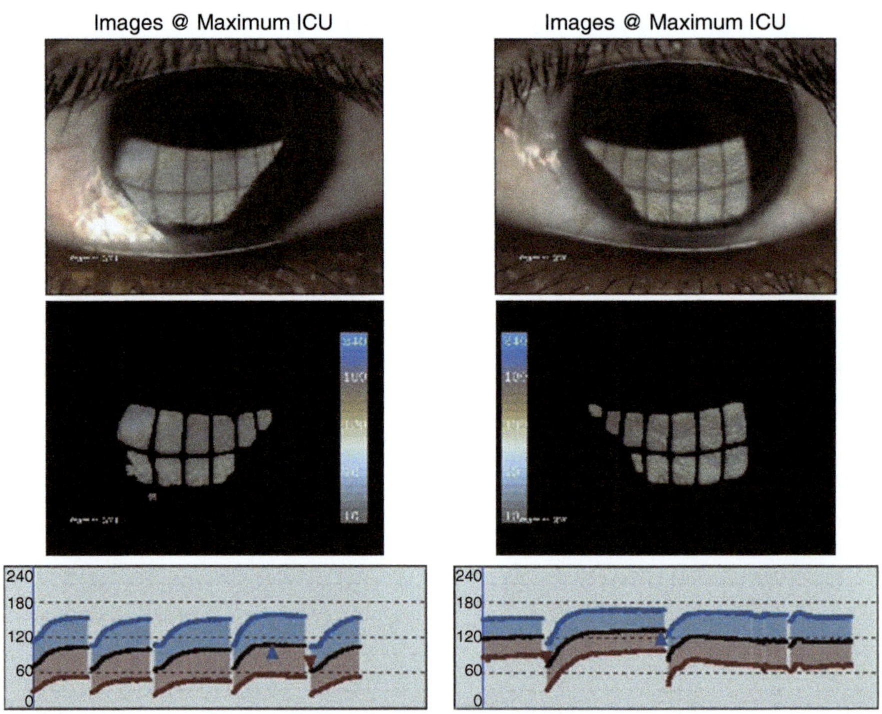

# Frames	507	Avg ICU	92
Max ICU	106 @ 374	Min ICU	61 @ 434
Std. Dev.	12	C-Factor	0.71

# Frames	569	Avg ICU	117
Max ICU	132 @ 276	Min ICU	70 @ 100
Std. Dev.	10	C-Factor	0.75

Fig. 2.2 LipiView scan of a normal patient (no dry eyes). In comparing the waveforms between each blink, this normal patient has increasing lipid tear thickness after each blink, not flat or "falling" waveforms

Looking at the Tear Film Interferometry Gives Part of the Picture, but Looking Directly at the Glands Would Help Determine If the Meibomian Glands Are Still Viable. What Technology Can Help Look at Meibomian Glands?

Meibography has been recently available as a clinical tool. In the past, infrared photography could be done, but it was time-consuming. Oculus Keratograph 5 and LipiView II can easily capture the meibomian glands for evaluation of gland architecture and atrophy.

Normal meibography shows long glands, extending across the height of the tarsus, and tiny grape-like clusters of acini around the length of the duct. Curved glands represent atrophy of adjacent glands.

This patient's meibography shows mild atrophy in both eyelids, up to 25 % shortening of the superior and inferior eyelid gland's length (Figs. 2.3 and 2.4).

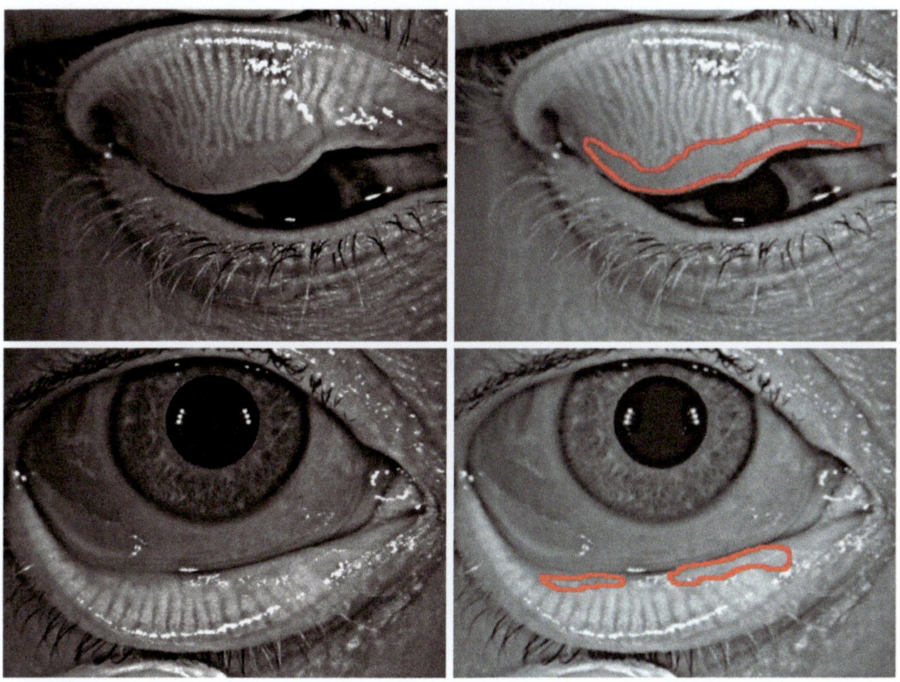

Fig. 2.3 Meibography of the right upper and lower lids. The *red lines* outline the areas where the glands have dropped out

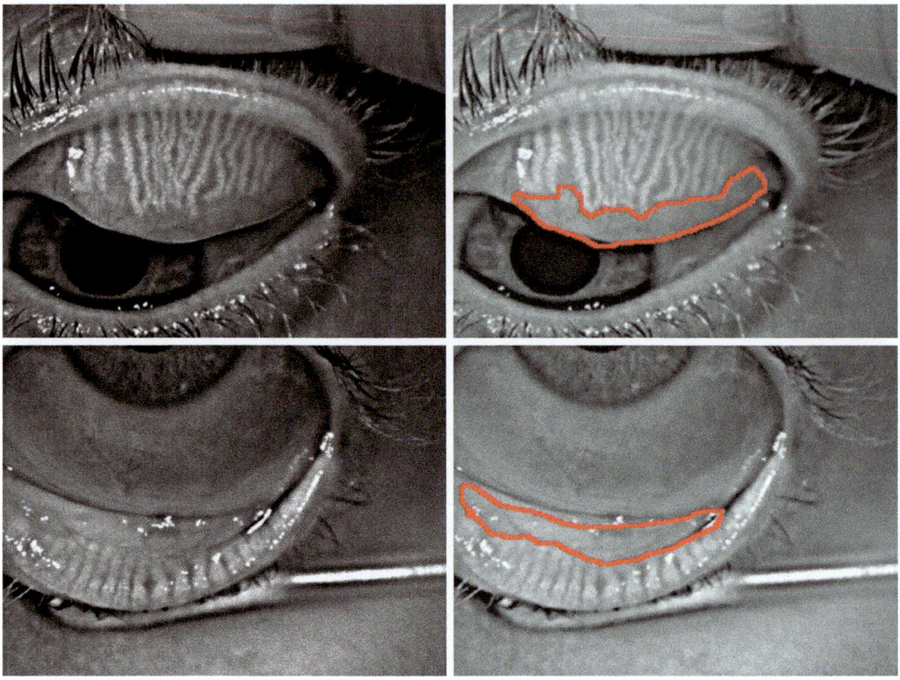

Fig. 2.4 Meibography of the left upper and lower lids. The *red lines* outline the areas where the glands have dropped out

The Patient Reported Tearing with His Work. How Do You Evaluate This?

A refraction can help determine if ciliary spasm with accommodation could contribute to tearing, in addition to probable reflex tearing from lipid tear deficiency. He has presbyopia and his vision improved to 20/20 with + 1.25 correction at near bilaterally. He was recommended to get a + 1.25 built into his procedural loupes.

Commonly, patients with lipid deficiency would expect to have bursts of reflex tearing that may overwhelm the nasolacrimal system and result in tearing. Epiphora, with tears actually rolling down the cheek, may indicate partial or complete nasolacrimal duct obstruction. Fortunately, this patient does not have epiphora and the tear meniscus is not high.

What Do You Recommend for This Patient?

Basic treatment that can help with meibomian gland deficiency consists of low-cost therapies with low risk of complications. Omega-3 fatty acids can be helpful. The dosing and exact combination of fatty acids has not been established. The NIH Dry

Eye Assessment and Management (DREAM) Clinical Trial will give answers on dosing in the future. Commonly 1–2 g of DHA (docosahexaenoic acid) and EPA (eicosapentaenoic acid) are suggested. Caution must be taken when prescribing in the context of blood thinners and risk of prolonging clotting mechanism beyond the 2 g range. Hot compresses are a mainstay of treatment to alleviate gland blockage with incomplete blinking.

How Are Patients Instructed To Do Hot Compresses? Is Eyelid Massage Recommended?

Hot compresses are an economical method of heating the lids that provide some relief and potentially can help warm meibum, making it easier to secrete through the meibomian gland orifices. Wet hot washcloth in the shower can be used for patients with seborrhea debris on the eyelids and lashes, but the intensity of the heat is limited in this application method. A homemade "rice in a gym sock" or commercially available cloth mask filled with polymer beads can be microwaved for 20–30 s (until hot but not burning to touch) and placed over the eyelids for at least 10 min. An AC or USB adaptor plugged-in heated eye masks can be more convenient for business travelers or patients without access to a microwave.

Ten minutes is recommended as a minimum duration since it is recognized that the meibomian glands need this amount of time to release meibum. Cornea ectasia has been reported in patients massaging after heat application. Therefore, at-home lid massage is only recommended with caution. Instead, blinking exercises (described below) may be considered.

The patient spends 4 weeks working on this basic treatment plan but returns with OSDI 40 and still symptomatic. The tearing is better with use of near correction, but he is still symptomatic.

What Other Treatment Can Be Offered?

He declines doxycycline due to problems with his stomach. He tries topical azithromycin but this does not help.

Antibiotics such as tetracyclines and macrolides can be used off-label to improve symptoms of ocular rosacea and dry eye in an economical fashion. Antibiotics are discussed before any out-of-pocket treatment is offered. The patient is an active participant in his/her treatment plan.

The anti-inflammatory effect of inhibition of matrix metalloproteinase-9 can certainly help many rosacea patients and some patients with mild ocular rosacea. Tetracyclines are inexpensive but patients are best warned about gastrointestinal upset, sunburn potential, yeast vaginitis, urinary tract infection, and rarely drug allergy. Most patients need 20–100 mg of doxycycline or minocycline daily for 3 months to see any effect. In patients, where cost is not an issue, the extended release preparations may be better tolerated; otherwise one preferred regimen is doxycycline monohydrate 50 mg twice/day, in part since it is minimizes the dose and is quite affordable (in US pharmacies). Once dry eye symptoms are resolved, then patients can try to stop the drug. Some patients need a 90-day treatment twice a year to maintain their comfort. Some patients prefer dosing every second day.

Azithromycin is a variety of dosing regimens that have been used by ophthalmologists: 5-day treatment vs. weekly maintenance dosing. Azithromycin may be more tolerated in term of GI upset experienced with tetracyclines. Topical daily azithromycin applied to the eyelid margins can be helpful for patients wishing to avoid systemic antibiotics, especially if they are on warfarin (drug-drug interactions) or have gastrointestinal disease. However, this drug may be expensive for patients to obtain for chronic use and its use for dry eye is off-label too.

Azithromycin is thought to have similar antimicrobial and anti-inflammatory effects like tetracyclines. However, there are also studies that have found that azithromycin can uniquely increase lipid accumulation and promote differentiation of meibomian gland epithelial cells in vitro.

His Exam Is Unchanged After 4 weeks. What Additional Treatment Option Can You Offer?

This patient is a candidate for LipiFlow automated thermal pulsation. LipiView is performed with marginal lid exfoliation with a golf club spatula prior to LipiFlow. Patient returns in 2 months.

He report his symptoms have improved; SPEED2 is 4 and OSDI 12. His grittiness symptom has resolved. TBUT has increased to 4 s OU. MGE improved to 11 OD and 12 OS. Patient is counseled that improvement of meibomian glands may not be permanent. He was encouraged to continue omega-3 fatty acids, hot compresses, and blink exercises and return for automated thermal pulsation expression of his eyelids when his symptoms recur.

What Are Blink Exercises?

Incomplete blinking is often observed at the slit lamp but quite noticeable on some dry eye patients on LipiView testing. Meibomian glands only secrete with the force of the orbicularis muscles pressing the eyelid margins together. Blink exercises are designed to help “retrain” a patient to develop the habit of complete blinking. Certainly some patients are more responsive to this habit development than others. Less success with retraining is expected with neuromuscular weakness, previous contact lens wear, or vertical lid shortening. Blink rate drops during dedicated visual activity (reading, watching TV, using the computer, or playing video games). While patients are performing dedicated visual activity, they are instructed to set a chime on a smartphone or timer every 10 min to remind them to take 4 s to perform the blink exercise. They are asked to close their eyelids for 2 s and then squeeze their eyelids tightly for 2 s, focusing on the sensation of the eyelids touching and squeezing together. This exercise is short and should not interfere with their visual activity. Blink exercises are thought to help keep open functioning meibomian glands.

Some Patients Do Not Respond to LipiFlow. What Else Can Be Offered If There Is Not Significant Meibomian Gland Atrophy?

Intense pulsed light combined with meibomian gland expression (IPL/MGX) is a protocol developed by Rolando Toyos MD for patients with ocular rosacea and dry eye symptoms. Our study shows that the majority of patients who fail to respond to LipiFlow can achieve improvement of symptoms with a series of four treatments of IPL/MGX. What is not yet clear is whether the MGX is producing the effect and what mechanism the IPL has on the dry eye symptoms. Further prospective studies are needed. An IPL/MGX series is more time-consuming and painful for the patient, as compared to a 12 min LipiFlow treatment.

Intraductal probing is offered for some patients to relieve the obstruction; however, it is also time-consuming and not comfortable for the patient. There is theoretical concern about causing acini damage from the probe itself or pushing surface secretions and microbes deep into the gland, nonetheless for select patients with MGD and evidence of blockage, this treatment has been shown to be beneficial.

Case 2

Patient is a 57-year-old hospital nurse manager who seeks additional opinion regarding her dry eyes for the past year. Her past medical history is significant for Crohn's disease in remission on biologics with past pancreatitis and facial rosacea. She has seasonal allergies and topical antihistamines work well. She has no family history of eye disease.

Past eyelid hygiene and artificial tears make her eyes worse and itchy. She takes 2000 mg of omega-3 fatty acids daily and places a microwaveable hot compress over her eyes at night for 10 min duration. She currently uses a preservative-free artificial tear five times a day in both eyes. Humidifiers did not improve her symptoms of dryness and burning. She had previously tried topical azithromycin and oral doxycycline and was intolerant of both. Her OSDI is 48.

On examination, her distance vision is 20/25 and near vision 20/20 in each eye with correction. Her pupils are reactive without an afferent pupillary defect. Her intraocular pressure is normal at 19 in both eyes. Evaluation of the periocular skin shows no evidence of allergic dermatitis, though she does have facial and ocular rosacea with lid margin telangiectasias. All four punctal are patent. There is no trichiasis or *Demodex* sleeving of lashes. There is no significant lid laxity or lagophthalmos. The meibomian glands show plugging and inspissation bilaterally. MGE shows three glands on the right lower lid yielding liquid secretions and eight glands on the left lower lid yielding toothpaste-consistency meibum. The eyelids margins are without notching. Her conjunctivae are moderately injected in both eyes. On upper and lower eyelid eversion, there is no significant papillary or follicular reaction or foreign bodies. Bulbar conjunctivae do not stain with lissamine green in either eye. No superior limbic keratoconjunctivitis is seen. Sclerae appear normal. Corneas have no punctate epithelial erosions and TBUT is 1 s in each eye. She has an ample tear meniscus and demonstrates reflex tearing while being examined at the slit lamp. Her anterior chambers are deep and quiet, and irides are normal bilaterally. Her crystalline lenses are clear bilaterally. Her optic nerve cup-to-disk ratio is 0.25 bilaterally. The remainder of her dilated fundus exam is normal.

What Diagnosis Do These Findings Suggest?

The patient appears to have meibomian gland dysfunction with low TBUT.

What Additional Testing Is Helpful?

MMP9 is positive in both eyes. Meibography was performed and shows severe atrophy in all four eyelids (Figs. 2.5 and 2.6).

Her basal tear secretion is high at 15 mm OD and 25 mm OS at 1 min.

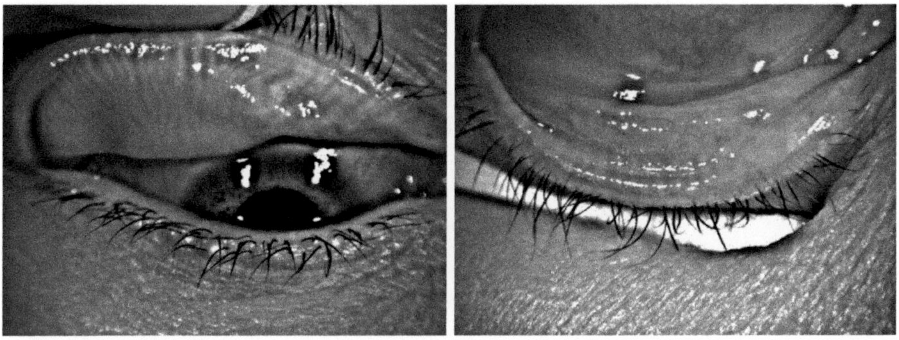

Fig. 2.5 Meibography of the right eye demonstrating significant drop out of the glands in both upper and lower lids

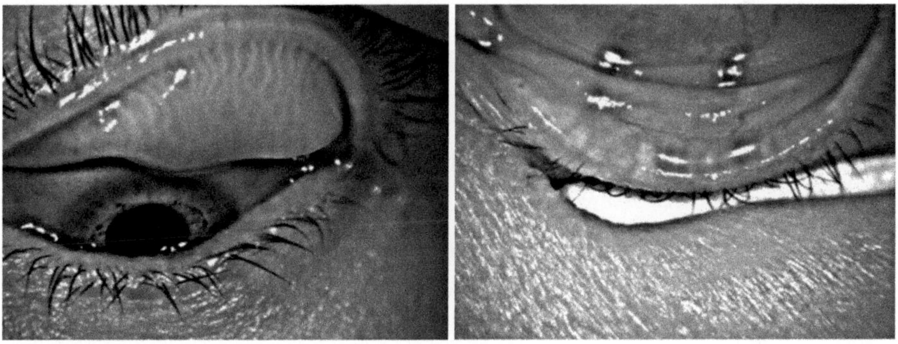

Fig. 2.6 Meibography of the left eye demonstrating significant drop out of the glands in both upper and lower lids

What Is Your Conclusion From These Additional Tests?

The positive MMP9 supports an inflammatory nature to her dry eye. The patient was started on topical cyclosporine BID OU. With the atrophy on meibography and high basal tear secretion, she has a severe meibum deficiency and has compensated with reflex tearing to protect her ocular surface.

She was previously intolerant to topical macrolide and oral doxycycline. At this current time, therapies for reviving atrophic meibomian glands is not available. Patient was recommend to try moisture chambers while she is using the computer or in highly ventilated areas. She declined this route and opted instead for fitting of scleral contact lenses for reduction in her symptoms.

Six months later, she is wearing scleral lenses full time with reduction of her OSDI score to 15.

What Caused Her Meibomian Gland Atrophy?

It is unknown what was the exact cause of the meibomian gland atrophy. Since meibography has not been clinically available in the past, no baseline tests are available for comparison. Facial rosacea and Crohn's disease likely contributed to the atrophy.

Final Thoughts

What Is the Role of Eyelid Hygiene (Cleaning the Lids/Lashes) in Meibomian Gland Disease?

Eyelid hygiene may play a role in "debulking" the antimicrobial load of the eyelid skin. This cleaning philosophy must be tempered with the fact that excessive washing is stressful to the epidermis. If patients have scurf and sleeving or residual makeup, I recommend lid hygiene.

Lid hygiene techniques are tapered to the individual. A nursing home patient who receives bathing only once a week may do better with a commercial lid wipe that can be used at the bedside. Baby shampoo has surfactants that may help relieve excessive amounts of oil and skin debris and may benefit those patients who can be upright or take a daily shower or bath. "Sulfate-free" baby shampoos are also available for patients who claim sensitivity to sodium lauryl sulfate products. If patients have clean appearing lid margins and lashes without eczematous changes, I usually will have them continue their present lid hygiene routine. If patients have eczematous changes to their skin, then I recommend backing off to allow the skin to heal, sometimes using topical steroid emollients for short-term control of dermatitis. A more recent commercial eyelid cleaning solution that some patients have found useful and nonirritating is hypochlorous acid (Avenova).

What Can Be Done About Demodex Infestation?

Demodex infestation can contribute to dry eye symptoms. It appears that *Demodex* mites have an etiologic role in some forms of anterior blepharitis and that treatment with tea tree oil is merited in these cases. However, it can be difficult to eradicate *Demodex* in eyelids even after confirming the diagnosis by viewing the parasite on sleeved eyelash under light microscopy.

Prior to commercially available tea tree oil wipes, I performed weekly eyelid treatments with tea tree oil on patients with severe sleeving at the base of the eyelashes based on Schaeffer Tseng's protocol. These treatments were difficult for patients to tolerate and time-consuming for us both. The majority of my patients who have used the commercial tea tree oil lid wipes had to eventually discontinue due to skin intolerance and pain with treatment or lack of improvement of symptoms. Interestingly, there is anecdotal suggestion that low glycemic diet can help reduce the proliferation rate of this opportunistic ectodermal parasite. Hypothetically, if there is less excess glucose available, then there would be less rapid growth of *Demodex*. Oral ivermectin (3–6 mg PO one dose—repeated in 2–4 weeks as needed) has been reported to be successful, while topical ivermectin (skin preparation commercially available as Soolantra), which has been shown to improve the skin disease in rosacea, has also been anecdotally reported to reduce *Demodex* when applied to the eyelids.

What Is the Role of Topical Corticosteroids in MGD?

In patients with signs of inflammation, steroids are useful especially as a short-term treatment. Soft steroids such as loteprednol 0.5% may be a good choice given their lower propensity to increase IOP and having no risk of inducing cataracts. In a patient who requires long-term anti-inflammatory therapy, either cyclosporine (Restasis), lifitegrast, or off-label use of tacrolimus ointment to the lids (dermatologic preparation 0.03%) may be considered.

Acknowledgments *Financial Disclosures*: The author has no financial disclosures regarding the contents discussed in this manuscript. *Conflict of Interest*: The author has no conflicts of interest with the contents discussed in this manuscript.

References

1. Nichols KK, et al. The international workshop on Meibomian gland dysfunction: executive summary. Invest Ophthalmol Vis Sci. 2011;52(4):1922–9. http://www.tearfilm.org.
2. 2007 Report of the International Dry Eye WorkShop (DEWS). Ocul Surf. 2007;5(2):67–199. www.tearfilm.org.
3. Vegunta S, Patel D, Shen JF. Combination therapy of intense pulsed light therapy and meibomian gland expression (IPL/MGX) can improve dry eye symptoms and meibomian gland function in refractory dry eye patients: a retrospective review. Cornea. 2016;35(3):318–22.
4. McMonnies CW, Korb DR, Blackie CA. The role of heat and rubbing and massage-related corneal deformation. Cont Lens Anterior Eye. 2012;35(4):148–54.

Chapter 3
Image-Guided Evaluation and Monitoring of Treatment Response in Patients with Ocular Surface Disease

Alessandro Abbouda, Nicholas Pondelis, and Pedram Hamrah

Introduction

The Dry Eye Workshop (DEWS), conducted in 2007, defined dry eye disease (DED) as "a multifactorial disease of the tears and ocular surface that results in symptoms of discomfort, visual disturbance, and tear film instability with potential damage to the ocular surface. It is accompanied by increased osmolarity of the tear film and inflammation of the ocular surface" [1]. In order to achieve successful DED treatment, there must be a precise diagnosis and careful management.

The application of new imaging methodology in the study of DED has resulted in the development of fascinating tools that each ophthalmologist should acknowledge when deciding to follow these patients. In vivo confocal microscopy (IVCM) is able to furnish data regarding lid, conjunctiva, and cornea modification in dry eye disease. This device also allows for the evaluation of meibomian gland density, duct morphology, gland enlargement, and the presence of fibrosis. Furthermore, IVCM can provide information regarding the density and the morphology of subepithelial immune cells and subbasal nerves in the cornea. Along with IVCM, anterior segment optical coherence tomography (AS-OCT) is another useful tool in DED treatment. Use of the AS-OCT can furnish data regarding tear meniscus height and depth, as well as meibomian gland length and width. Together, these instruments offer more sophisticated examination options than have ever been available to

A. Abbouda, MD • P. Hamrah, MD, FRCS (✉)
Cornea Service, New England Eye Center, Boston, MA 02111, USA

Department of Ophthalmology, Center for Translational Ocular Immunology, Tufts Medical Center, Tufts University School of Medicine, Boston, MA 02111, USA
e-mail: PHamrah@tuftsmedicalcenter.org

N. Pondelis, BA
Department of Ophthalmology, Center for Translational Ocular Immunology, Tufts Medical Center, Tufts University School of Medicine, Boston, MA 02111, USA

A.R. Djalilian (ed.), *Ocular Surface Disease*,
https://doi.org/10.1007/978-3-319-15823-5_3

clinicians seeking to find relief for their DED patients. The cases presented below will explore the various aspects of DED and will highlight how these new imaging techniques facilitate the evaluation and treatment of this ocular surface disease.

Case 1

LC is a 73-year-old female referred to our center with a diagnosis of *aqueous-deficient dry eye*. She underwent punctual plug occlusion 1 year prior to her referral, which provided partial relief from her symptoms. She reports having significant tearing and difficulty reading due to blurry vision. Her symptoms began 6 months before her visit. Her past medical history was significant for dyslipidemia and neurological transient ischemic attack. She does not have significant ocular family history. She was prescribed clopidogrel 75 mg per day and atorvastatin. She was not able to tolerate cyclosporine drops.

What Diagnosis Do These Symptoms Suggest?

Based on abnormalities of the tear film composition, DED has been classified into two categories: aqueous-deficient dry eye (ADDE) and evaporative dry eye (EDE). These two classifications correspond to disorders of the lacrimal system (resulting in ADDE) and meibomian glands (resulting in EDE). Aqueous-deficient dry eye can further be classified into Sjögren's syndrome (SS) and non-Sjögren's syndrome (NSS) dry eye. Similarly, evaporative dry eye can be classified into intrinsic and extrinsic causes, with meibomian gland dysfunction (MGD) being the most common cause of EDE. ADDE and EDE are not mutually exclusive and often act together to result in typical DED signs and symptoms [1, 2]. This overlap of etiology makes it challenging to identify pure cases of EDE or ADDE. A distinction between the two is further made difficult by the reality that both fall together under the same broad diagnosis of DED according to the current system of classification. In the above example, if relying exclusively on the patient's symptoms for information, it would be easy to conclude that the excessive tearing was related to plug occlusion. This thought process may lead to a conclusion that the best treatment option is removal of the punctual plugs. Thorough testing and examination must be done first, however, as meibomian gland disease could be causing her uncomfortable symptoms.

Her corrected visual acuity at the time of her visit was 20/20 in both eyes. Near corrected vision was J1+ in both eyes. Evaluation of the periocular skin gave no evidence of rash or other lesions. There was no evidence of trichiasis. There was no significant presence of lid laxity or lagophthalmos. Her meibomian glands and the eyelid margin presented a Marx's line running through the meibomian orifices, along with telangiectasia over the lid rim. Her conjunctiva was normal. Slit-lamp examination revealed trace superficial punctate keratopathy. Schirmer's test was 9 mm/5 min in both eyes and she had a TBUT of 6 s in both eyes. Intraocular pressure and fundus examination were normal.

What Are Your Next Diagnostic Steps?

The recent 2011 International Workshop on Meibomian Gland Dysfunction (IWMGD 2011) defined MGD as "a chronic, diffuse abnormality of the meibomian glands, commonly characterized by terminal duct obstruction and/or qualitative/quantitative changes in the glandular secretion. It may result in alteration of the tear film, symptoms of eye irritation, clinically apparent inflammation, and ocular surface disease" [3, 4]. The clinical examination of our patient showed a clear condition of meibomian gland disease, but we need to understand how much this condition impacts her symptoms to fully treat her. It is also necessary to quantify MG inflammation in order to devise a successful treatment regimen. To gather this critical clinical information, an IVCM examination and an AS-OCT were performed to evaluate MG function and morphology.

IVCM revealed significant intrapalpebral scarring, MG ductal dilatation, and glandular obstruction (Fig. 3.1a–d). AS-OCT showed an enlargement of MG ducts and areas devoid of glands, especially in the upper lids (Fig. 3.1e, f). These findings are all associated with intraductal meibomian gland inflammation.

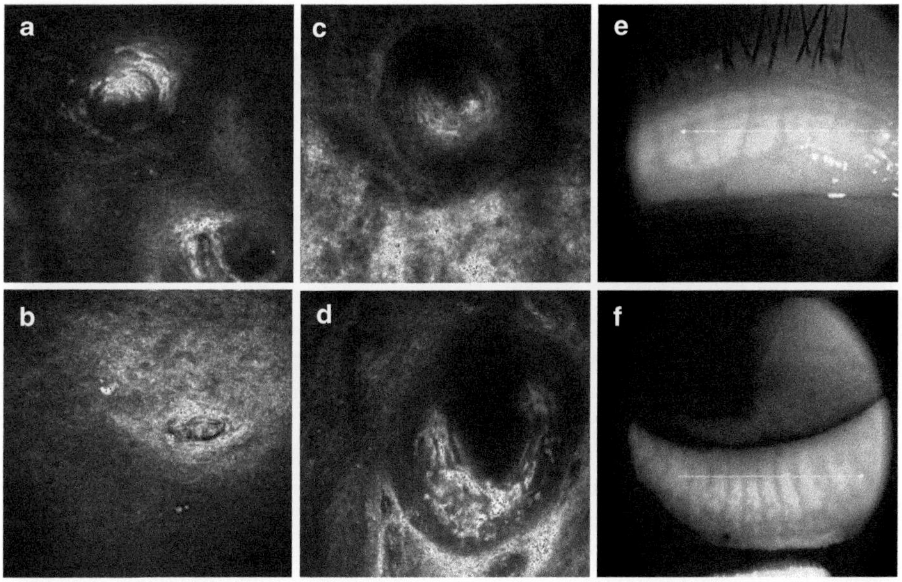

Fig. 3.1 IVCM meibomian gland evaluation (**a–d**). At the time of diagnosis, IVCM scans of upper lids reveal obstruction of meibomian gland ducts close to the orifices (**a–b**), progressive intraductal obstruction along the length of the glands (**c**), and the presence of inflammatory cells adjacent to the duct walls (**d**). AS-OCT meibography of the patient's upper lid displays enlargement of meibomian gland ducts and reduction in length (**e**). In the lower lid, there is an obvious obstruction near the meibomian orifices that prevents gland secretions from reaching the ocular surface (**f**)

What Diagnosis Do These Findings Suggest?

IVCM and AS-OCT of MGs furnish objective parameters regarding the amount of orifices and their diameter, as well as the number of MG, their length, and their width. The AS-OCT is also able to give an overview of MG distribution in the upper and lower eyelid [5]. These imaging technologies have potential to guide physicians in the management of MGD therapy. The choice between topical and systemic therapy is guided by live imaging of the glands themselves. Visualization of intraductal inflammatory cells and fibrosis are fundamental pieces of information that can be obtained from IVCM and AS-OCT. It should be noted that near-infrared imaging of the meibomian glands with devices such as LipiView™ or Keratograph 5M™ can now provide very nice images and information about the morphology of the glands (higher quality than AS-OCT images); however, they cannot provide cellular level detail about inflammatory cells which can only be provided by IVCM. In this case, the findings are an indicator for the success of intraductal meibomian gland probing as a measure to improve symptoms attributable to glandular obstruction [6].

Intraductal MG probing was performed with 1 mm and 2 mm probes for all glands, after a 2% lidocaine local injection (into the upper lid) and proparacaine eyedrops were applied. Additionally, the lids were expressed with a meibomian gland expresser. The patient tolerated the procedure well. Further treatment included systemic treatment of doxycycline 100 mg two times per day, azithromycin ophthalmic solution 1% one application at night to eyelids, prednisolone 0.12% drops twice per day, and hot compresses along with lid massage. Flaxseed oil supplement was also prescribed.

What Are Your MGD Treatment Recommendations?

Treatment of MGD can include a surgical approach, medical therapy, or a combination of both. Invasive orifice penetration and intraductal probing is a relatively new and successful application to consider when you have to manage recurrent and severe MGD caused by intraductal fibrosis. This approach yields results immediately and is effective in relieving symptoms that accompany dry eye disease. AS-OCT and IVCM can guide this approach to therapy. These instruments are able to visualize the number of atrophic glands that are not candidates for probing. Moreover, these instruments furnish information that can reveal the length of MG ducts. This data can then be used to select the appropriate length probes before the procedure. Medical treatments include systemic tetracyclines (doxycycline, minocycline) and topical macrolides (1% azithromycin) [7–11]. These drugs have anti-inflammatory properties, such as inhibiting microbial lipase production, reducing the activity of tissue matrix metalloproteinases (MMP), and lowering the release of pro-inflammatory-free fatty acids and diglycerides onto the lid margin [12–16].

At her last follow-up, 1 year after MG probing, the patient reported a remarkable improvement in her symptoms. She does not complain anymore about excessive tearing. She has followed her treatment instructions of maintaining lid hygiene, using hot compresses, performing lid massages, and taking flaxseed oil supplement. She stopped systemic anti-inflammatory treatment after 6 months. Ophthalmic examination showed some isolated meibomian glands occluded and a marked decrease of lid hyperemia. Her conjunctiva was normal. Slit-lamp examination revealed a normal ocular surface. Schirmer's test was 10 mm/5 min in both eyes, and a TBUT of 8 s was found in both eyes.

Her latest IVCM scans showed MG ducts were more prevalent than before treatment and did not show inflammation in the meibomian ducts (Fig. 3.2a). IVCM results indicated that some areas of fibrosis persisted, but obstruction was significantly reduced (Fig. 3.2b). AS-OCT of upper and lower lids revealed a change from abnormal gland morphology (Fig. 3.1e, f) to a more normal state (Fig. 3.2c, d).

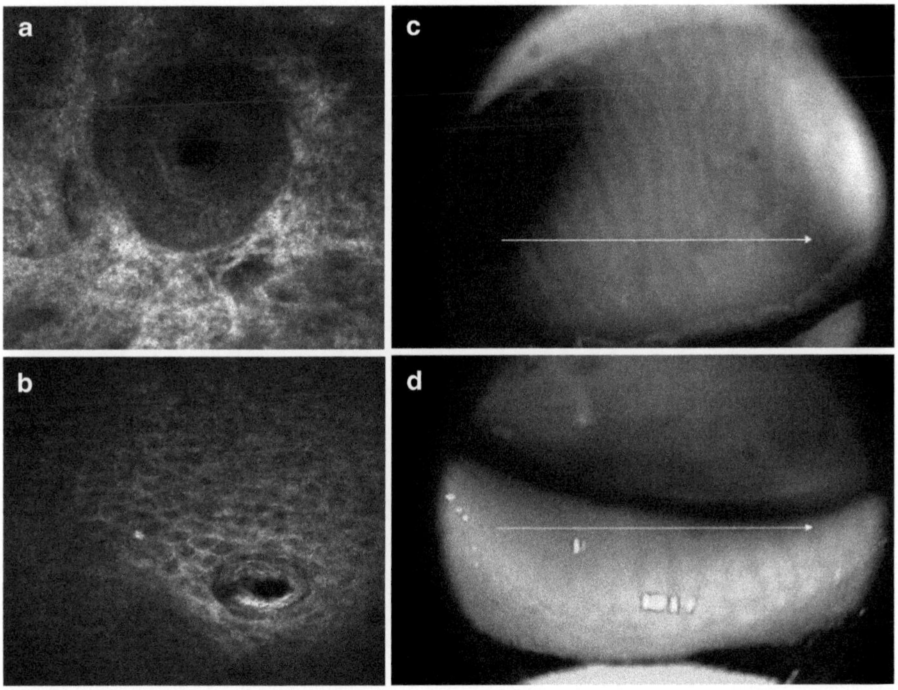

Fig. 3.2 One year after MG probing, IVCM scans of the upper lid reveal open meibomian glands, although ducts remain smaller than normal (**a**). Some areas of fibrosis remain in the duct walls, especially close to the orifices (**b**). AS-OCT at 1 year after meibomian gland probing demonstrates a clear reduction in duct width and an elongation of gland length (**c**). The lower lid displays recanalization of the meibomian gland ducts along the entire length of the lid, up to the previously sealed orifices (**d**)

Case 2

JO is a 38-year-old female referred to our center with a diagnosis of dry eye disease. She complained of light sensitivity and pain in both eyes. She was put on artificial tears for 6 months without noticing any improvement. The patient denied having any significant disease or surgery in the past. Her visual acuity was 20/20, and her near vision was J1+ in both eyes. Her meibomian glands and eyelid margin appeared normal, as did her conjunctiva. Slit-lamp examination revealed a normal ocular surface with normal tear breakup time and without a staining. Intraocular pressure and fundus examination were normal.

How Would You Proceed at This Stage?

In all patients with a significant discrepancy between symptom and ocular surface condition, it is likely that the patient's troubles are caused by some form of corneal neuropathy. Chronic and persistent ectopic activity of injured corneal nerves can cause pain in response to both innocuous stimulation (allodynia) and noxious stimuli (hyperalgesia) [17–19]. Photoallodynia is an important symptom associated with neuropathy in the cornea. If the ocular surface does not justify the light sensitivity, it is quite common to identify nerve abnormalities. Very recently, IVCM has demonstrated the ability to detect corneal subbasal nerve damage and aberrant nerve regeneration. The tests also image the formation of neuromas and neurite sprouting in patients with photoallodynia [20].

In vivo confocal microscopy was performed on this patient. The test showed nerves with severe tortuosity, nerve beading, and frequent microneuromas (Fig. 3.3a, b). These findings led to a diagnosis of corneal neuropathy.

What Are Your Next Diagnostic Steps?

The first thing to do after you diagnose corneal neuropathy is spend some time with your patient in order to fully explain this disorder. Most will be relieved to know that there is an explanation for their symptoms. Many of these patients have had years of frustration searching for a solution to painful symptoms and are familiar with having their complaints written off. Now, the next step is to understand if the pain is localized peripherally (peripheral sensitization) or if there is a central component (central sensitization). The best way to determine this is with the installation of proparacaine drops.

A significant amount of pain relief was obtained from proparacaine drops.

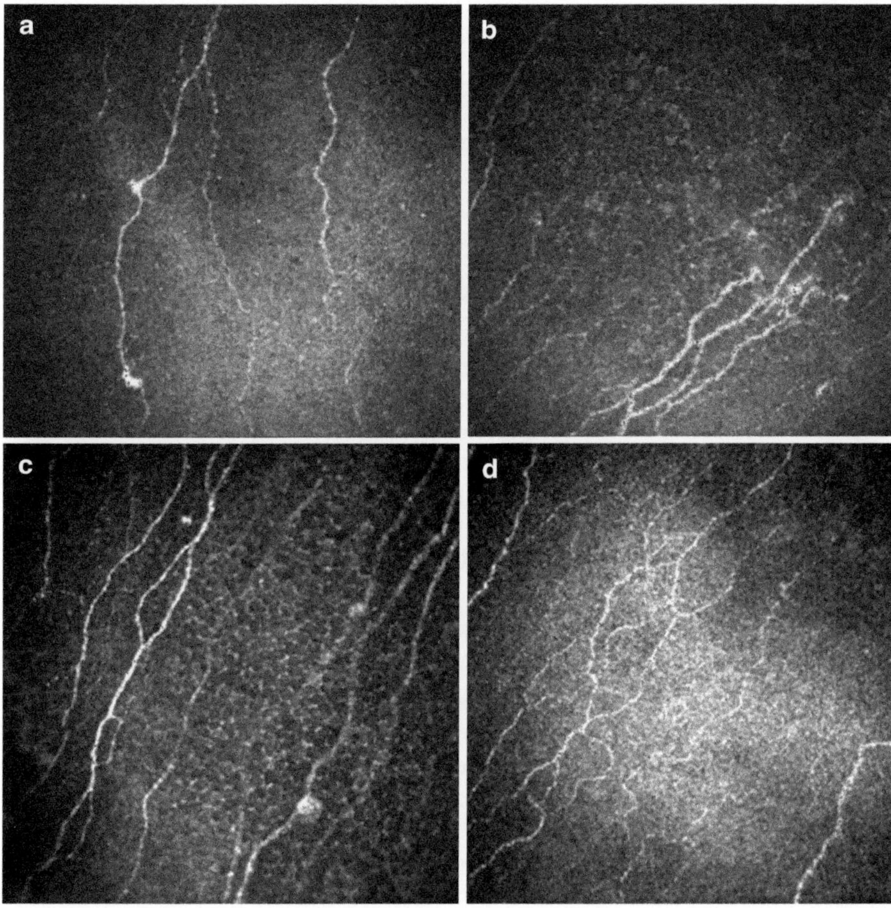

Fig. 3.3 Peripheral corneal neuropathy in the subbasal nerve plexus. The IVCM scans display an abnormal arrangement of subbasal plexus nerves, reduction of nerve density, the presence of neuromas, nerve beading, and nerve sprouting (**a**, **b**). IVCM scans taken 8 months after treatment reveal a less aberrant subbasal layer. Visible differences include a marked decrease of neuromas, the disappearance of sprouting, and an increase in nerve density (**c**, **d**)

What Are Your Treatment Recommendations?

To establish the best treatment for a patient with corneal neuropathy, we need to consider several factors. The proparacaine challenge is the first step to take, as any central component of pain requires different treatment from neuropathy originating in peripheral nerves alone. Patients with a central component need systemic treatment, such as with a tricyclic antidepressant, which has proven to be effective in pain remodulation. However, a systemic treatment could also be called for in a patient with peripheral pain only, if other treatments are not effective.

Peripheral corneal neuropathy can result from nerve dysfunction alone, but another factor potentially contributing to pain is corneal inflammation. IVCM can locate areas of the cornea experiencing an increased presence of activated dendritic cells and thus justify an anti-inflammatory treatment for your patient. Regardless of the cause, in patients with peripheral cornea pain, the goal in treatment is to restore both frequency and distribution of nerves in the subbasal nerve plexus, as well as functional recovery of the nerves. Autologous serum tear (AST) drops 20% are the first choice for therapy in cases of corneal neuropathy as a neuro-regenerative therapy [20]. After the application of ASTs, for a mean duration of 4 months, many patients have demonstrated a significant reduction in the severity of their symptoms. Follow-up IVCM imaging of these patients clearly shows a significant reversal of morphological nerve alterations and reversal of symptoms.

In this case, AST (20%) were prescribed for 6 months at the dose of eight drops per day. Additionally, the patient was instructed to administer loteprednol etabonate 0.5% drops four times a day for a week, tapering to a drop each week for 3 months. IVCM at 8 months posttreatment showed a reduction in the frequency of neuromas compared to the first visit, as well as an increase in nerve density (Fig. 3.3c, d). The patient subsequently reported a complete resolution of photoallodynia.

Case 3

PC is a 57-year-old woman with a severe keratoconjunctivitis sicca associated with her diagnosis of *Sjögren's syndrome*. She underwent punctual plug occlusion, followed by punctual cautery, in both eyes 1 year before her visit. These interventions afforded partial relief from symptoms. Her past medical history included breast cancer. Her current ocular medications included various artificial tears and contact lenses.

At her first visit visual acuity was 20/20 in the right eye and 20/40 in the left eye. Her lids were in normal position. Slit-lamp examination did not reveal any signs of blepharitis. The central cornea showed diffuse punctate epithelial keratitis. Schirmer's test was 2 mm/5 min in the right eye and 0 mm/5 min in the left eye. Tear breakup time was 2 s, and tear meniscus was reduced. She had PC-IOLs in both eyes, and no signs of intraocular inflammation. Fundus examination was normal.

What Is Your Examination Approach to Chronic Dry Eye?

In the case of dry eye disease occurring along with another condition, it is important to establish the amount of inflammation in the cornea. According to a recent paper, aqueous-deficient DED with underlying systemic immune disease (Sjögren's syndrome and graft-versus-host disease) showed significantly higher dendritic cell density, size, and digitation, compared to DED not associated with immune conditions [21]. IVCM is able to determine if this is true for your patient and provides objective measures in the management of such a case.

IVCM showed an elevated number of dendritic cells in the subepithelial layer in both eyes. Most of the dendritic cells projected dendrites and were of increased size. In addition, nerve density was very low (Fig. 3.4a).

What Are Your Ocular Treatment Recommendations?

The IVCM findings in this case indicate the presence of active inflammation in the corneal. Therefore, it is important to explain to the patient the role of inflammation in her disease and how the steroid treatment should help effectively treat her. Thanks to IVCM, it was possible to visualize the inflammation and to precisely modify the patient's treatment according to the presence of inflammation. The use of IVCM in this case was fundamental, not only for its role in informing treatment strategy but as a visual too when emphasizing treatment compliance to your patient. The ability to show this patient exactly the reason for her symptoms, and the rationale for the suggested therapies, was critical in this situation. Neither the precise treatment program nor the cooperation of the patient would have been possible without the use of advanced imaging techniques.

The patient was prescribed ASTs eight times a day, as well as loteprednol etabonate 0.5% drops four times a day for a week, tapering to a drop each week for 4 weeks. IVCM at 2 months posttreatment discovered a significant reduction in the number of DCs but no change in the patient's nerve density (Fig. 3.4b). The patient continued her AST regimen, but loteprednol was switched to cyclosporine 0.05% drops twice a day for 4 months. IVCM at 6 months after the first visit showed a regeneration of subbasal plexus nerves and inflammation firmly under control (Fig. 3.4c).

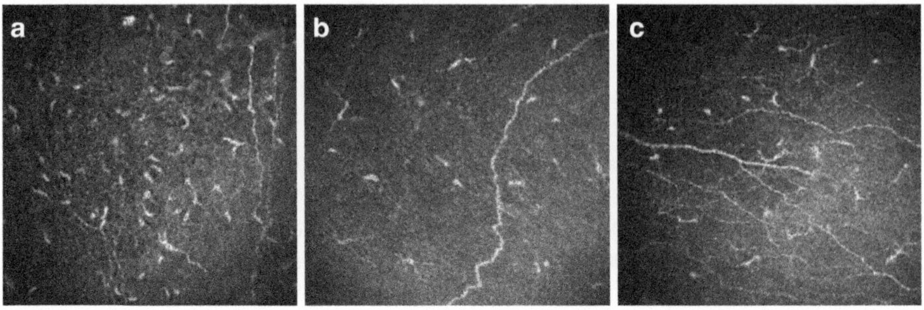

Fig. 3.4 Inflammation in the subbasal nerve plexus. At the time of diagnosis, IVCM scans show a substantial decrease in nerve density and a considerable number of dendritic cells. Most of these cells are large in size and project dendrites, indicating that they are in an active state (**a**). IVCM scans taken 2 months into treatment reveal markedly fewer dendritic cells. Nerve density seems unchanged, although some nerves appear healthier. Some indicators of unhealthy nerves are tortuosity and beading, and a lack thereof is a sign that a nerve is healthy (**b**). IVCM scans taken 6 months into treatment display significant regeneration of subbasal plexus nerves. Dendritic cells are fewer in number than before treatment but are still present (**c**)

References

1. The definition and classification of dry eye disease: report of the definition and classification Subcommittee of the International dry eye WorkShop. Ocul Surf. 2007;5:75–92.
2. Shimazaki J, Goto E, Ono M, Shimmura S, Tsubota K. Meibomian gland dysfunction in patients with Sjogren syndrome. Ophthalmology. 1998;105:1485–8.
3. Nelson JD, Shimazaki J, Benitez-del-Castillo JM, Craig JP, McCulley JP, Den S, Foulks GN. The international workshop on meibomian gland dysfunction: report of the definition and classification subcommittee. Invest Ophthalmol Vis Sci. 2011;52:1930–7.
4. Nichols KK, Foulks GN, Bron AJ, Glasgow BJ, Dogru M, Tsubota K, Lemp MA, Sullivan DA. The international workshop on meibomian gland dysfunction: executive summary. Invest Ophthalmol Vis Sci. 2011;52:1922–9.
5. Liang Q, Pan Z, Zhou M, Zhang Y, Wang N, Li B, Baudouin C, Labbé A. Evaluation of optical coherence tomography meibography in patients with obstructive Meibomian gland dysfunction. Cornea. 2015;34(10):1193–9.
6. Maskin SL. Intraductal meibomian gland probing relieves symptoms of obstructive meibomian gland dysfunction. Cornea. 2010;29:1145–52.
7. Sanchez J, Somolinos AL, Almodovar PI, Webster G, Bradshaw M, Powala C. A randomized, double-blind, placebo-controlled trial of the combined effect of doxycycline hyclate 20-mg tablets and metronidazole 0.75% topical lotion in the treatment of rosacea. J Am Acad Dermatol. 2005;53:791–7.
8. Frucht-Pery J, Sagi E, Hemo I, Ever-Hadani P. Efficacy of doxycycline and tetracycline in ocular rosacea. Am J Ophthalmol. 1993;116:88–92.
9. Yoo SE, Lee DC, Chang MH. The effect of low-dose doxycycline therapy in chronic meibomian gland dysfunction. Korean J Ophthalmol. 2005;19:258–63.
10. Theobald K, Bradshaw M, Leyden J. Anti-inflammatory dose doxycycline (40 mg controlled-release) confers maximum anti-inflammatory efficacy in rosacea. Skinmed. 2007;6:221–6.

11. Del Rosso JQ, Webster GF, Jackson M, Rendon M, Rich P, Torok H, Bradshaw M. Two randomized phase III clinical trials evaluating anti-inflammatory dose doxycycline (40-mg doxycycline, USP capsules) administered once daily for treatment of rosacea. J Am Acad Dermatol. 2007;56:791–802.
12. Dougherty JM, McCulley JP. Bacterial lipases and chronic blepharitis. Invest Ophthalmol Vis Sci. 1986;27:486–91.
13. Dougherty JM, McCulley JP, Silvany RE, Meyer DR. Thenrole of tetracycline in chronic blepharitis. Inhibition of lipase production in staphylococci. Invest Ophthalmol Vis Sci. 1991;32:2970–5.
14. Duerden JM, Tiffany JM. Lipid synthesis in vitro by rabbit meibomian gland tissue and its inhibition by tetracycline. Biochim Biophys Acta. 1990;1042:13–8.
15. Shine WE, McCulley JP, Pandya AG. Minocycline effect on meibomian gland lipids in meibomianitis patients. Exp Eye Res. 2003;76:417–20.
16. Souchier M, Joffre C, Gregoire S, Bretillon L, Muselier A, Acar N, Beynat J, Bron A, D'Athis P, Creuzot-Garcher C. Changes in meibomian fatty acids and clinical signs in patients with meibomian gland dysfunction after minocycline treatment. Br J Ophthalmol. 2008;92:819–22.
17. Borsook D, Rosenthal P. Chronic (neuropathic) corneal pain and blepharospasm: five case reports. Pain. 2011;152:2427–31.
18. Rosenthal P, Baran I, Jacobs DS. Corneal pain without stain: is it real? Ocul Surf. 2009;7:28–40.
19. Rosenthal P, Borsook D. The corneal pain system. Part I: the missing piece of the dry eye puzzle. Ocul Surf. 2012;10:2–14.
20. Aggarwal S, Kheirkhah A, Cavalcanti BM, Cruzat A, Colon C, Brown E, Borsook D, Prüss H, Hamrah P. Autologous serum tears for treatment of photoallodynia in patients with corneal neuropathy: efficacy and evaluation with in vivo confocal microscopy. Ocul Surf. 2015;13(3):250–62.
21. Kheirkhah A, Rahimi Darabad R, Cruzat A, Hajrasouliha AR, Witkin D, Wong N, Dana R, Hamrah P. Corneal epithelial immune dendritic cell alterations in subtypes of dry eye disease: a pilot in vivo confocal microscopic study. Invest Ophthalmol Vis Sci. 2015;56(12):7179–85.

Chapter 4
Management of Ocular Surface Disease in Cataract and Refractive Surgery Patients

Giancarlo A. Garcia and Marjan Farid

Introduction

The health of the ocular surface must be thoroughly evaluated before a patient undergoes cataract or refractive surgery. Integrity of the tear film is essential for proper visual function, corneal protection and health, and patient comfort. Tear film irregularities and an imbalance in tear composition can result in significant optical aberrations that can compromise vision. Ocular surface disease (OSD), including dry eye syndrome (DES) and meibomian gland dysfunction (MGD), is one of the most commonly seen ophthalmologic conditions that can have significant negative impacts on surgical outcomes and patient satisfaction. Refractive procedures such as cataract surgery and laser vision correction are especially susceptible to the potential negative visual outcomes from OSD, as the tear film is the first refractive component that light hits as it enters the eye.

The presence of OSD in refractive surgery cases can significantly affect preoperative assessments, intraoperative management, and postoperative outcomes and monitoring. Detection and treatment of OSD before surgery and preoperative measurements is therefore essential. Careful preoperative evaluation of the ocular surface should be performed even in patients without active dry eye complaints, as many patients with clinical signs of dry eye may be asymptomatic [1]. Furthermore, a review of past medical and ocular history looking for risk factors can aid in the identification of OSD. Lifestyle factors such as hours of screen time, chronic contact lens use, or use of hormonal replacement therapy may be clues that the patient needs to be screened for OSD. Many simple yet effective diagnostic techniques and treatment regimens for DES and MGD can be utilized to improve ocular surface health and ultimately improve surgical outcomes.

G.A. Garcia, MS • M. Farid, MD (✉)
Gavin Herbert Eye Institute, UC-Irvine, 850 Health Sciences Road, Irvine, CA 92697, USA
e-mail: mfarid@uci.edu

A.R. Djalilian (ed.), *Ocular Surface Disease*,
https://doi.org/10.1007/978-3-319-15823-5_4

Case 1

A 75-year-old man is being evaluated for cataract surgery. He is unhappy with the quality of his vision and reports difficulty with driving and reading. Over the past 2 years, he has experienced progressively worsening redness of his eyes and eyelids and visual fluctuations in conjunction with blinking. He has used saline eye drops several times daily for the past few months without relief. His past medical history includes hypertension, for which he is taking lisinopril and hydrochlorothiazide. He is a retired schoolteacher with no other significant social history.

On clinical examination, best-corrected visual acuity (BCVA) is 20/60 OU. Intraocular pressure is 17 mmHg OD and 15 mmHg OS. On slit lamp examination, hyperemia and scattered telangiectasias of the upper and lower lid margins are noted bilaterally. Lid margin debris is prominent on both lower lids. The corneas are clear bilaterally, and both eyes demonstrate grade 3 lens opacities in accordance with the Lens Opacification Grading System III (LOCS) scale. Dilated fundoscopic exam reveals no abnormalities.

What Risks Does Cataract Surgery Pose to Individuals with OSD?

Patients with pre-existing OSD have a high likelihood of experiencing postoperative exacerbation of dry eye [2]. The pathogenesis of this phenomenon is likely multifactorial. Damage to corneal nerves can disrupt corneal sensation, resulting in decreased feedback stimulation of the lacrimal gland and subsequent aqueous deficiency. Corneal hypoesthesia can also reduce blink rate, leading to increased tear evaporation. In addition, inflammation from tissue manipulation and ocular surface irritation can lead to further corneal damage and decreased tear production.

Other factors such as application of topical anesthesia, microscope light exposure, aggressive irrigation of the tear film, use of preserved eye drops postoperatively, and goblet cell loss may increase dry eye incidence and severity postsurgically [3–6]. Additionally, Han et al. report that cataract surgery is associated with postoperative decline in MG function, though the mechanism of this impairment is unclear [7].

As a result of poor ocular surface health, patients with dry eye are at higher risk of developing postoperative complications such as epithelial defects, corneal melts, infection, and impaired visual outcome [8].

What Testing Should Be Performed to Evaluate This Patient's OSD?

Detection and management of OSD in all patients before any cataract/refractive surgery is critical, as the health of the tear film can have significant effects on postoperative visual outcomes. Advanced age is a risk factor for dry eye syndrome, and thus elderly individuals, in particular, must have a thorough ocular surface evaluation prior to surgery.

This elderly patient demonstrates evidence of visually significant cataracts and OSD secondary to MGD. MGD is often associated with varying degrees of eyelid inflammation, lid margin erythema, inspissated gland orifices, and thickened or absent oil secretions. The presence of debris at the base of the lashes may indicate concomitant anterior blepharitis that may be bacterial or secondary to *Demodex* mite infestation.

A simple slit lamp evaluation of the eyelid health can be performed. Using a cotton tip applicator, gentle pressure on the eyelid margins reveals the ease of oil flow as well as the constitution of the meibum. Expressibility—a reflection of meibomian gland (MG) function—refers to the ease with which secretion can be physically expelled from MGs of the lower lid with either digital pressure or other expression instrument. In this assessment, a lower number of MGs yielding liquid secretion correlate with higher dry eye symptom severity [9]. No flow indicates severe disease.

Meibography imaging of the everted lids can be used to evaluate gland density, architecture, and degree of atrophy or dropout (Fig. 4.1). Imaging of the glands also allows patients to witness the severity of the disease and help them understand the necessity for treatment.

Evaporative dry eye and aqueous-deficient dry eye frequently co-occur, and as such, patients must be assessed for both [10]. Ocular surface staining with vital dyes such as Lissamine green helps assess the degeneration of conjunctival and corneal epithelial cells and is a sign of late-stage disease. Fluorescein staining may also be used but will only pick up microerosions from areas of cell loss and exposed basement membrane. A low tear breakup time (TBUT) correlates well with MGD and shows the instability of the tear film. Patients with decreased TBUT often complain of rapid loss of clear vision between blinks and visual fluctuations.

Newer point of care testing for tear film analysis is now available as simple in-office tests to help guide diagnosis and treatment. Tear film osmolarity can be rapidly obtained using test cards with a minimal tear sample as part of the routine in-office workup for these patients. A tear film osmolarity score will help categorize the severity of dryness [11]. Tear hyperosmolarity has been demonstrated to be an accurate indicator of dry eye as compared to traditional

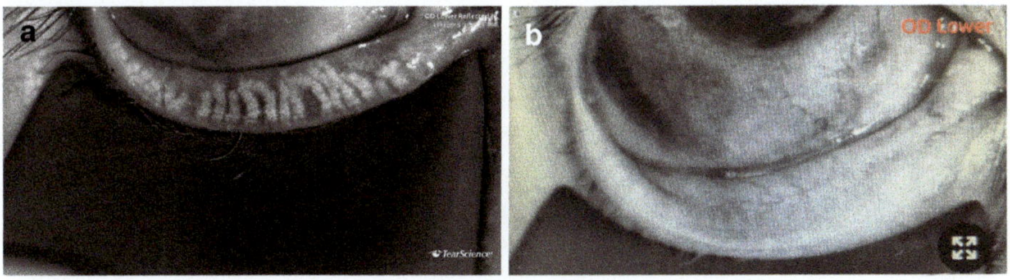

Fig. 4.1 Meibography imaging of the everted lids can be used to evaluate gland density, architecture, and degree of atrophy or dropout. (**a**) Moderate disease with gland shortening and partial dropout. (**b**) Severe disease with near total dropout

Schirmer's testing [12]. An osmolarity value of ≥308 mOsms/L or a variability of >8 mOsms/L between the eyes is significant for dry eye. Another rapid in-office tear film test looks for the presence of matrix metalloproteinase 9 (MMP-9), an inflammatory cytokine that can be used as a biomarker to detect ocular surface inflammation. The high sensitivity and specificity for detection of elevated levels of MMP-9 (>40 mg/mL) in the tears of individuals with dry eye make this test valuable for identifying patients that may need the addition of an anti-inflammatory therapeutic [13].

Corneal sensation can also be tested preoperatively, especially in patients who are at risk for neurotrophic corneal disease, such as diabetics. These individuals have a higher likelihood of postoperative dry eye, as further damage to corneal nerves from surgery can exacerbate symptoms.

Fluorescein staining in this patient reveals 2+ inferior punctate corneal epithelial erosions and a TBUT of 3 s in both eyes. The tear film osmolarity test reads 318 mOsms/L OD and 307 mOsms/L OS, and InflammaDry testing demonstrates elevated levels of MMP-9 in both eyes. Meibomian glands are poorly expressible with 2–3 expressible glands per lid showing thickened "toothpaste"-like secretions. Meibography demonstrates significant truncation of meibomian glands with 50% gland dropout.

What Treatments Should Be Initiated in This Patient?

Treatment of MGD and blepharitis is particularly important prior to surgery. Blepharitis is a common cause of cataract surgery cancelation and is a major risk factor for postoperative endophthalmitis [14].

Treatment of MGD can be initiated with regular warm compresses at home. Expression of glands at home is often difficult to perform adequately especially in the elderly. Bacterial blepharitis should be cleared with the use of regular lid cleaning soaps. Baby shampoo is often used in clinical practice but can lead to skin irritation in some. In cases of *Demodex* mite infection, lid scrubs with the addition of a tea tree oil component can produce significant improvement [15]. Patients need to be counseled not to use direct tea tree oil on the lids as it can cause severe burning and discomfort.

As warm compresses used at home often do not reach adequately high enough temperatures for enough time, the use of in-office thermal pulsation treatments are very beneficial in patients who are unable to achieve success with home therapy alone. At this time, the only FDA-approved system for thermal pulsation is LipiFlow (TearScience, Morrisville, North Carolina, U.S.A.), which is a 12-min procedure for heat and expression of the glands in-office [16].

Moderate to severe cases of lid margin disease can be managed with topical antibiotic ointments or oral tetracyclines [17]. Doxycycline is particularly useful, not only for control of deleterious free fatty acids and bacterial overgrowth but also for its inhibition of tear film cytokines including, most notably, MMP-9 [18]. Treatment with antibiotics will likely be required for at least 1 month before the patient has improved and is eligible for further cataract surgery evaluation [8]. Increasing dietary intake of omega-3 fatty acids will also improve lid health by reducing inflammation and improving the quality of oil secretions from the glands [19].

Tear film inflammation can be further suppressed with short-term use of topical steroids. Although topical steroids have immediate effectiveness in decreasing tear film inflammatory cytokines, their long-term use is limited due to known side effects. In the preoperative setting, where rapid rescue and improvement of the ocular surface is needed, steroids may play an important role. Clinicians can therefore have a lower threshold for initiation of steroids in cataract surgery candidates with OSD than they would for other patients with dry eye. Long-term control of surface inflammation can be maintained with the use of topical cyclosporine A (CsA). CsA 0.05% used twice daily with an adjunctive topical corticosteroid has been reported effective in managing dry eye patients in the cataract setting, with symptomatic and clinical amelioration in as few as 2 weeks [20]. Newer anti-inflammatories targeting the specific inflammatory cascade in DES, such as lifitegrast, can also play an important role in long-term control of symptoms and signs of DES.

Aggressive lubrication with preservative-free artificial tears (PFATs) should be initiated in this patient. Preserved eye drops should be avoided—especially if used more than four times daily—as preservatives often promote further surface irritation and corneal damage [5]. Autologous serum eye drops have also shown to significantly improve ocular surface punctate erosions and improve the tear film [21].

Before Cataract Surgery, What Preoperative Testing Should Be Performed in This Patient to Ensure Improvement and Stability in the Ocular Surface?

As light enters the eye, the most powerful refraction or bending of light occurs at the air-tear film interface. This is the point with the greatest change in refractive index from 1.00 in air to 1.34 in tear film [22]. Montés-Micó estimated that small changes to the anterior radius of curvature of the tear film in DES can result in refractive power changes as high as 1.3 diopters [23]. Individuals with a hyperosmolar tear film can have significant variability of repeated keratometry measurements, with corresponding variation in astigmatism and intraocular lens (IOL) power calculations [24]. Hence, disturbances to the tear film in DES can interfere with refraction and potentially yield inaccurate preoperative measurements used for IOL selection and surgical planning. Stability of refractions, decrease in ocular surface staining, increase in TBUT, and normalization of the hyperosmolar and inflammatory marker tests in the tear film will be positive indicators of improvement.

Imaging modalities that can be used to assess tear film include topography and wavefront imaging. These tests are usually obtained during the workup of cataract or laser refractive patients and can be a first indication to the physician that there is irregularity of the tear film. The mires rings from the Placido images on topography can be irregular and show patches of missing rings when there is significant tear film disturbance. A Hartmann-Shack spot distortion can also be seen when trying to capture the wavefront image when there is tear film irregularity (Fig. 4.2). For optimal preoperative measurements, accurate biometry, and postoperative outcomes, these imaging tools can be used to ensure improvement of the tear film prior to proceeding with surgical planning.

The patient discontinues saline eye drops and switches to lipid-based PFATs an average of six to eight times daily. He adheres to daily lid hygiene measures and begins treatment with topical cyclosporine 0.05% BID and oral doxycycline 50 mg BID. At a 1-month follow-up, signs of lid margin disease have significantly improved. However, topography (Fig. 4.3) reveals tear film abnormalities with Placido disc rings demonstrating significant irregularities. After continuing therapy for an additional 6 weeks, repeat topography demonstrates smooth rings and regular corneal curvatures, and all other preoperative indices remain stable. Accordingly, the decision is made to schedule cataract surgery in the patient's right eye.

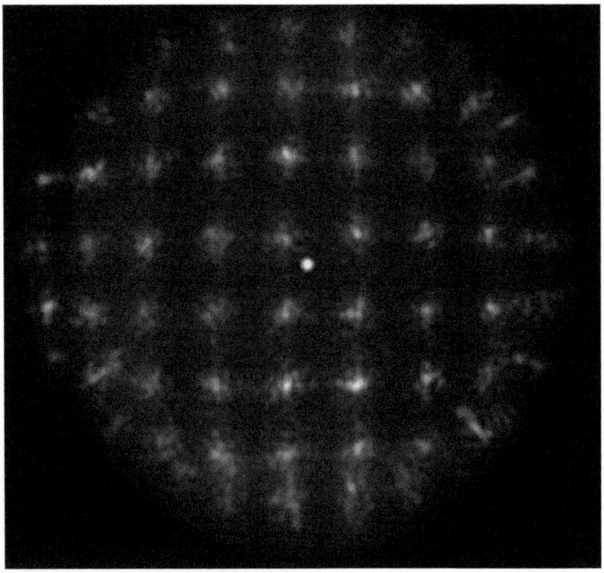

Fig. 4.2 A Hartmann-Shack spot distortion can be seen when trying to capture the wavefront image as a consequence of tear film irregularity

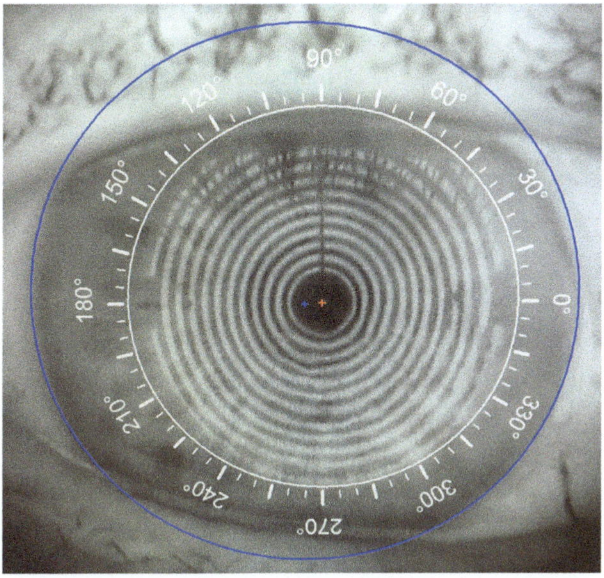

Fig. 4.3 Topography reveals tear film abnormalities with Placido disc rings demonstrating significant irregularities

What Intraoperative Considerations Should Be Taken into Account in a Patient with a History of OSD?

Various intraoperative measures can be taken to minimize surface damage and forestall the risk of postoperative dry eye. Anesthetic eye drop application and exposure to light from the operating microscope should be minimized. Use of light filters, delicate handling of the ocular surface, and avoidance of overly vigorous irrigation techniques may further mitigate the likelihood of postoperative dryness [4].

There is some evidence that the construction of grooved corneal incisions have been associated with persistent foreign body sensation, as well as pooling of mucus and debris in the groove [25]. Cho et al. noted an increase in the severity of postoperative dry eye after grooved incisions compared to single-plane incisions [2]. However, this was only significant in patients without pre-existing dry eye. The choice of incision architecture should be weighed against other important factors, such as the greater wound strength that can be achieved with grooved incisions. Additionally, a study by Donnenfeld et al. showed a decrease in corneal sensation in eyes that got limbal relaxing incisions at the 3 and 9 o'clock site that can result in worsening dry eye [26].

Femtosecond laser-assisted cataract surgery may also temporarily worsen postoperative dry eye symptoms when compared to conventional techniques [27]. This may be related to the patient interface used, and various platforms may have varying degrees of impact on the conjunctival goblet cells. Long-term effects have not been studied, and therefore the choice to use a femtosecond laser to improve refractive outcomes can be weighed against this potential short-term worsening in the dry eye symptoms.

Successful conventional cataract extraction and monofocal IOL implantation is performed in the patient's right. Corneal clarity is maintained throughout the case, and the patient tolerates the procedure well.

What Postoperative Measures Will Promote Ocular Surface Health?

Dry eye symptoms can worsen after cataract surgery—even in patients who have reestablished ocular surface health before surgery. Signs and symptoms of dryness tend to peak from as early as the first day through the first month postoperatively [4, 28]. Patients should continue therapy with PFATs, and individuals with MGD should maintain appropriate lid hygiene. The standard postoperative eye drop regimen may need to be modified in these patients. The use of preservative-free drops or newer formulations of NSAIDs and antibiotic drops with decreased ocular surface effects should be employed. As intracameral medications for cataract surgery develop and become mainstream, this postoperative drying effect from the preserved postoperative regimens may decline. Postoperative cyclosporine 0.05% twice daily, in particular, has been effective in limiting dry eye severity [29].

A postoperative regimen of prednisolone 1% and moxifloxacin 0.30% is prescribed for the patient; an NSAID eye drop is not used. Adjunctive cyclosporine 0.05% is continued. The patient continues the use of PFATs and lid hygiene measures. He is adherent to this postoperative regimen, though reports a mild increase in dryness, redness, and visual fluctuation during the first month. At his 1 month postoperative visit, uncorrected distance VA in the operated eye is 20/25. This VA remains stable over the first 6 months, and the patient is satisfied with the surgical result.

Case 2

A 34-year-old woman with visually significant myopia is interested in LASIK. She has been a soft contact lens (CTL) wearer for the past 25 years. She uses daily-wear CTLs all day and sometimes sleeps in them. The patient reports worsening irritation with CTLs and no longer wishes to use them. In particular, she describes 3 months of persistent bilateral redness and frequent episodes of tearing, burning, foreign body sensation, and visual fluctuation. She recently saw another ophthalmologist, who recommended artificial tears and prescribed antivirals for presumed herpes simplex keratitis. Neither of these have alleviated her symptoms. Her past medical history is unremarkable, and she is taking no other medications. She is an attorney and spends the majority of the day working at a computer.

Her vision is poor without CTLs, and she prefers not to switch to glasses as her visual quality is not as good with glasses. You proceed to evaluate her as a

candidate for LASIK. Uncorrected distance VA is 20/100 OD and 20/80 OS. BCVA is 20/20 OU. IOP is 14 mmHg OU. Slit lamp examination shows no lenticular opacities, and dilated fundus exam is unremarkable.

For a Chronic CTL Wearer with CTL-Related Discomfort, What Preoperative Considerations Should Be Taken into Account?

Long-standing CTL use may predispose patients to the development of various ocular surface disorders. Contact lens-associated keratopathy is a common cause of ocular surface disease in chronic CTL wearers. Timing of onset is highly variable among individuals, with cases occurring anywhere from 1 to 30 plus years after initiation of CTL use [30].

Chronic CTL wear may alter corneal metabolism and physiology as a result of injury to limbal stem cells (LSCs) [31]. LSCs are required for normal corneal epithelial cell turnover and repair of epithelial defects. However, CTLs can create a hypoxic environment, resulting in limbal stem cell strain and dysfunction with subsequent epithelial instability. Poorly fitting lenses may lead to additional mechanical irritation at the limbus and cause further damage to the stem cell population [32]. Chronic inflammation likely plays a role in limbal stem cell dysfunction (LSCD) from CTL overwear [33].

Pre-LASIK evaluation of this patient for LSCD is imperative. Irregularity of the corneal epithelium can result in instability of refractions and incorrect treatment measurements. Furthermore, wound healing requires proper LSC health and function to allow a smooth reepithelialization of the ocular surface. In addition, because LSCD predisposes individuals to corneal erosions or abrasions, these must be ruled out before surgery.

Prolonged CTL wear may also promote or exacerbate dry eye syndrome (DES), particularly in individuals with subclinical or pre-DES. DES is the most common reason for CTL intolerance and discontinuation [34]. Ocular irritation and discomfort in this patient may therefore be a sign of chronic dry eye. Though the exact mechanisms of CTL-associated DES are unknown, potential causes include chronic inflammation, hypoxic environment, corneal hyposensitivity, and adverse reaction to lens solution [34–37]. Subsequent tear film insufficiency increases the risk of corneal damage, and the resulting inflammation exacerbates both dry eye and LSCD. Reduced healing capacity secondary to LSCD further increases risk of corneal injury and inflammation, promoting a vicious cycle. DES certainly worsens in patients following LASIK [38], and as such, this patient must be thoroughly evaluated and treated for dry eye disease before undergoing surgery.

Preoperative pachymetry and corneal topography evaluation are essential in all LASIK candidates and are particularly relevant in chronic CTL wearers. Long-term use of CTLs often alters corneal topography—a phenomenon that was historically exploited by practitioners of orthokeratology. Continuous CTL wear can increase central and peripheral corneal thickness within periods as short as 30 days [31]. Further, CTL-induced warpage may mask subclinical keratoconus, and artificially thick pachymetry measurements prior to LASIK may increase the risk of postoperative ectasia [39].

What Symptoms in This Patient Elevate Your Suspicion for Limbal Stem Cell Strain or Deficiency?

Patients with LSCD often have nonspecific complaints of irritation, with symptoms similar to those of DES [40]. LCSD and DES cannot be differentiated based on symptomatology alone, and the patient may demonstrate elements of both conditions concurrently. Individuals with mild or partial LSCD may be asymptomatic. As the deficiency progresses, however, patients can present with chronic redness, tearing, burning, foreign body sensation, blepharospasm, and visual fluctuation. LSCD can predispose to persistent epithelial defects or recurrent epithelial erosions and abrasions, which can lead to severe pain, photophobia, and further compromise visual acuity. These features can masquerade as herpes keratitis. This particular patient's failure to improve with antivirals, however, renders herpes keratitis less likely. Importantly, treatment with topical antivirals can cause further insult to LSCs and thus exacerbate symptoms.

How Do You Diagnose OSD in a Chronic CTL Wearer?

Clinical examination of these patients should involve multiple modalities. Slit lamp biomicroscopy with fluorescein staining may reveal characteristic, albeit nonspecific, features of LSCD. Late fluorescein staining may be apparent secondary to loss of intercellular tight junctions with subsequent basement membrane staining. A whorled epithelial keratopathy can be seen at the superior and inferior limbus, and severe cases can extend into the visual axis and cause significant visual dysfunction (Fig. 4.4). Other typical features that may be apparent early in the course of LSCD

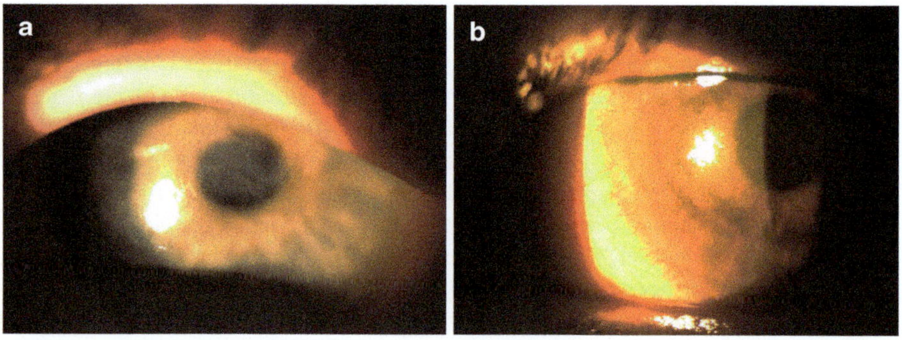

Fig. 4.4 As a consequence of limbal stem cell deficiency, (**a**) a whorled epithelial keratopathy can be seen in the visual axis approaching from the limbus, and (**b**) loss of normal limbal architecture with invading neovascularization can be visualized

include conjunctival hyperemia and a loss of limbal architecture with obscuration of the palisades of Vogt [41]. The superior limbus may be more susceptible to mechanical rubbing or hypoxia from CTLs, and as such, focal LSCD is more common superiorly than inferiorly [30].

Limbal stem cells serve as a physiologic barrier separating the cornea from adjacent conjunctiva. Disruption of this barrier may therefore result in conjunctivalization of the cornea. Early on this may be seen as an opaque sheet of cells indicating encroachment of conjunctival tissue onto the corneal surface and later may develop into superficial vascularization onto the peripheral cornea [31]. In severe disease, a fibrovascular pannus can result in corneal scarring or keratinization of the ocular surface. Mild LSCD typically demonstrates focal or sectoral corneal involvement, whereas advanced disease can affect most or all of the corneal surface.

Advanced LSCD is often characterized by the presence of poorly healing or recurrent epithelial erosions; ulceration, melting, and perforation can also occur [32]. CTL-induced keratoconjunctivitis resembling superior limbic keratoconjunctivitis can also be a sequela of long-term CTL use [32].

Although LSCD is diagnosed clinically on the basis of the characteristic examination features described above, in cases where the diagnosis is in doubt, impression cytology can be used for histologic confirmation of the presence of goblet cells on the cornea [42].

In vivo confocal microscopy may also be useful in the diagnosis of LSCD. For example, detection of decreased limbal basal epithelial cell density may be a sign of early disease [43]. Assessment of epithelial thickness may be a further diagnostic measure to detect LSCD, as epithelial thinning may be a consequence of LSCD that correlates with the severity of the deficiency [36].

Evaluation for DES in the context of a chronic contact lens wearer may also involve multiple modalities, as outlined in **Case 1**. Inspection of the eyelids should also be performed to evaluate for evidence of blepharitis, MGD, or CTL-associated giant papillary conjunctivitis [44]. Tear osmolarity and MMP-9 levels may also be elevated and can help to guide treatment decisions.

This patient's symptoms are suggestive of early LSCD with comorbid DES. Laser refractive surgery would not only exacerbate her dry eye symptoms and place her at risk for problems with wound healing but would also likely result in a poor refractive outcome given the unreliability of her preoperative refractions and her unstable surface disease.

The patient's exam reveals evidence of bilateral conjunctival injection. The patient demonstrates evidence of partial LSCD bilaterally. An inferior and superior whorl-like epitheliopathy extending into the visual axis is noted along with late fluorescein staining, greater in the right eye compared to the left (Fig. 4.5). There is no evidence of superficial neovascularization or corneal conjunctivalization. Tear film osmolarity and MMP-9 levels are elevated bilaterally.

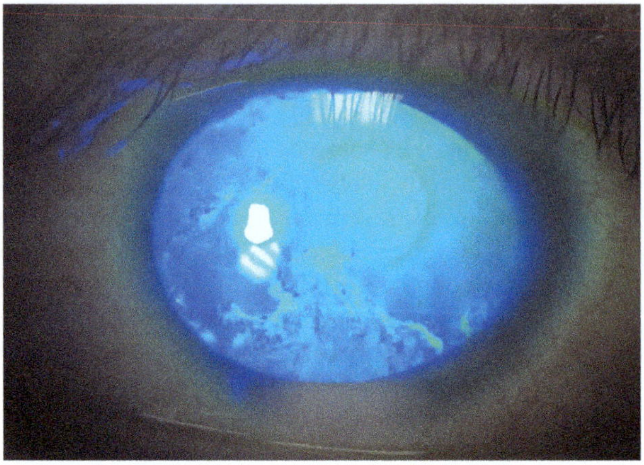

Fig. 4.5 Fluorescein staining shows a prominent whorl-like irregular extending onto the visual axis

How Do You Treat OSD in a Chronic CTL Wearer?

Effective treatment of LSCD requires a multifaceted strategic approach. First, the inciting agent (i.e., contact lens use) must be immediately withdrawn. Subsequent therapy must then seek to restore a normal, nutritious ocular surface environment and treat the inflammation. Dry eye can exacerbate LSCD, and thus management of concurrent DES, as described in **Case 1**, is important in order to provide an optimal environment for the remaining LSCs to survive.

Asymptomatic or mild cases with partial LSCD may resolve with time once contact lens wear is suspended. However, more advanced cases, as well as patients desirous of keratorefractive surgery, should be treated more aggressively. Conservative therapy involves cessation of CTL use and frequent administration of preservative-free artificial tears. Preservative-containing eye drops are relatively contraindicated due to potential cytotoxic effects to LSCs and association with further corneal damage and surface irritation [6]. In eyes with elevated inflammatory markers, the role of topical steroids should not be underestimated. Topical steroids with lower side effect profiles such as loteprednol or a non-preserved topical formulation of methylprednisolone or dexamethasone can be employed. These have a lower intraocular pressure rising effect and can be used in short-term pulsing, while other anti-inflammatory treatments are taking effect. Initiation of these topical steroids may be used as frequently as every 2 h to BID dosing depending on the severity of the presenting ocular surface disease and degree of inflammation. Once a generalized and fast-acting topical steroid has been initiated, a long-term treatment to target the dry eye inflammatory cascade should also be employed. Topical cyclosporine, with its preservative-free formulation and BID dosing, makes it ideal for these cases. Studies on the new integrin inhibitor, lifitegrast, have shown potent effects at blocking the dry eye inflammatory cycle at multiple points; lifitegrast may therefore be another key treatment for these patients once it is available [45].

Autologous serum eye drops and nightly application of vitamin A ointment may be included as an adjunct to anti-inflammatory therapy to further enhance epithelial and tear film health [33]. The use of autologous serum drops in dry eye disease has been studied, and its superiority to preservative-free artificial tears in ocular surface healing has been demonstrated [21]. Autologous serum drops may help provide the additional growth factor and nutritional support essential to boost the health of the remaining limbal stem cells and help restore the limbal niche. Refractory cases may benefit from the use of the PROSE scleral lens [46].

The patient should be advised that resolution and ocular surface stability typically requires several months of medical management. The patient needs to stay out of CTL wear during this time. Careful education is required for these patients as they are very dependent on their CTLs and having to wear glasses is often not an appealing alternative to them. Kim et al. reported that a mean of 15 months of treatment may be required for abatement of symptoms and restoration of ocular surface health [33]. Regular follow-up should be scheduled over this period to assess for gradual symptomatic improvement and refractive stabilization.

Once Treatment Has Been Initiated and the Limbal Stem Cell Deficiency Has Improved, What Preoperative Testing and Imaging Is Required?

Routine preoperative LASIK evaluations should be performed, including assessment of tear film regularity, pupil size, pachymetry, keratometry, corneal topography, manifest and cycloplegic refraction, and wavefront analysis.

Topography and pachymetry may take the longest to yield preoperative consistency. Stability of these measures often requires 4–6 weeks after suspension of soft CTL use and up to 20 weeks after cessation RGP use [47]. However, these time periods are highly variable among individuals, and preoperative measurements may thus need to be repeated multiple times before scheduling LASIK. Patients should be evaluated at follow-up visits approximately 2–3 weeks apart until stable measurements are demonstrated at two consecutive visits. Chronicity of CTL wear may correlate with more profound corneal warpage and longer interval to achieve preoperative stability.

Placido disc topographical assessment in this patient demonstrates irregularities consistent with ocular surface disease and possible CTL-related warpage. The patient discontinues CTL wear and begins therapy with PFATs, topical loteprednol, and topical cyclosporine 0.05%. The topical steroid is tapered over 2 months, and cyclosporine is continued. The positive MMP-9 tear test becomes negative after 3 months. After 9 months, the patient demonstrates significant improvement and returns for preoperative refractive measurements. Her whorled keratopathy has significantly regressed, and only minimal punctate staining is seen at the superior limbus. The central

corneal epithelium is smooth. Manifest refraction is −3.00 −1.00 ×80 OD and −2.50 −1.25 ×45 OS. Topography demonstrates regularity and improved Placido disc mires in both eyes. Wavefront refractions correlate with manifest refractions, and stability is established. Repeat measurements show consistent and stable refractions, and LASIK is subsequently performed in both eyes without complication. The patient is instructed to continue aggressive ocular surface management as above for at least 6 months to a year following her LASIK.

Case 3

A 55-year-old woman is being evaluated for cataract surgery. Two years ago, the patient was told she was developing mild cataracts. She complains of fluctuating vision while reading and at the computer and is concerned that her cataracts are becoming worse. The patient denies any irritation or burning. She typically works at her computer for several hours daily, and her desk is immediately beneath the air conditioning/fan vent. The patient is myopic and has used glasses for distance vision since she was a child. She now would like complete spectacle independence and thus desires a multifocal IOL. She has not had any prior ocular surgeries. Her past medical history includes osteopenia, for which she is taking alendronate.

BCVA is 20/30 OU. This decreases to 20/40 OU with a brightness acuity test. Slit lamp examination demonstrates no evidence of lid margin disease and reveals LOCS grade 1 cataracts in both eyes.

What Other Testing Should Be Performed on This Patient?

The patient's visual fluctuations while reading and using the computer are highly suggestive of dry eye syndrome (DES). In addition to a complete slit lamp exam with assessment of lids, vital dye staining and TBUT, point of care tear film tests, and meibography may help cinch the diagnosis and allow the patient to see the objective evidence of dry eye disease.

Lissamine green staining demonstrates temporal and nasal 1+ punctate epithelial erosions of the interpalpebral conjunctiva OU. Fluorescein staining is positive for inferior punctate erosions of both corneas. TBUT is 5–6 s OU. Tear film osmolarity readings are 309 mOsms/L OD and 319 OS mOsms/L, and MMP-9 levels are elevated in both eyes.

This patient's examination and workup demonstrate hallmarks of moderate-severe DES including instability of the tear film as demonstrated by decreased TBUT and positive inflammatory markers. The tear film instability causes degradation of visual quality between blinks, which this patient has interpreted as an effect of cataracts. Her glare disability is more likely a consequence of ocular surface irregularity than her mild lens opacification. The lack of eye irritation, burning, or pain does not rule out DES, as symptoms do not always correlate with signs of disease severity [1].

What Factors Likely Promote Dry Eye in This Patient?

The etiology of this patient's dry eye is likely multifactorial. Peri- and postmenopausal women are at increased risk for dry eye secondary to inflammatory changes and hormonal imbalance [48]. Disturbances to estrogen levels are believed to disrupt ocular surface conditions, though the mechanism is unknown. Estrogen is believed to influence ocular surface physiology via receptors on the cornea, conjunctiva, and meibomian glands [49]. Further, the patient's prolonged computer use and environmental conditions while at work likely exacerbate her dry eye as a result of reduced blink rate and increased tear evaporation.

How Should This Patient's Dry Eye Be Managed?

Although the use of lipid-based preservative-free artificial tears (PFATs) can be initiated primarily, these will not be sufficient to treat her DES. Anti-inflammatory treatment is required as inflammatory markers are elevated in this patient's tear film. The concurrent initiation of a short course of steroids along with a long-term cyclosporine A (CsA) 0.05% BID (or lifitegrast once available) will affect the underlying pathology. The patient should be advised that restoring ocular surface health will take time and persistence and improvement with CsA may take several months for some individuals. The addition of oral omega-3 fatty acid supplements as well as warm compresses will also help to normalize her lipid layer.

She should also be instructed to take regular breaks from computer usage and consider altering her work environment conditions to reduce direct air blowing into her face. The breaks can also serve as reminders to instill artificial tears. Additionally, the use of exogenous hormone replacement therapy (HRT) should be left at the discretion of her gynecologist. The exact role of HRT in the treatment of DES is unclear, and dosage alterations may have some impact on symptoms and signs of DES [50, 51].

The patient begins therapy with CsA and frequent administration of PFATs. She uses PFATs "every time she remembers." She begins omega-3 fatty acid supplementation and nightly warm compresses. She also adjusts her desk location at work and takes breaks while working at the screen. At a 3-month follow-up, she reports substantial improvement in visual fluctuations, which now occur much less frequently. She is encouraged to continue treatment and have her mild cataract observed for the time being.

How Should This Patient Be Counseled Regarding Eventual Cataract Surgery?

Once her cataract is ready for surgical intervention, this patient should consider the implications of DES in presbyopia correcting IOLs, specifically multifocal IOLs. Although multifocal optics may increase the likelihood of spectacle independence, they can impair visual function by decreasing contrast sensitivity and causing glare [52]. These effects are particularly relevant in the context of OSD, as dry eye itself is associated with glare disability and diminution in contrast sensitivity [53, 54]. Her dry DES needs to be in optimal control to minimize the potential for exacerbation of visual disturbances.

She should be advised that ocular surface health is critical to achieve optimal refractive goals post-cataract surgery. Inaccuracy of preoperative biometric measurements as a result of OSD can impact IOL power calculations and evaluation of astigmatism. This can especially confound refractive result should the patient elect a complex optical system such as a multifocal IOL. As such, this patient should continue her dry eye treatment pre- and post-cataract surgery. The ocular surface needs to be in very good shape for a multifocal lens, and in cases where the tear film quality cannot be improved despite maximal medical therapy, we advise against multifocal IOLs.

Acknowledgment *Financial Disclosures*: Dr. Farid is a consultant to AMO, Shire, Allergan, RPS, and TearScience.

References

1. Trattler W, Reilly C, Goldberg D, et al. Cataract and dry eye: prospective health assessment of cataract patients ocular surface study. American Society of Cataract and Refractive Surgery annual meeting. San Diego, CA, USA; 2011.
2. Cho YK, Kim MS. Dry eye after cataract surgery and associated intraoperative risk factors. Korean J Ophthalmol. 2009;23:65–73.
3. Li XM, Hu L, Hu J, et al. Investigation of dry eye disease and analysis of the pathogenic factors in patients after cataract surgery. Cornea. 2007;26:S16–20.
4. Kasetsuwan N, Satitpitakul V, Changul T, Jariyakosol S. Incidence and pattern of dry eye after cataract surgery. PLoS One. 2013;8(11):e78657.
5. Cha SH, Lee JS, Oum BS, Kim CD. Corneal epithelial cellular dysfunction from benzalkonium chloride (BAC) in vitro. Clin Exp Ophthalmol. 2004;32(2):180–4.
6. Lin JC, Rapuano CJ, Laibson PR, Eagle RC Jr, Cohen EJ. Corneal melting associated with use of topical nonsteroidal anti-inflammatory drugs after ocular surgery. Arch Ophthalmol. 2000;118(8):1129–32.
7. Han KE, Yoon SC, Ahn JM. Evaluation of dry eye and meibomian gland dysfunction after cataract surgery. Am J Ophthalmol. 2014;157(6):1144.e1–50.e1.
8. Afsharkhamseh N, Movahedan A, Motahari H, Djalilian AR. Cataract surgery in patients with ocular surface disease: an update in clinical diagnosis and treatment. Saudi J Ophthalmol. 2014;28(3):164–7.
9. Korb DR, Blackie CA. Meibomian gland diagnostic expressibility: correlation with dry eye symptoms and gland location. Cornea. 2008;27(10):1142–7.

10. The definition and classification of dry eye disease: report of the Definition and Classification Subcommittee of the International Dry Eye WorkShop (2007). Ocul Surf. 2007;5:75–92.
11. Sullivan BD, Whitmer D, Nichols KK, et al. An objective approach to dry eye disease severity. Invest Ophthalmol Vis Sci. 2010;51(12):6125–30.
12. Tomlinson A, Khanal S, Ramaesh K, et al. Tear film osmolarity: determination of a referent for dry eye diagnosis. Invest Ophthalmol Vis Sci. 2006;47(10):4309–15.
13. Sambursky R, Davitt WF III, Latkany R, et al. Sensitivity and specificity of a point-of-care matrix metalloproteinase 9 immunoassay for diagnosing inflammation related to dry eye. JAMA Ophthalmol. 2013;131(1):24–8.
14. Speaker MG, Milch FA, The SMK. role of external bacterial flora in the pathogenesis of acute postoperative endophthalmitis. Ophthalmology. 1991;98:639–49.
15. Gao YY, Di Pascuale MA, Elizondo A, Tseng SC. Clinical treatment of ocular demodecosis by lid scrub with tea tree oil. Cornea. 2007;26(2):136–43.
16. Lane SS, DuBiner HB, Epstein RJ, et al. A new system, the LipiFlow, for the treatment of meibomian gland dysfunction. Cornea. 2012;31(4):396–404.
17. Geerling G, Tauber J, Baudouin C, et al. The international workshop on meibomian gland dysfunction: report of the subcommittee on management and treatment of meibomian gland dysfunction. Invest Ophthalmol Vis Sci. 2011;52(4):2050–64.
18. De Paiva CS, Corrales RM, Villarreal AL, et al. Corticosteroid and doxycycline suppress MMP-9 and inflammatory cytokine expression, MAPK activation in the corneal epithelium in experimental dry eye. Exp Eye Res. 2006;83(3):526–35.
19. Bhargava R, Kumar P, Kumar M, et al. A randomized controlled trial of omega-3 fatty acids in dry eye syndrome. Int J Ophthalmol. 2013;6(6):811–6.
20. Donnenfeld ED, Solomon R, Roberts CW, et al. Cyclosporine 0.05% to improve visual outcomes after multifocal intraocular lens implantation. J Cataract Refract Surg. 2010;36(7):1095–100.
21. Kojima T, Ishida R, Dogru M, et al. The effect of autologous serum eyedrops in the treatment of severe dry eye disease: a prospective randomized case-control study. Am J Ophthalmol. 2005;139(2):242–6.
22. Tutt R, Bradley A, Begley C, Thibos LN. Optical and visual impact of tear break-up in human eyes. Invest Ophthalmol Vis Sci. 2000;41(13):4117–23.
23. Montés-Micó R. Role of the tear film in the optical quality of the human eye. J Cataract Refract Surg. 2007;33(9):1631–5.
24. Epitropoulos AT, Matossian C, Berdy GJ, et al. Effect of tear osmolarity on repeatability of keratometry for cataract surgery planning. J Cataract Refract Surg. 2015;41(8):1672–7.
25. Fine IH, Hoffman RS, Packer M. Profile of clear corneal cataract incisions demonstrated by ocular coherence tomography. J Cataract Refract Surg. 2007;33:94–7.
26. Donnenfeld E. Multicenter prospective evaluation of effects of cataract extraction and limbal relaxing incisions on corneal sensation and dry eye. American Society of Cataract and Refractive Surgery annual meeting. San Diego, CA; 2011.
27. Yu Y, Hua H, Wu M, et al. Evaluation of dry eye after femtosecond laser-assisted cataract surgery. J Cataract Refract Surg. 2015;41(12):2614–23.
28. Cetinkaya S, Mestan E, Acir NO, et al. The course of dry eye after phacoemulsification surgery. BMC Ophthalmol. 2015;15:68.
29. Chung YW, TH O, Chung SK. The effect of topical cyclosporine 0.05% on dry eye after cataract surgery. Korean J Ophthalmol. 2013;27(3):167–71.
30. Jeng BH, Halfpenny CP, Meisler DM, Stock EL. Management of focal limbal stem cell deficiency associated with soft contact lens wear. Cornea. 2011;30(1):18–23.
31. Yeniad B, Adam YS, Bilgin LK, Gözüm N. Effect of 30-day continuous wear of silicone hydrogel contact lenses on corneal thickness. Eye Contact Lens. 2004;30(1):6–9.
32. Bloomfield SE, Jakobiec FA, Theodore FH. Contact lens induced keratopathy: a severe complication extending the spectrum of keratoconjunctivitis in contact lens wearers. Ophthalmology. 1984;91(3):290–4.
33. Kim BY, Riaz KM, Bakhtiari P, et al. Medically reversible limbal stem cell disease: clinical features and management strategies. Ophthalmology. 2014;121(10):2053–8.

34. Sindt CW, Longmuir RA. Contact lens strategies for the patient with dry eye. Ocul Surf. 2007;5(4):294–307.
35. Nichols JJ, Sinnott LT. Tear film, contact lens, and patient-related factors associated with contact lens-related dry eye. Invest Ophthalmol Vis Sci. 2006;47(4):1319–28.
36. Chan EH, Chen L, Yu F, Deng SX. Epithelial thinning in limbal stem cell deficiency. Am J Ophthalmol. 2015;160(4):669.e4–77.e4.
37. Pisella PJ, Malet F, Lejeune S, et al. Ocular surface changes induced by contact lens wear. Cornea. 2001;20:820–5.
38. EY Y, Leung A, Rao S, Lam DS. Effect of laser in situ keratomileusis on tear stability. Ophthalmology. 2000;107(12):2131–5.
39. Leroux Les Jardins S. Contact lens wearers as candidates for LASIK surgery: two pitfalls to avoid. J Fr Ophtalmol. 2002;25(1):71–7.
40. Espana EM, Grueterich M, Romano AC, et al. Idiopathic limbal stem cell deficiency. Ophthalmology. 2002;109(11):2004–10.
41. Sacchetti M, Lambiase A, Cortes M, et al. Clinical and cytological findings in limbal stem cell deficiency. Graefes Arch Clin Exp Ophthalmol. 2005;243(9):870–6.
42. Joussen AM, Poulaki V, Mitsiades N, et al. VEGF-dependent conjunctivalization of the corneal surface. Invest Ophthalmol Vis Sci. 2003 Jan;44(1):117–23.
43. Chan EH, Chen L, Rao JY, Yu F, Deng SX. Limbal basal cell density decreases in limbal stem cell deficiency. Am J Ophthalmol. 2015;160(4):678.e4–84.e4.
44. Donshik PC. Giant papillary conjunctivitis. Trans Am Ophthalmol Soc. 1994;92:687–744.
45. Sun Y, Zhang R, Gadek TR, et al. Corneal inflammation is inhibited by the LFA-1 antagonist, lifitegrast (SAR 1118). J Ocul Pharmacol Ther. 2013;29:395–402.
46. Rosenthal P, Cotter J. The Boston Scleral Lens in the management of severe ocular surface disease. Ophthalmol Clin North Am. 2003;16:89–93.
47. Wilson SE, Lin DT, Klyce SD, Reidy JJ, Insler MS. Topographic changes in contact lens-induced corneal warpage. Ophthalmology. 1990;97(6):734–44.
48. The epidemiology of dry eye disease: report of the epidemiology subcommittee of the international dry eye workshop. Ocul Surf. 2007;5:93–107.
49. Versura P, Campos EC. Menopause and dry eye. A possible relationship. Gynecol Endocrinol. 2005;20(5):289–98.
50. Schaumberg DA, Buring JE, Sullivan DA, Dana MR. Hormone replacement therapy and dry eye syndrome. JAMA. 2001;286(17):2114–9.
51. Erdem U, Ozdegirmenci O, Sobaci E, et al. Dry eye in post-menopausal women using hormone replacement therapy. Maturitas. 2007;56(3):257–62.
52. Leyland M, Zinicola E. Multifocal versus monofocal intraocular lenses in cataract surgery: a systematic review. Ophthalmology. 2003;110(9):1789–98.
53. Huang FC, Tseng SH, Shih MH, Chen FK. Effect of artificial tears on corneal surface regularity, contrast sensitivity, and glare disability in dry eyes. Ophthalmology. 2002;109(10):1934–40.
54. Puell MC, Benítez-del-Castillo JM, Martínez-de-la-Casa J, et al. Contrast sensitivity and disability glare in patients with dry eye. Acta Ophthalmol Scand. 2006;84(4):527–31.

Chapter 5
Diagnosis and Management of Ocular Involvement in Sjögren's Syndrome

Vatinee Y. Bunya, Nicole M. Fuerst, Stephen E. Orlin, Mina Massaro-Giordano, Frederick B. Vivino, and Michael E. Sulewski

Introduction

Sjögren's syndrome (SS) is a chronic, debilitating, potentially life-threatening autoimmune disorder that causes irreversible damage to the lacrimal and salivary glands resulting in a loss of tear and saliva production, severely impairing quality of life [1]. SS is estimated to affect between two and four million Americans, with half of SS patients remaining undiagnosed due to the nonspecific nature of early clinical manifestations and an average delay in diagnosis of up to 7 years from the onset of symptoms [2–6]. Early diagnosis of SS is critical to enable surveillance for serious systemic complications such as lymphoma and to facilitate early treatment to lessen the morbidity of the disease [7].

It is important to have a low threshold for referring dry eye patients for SS work-ups, and there are special considerations for intraocular surgery and for the management of complications of severe ocular surface disease. The cases presented will review various aspects of the ophthalmologic evaluation and management of SS patients.

V.Y. Bunya, MD (✉) • N.M. Fuerst, MD • S.E. Orlin, MD
M. Massaro-Giordano, MD • M.E. Sulewski, MD
Department of Ophthalmology, Scheie Eye Institute, University of Pennsylvania,
51 N. 39th Street, Philadelphia, PA 19104, USA
e-mail: vatinee.bunya@uphs.upenn.edu

F.B. Vivino, MD, MS
Department of Rheumatology, University of Pennsylvania, Philadelphia, PA, USA

A.R. Djalilian (ed.), *Ocular Surface Disease*,
https://doi.org/10.1007/978-3-319-15823-5_5

Case 1

A 55-year-old Caucasian woman presents for a second opinion regarding eye irritation. Her local ophthalmologist recommended that she use bottled artificial tears every hour. She feels that she is getting worse on this regimen and came seeking a second opinion.

What Are Your Initial Thoughts?

Bottled artificial tears contain preservatives that can exacerbate ocular surface disease. As a result, they should not be used more than four times a day, and if a patient has moderate or severe dry eye, we recommend avoiding bottled artificial tears completely. Instead, we recommend the use of preservative-free artificial tears in individual vials that can be used as frequently as needed.

What Additional Questions Should You Ask?

It is important to always conduct a review of systems for dry eye patients to determine if there are any symptoms that could indicate the presence of SS. Specifically, we recommend including questions that cover the following: the presence of dry mouth, swelling of the major salivary glands, frequent dental caries, difficulty swallowing foods without liquid, fatigue, Raynaud's phenomenon, constipation, vaginal dryness, and joint pain [8].

On further questioning, the patient reports that she has had some dry mouth symptoms for the past few months, but she recently started a new blood pressure medication and is unsure if her dry mouth is a side effect of that medication. She is a nurse and has been unable to work and stopped driving due to the ocular discomfort.

What Components Are Important to Include on the Exam?

Initial evaluation should include examination of the face for signs of rosacea and of the patient's hands for signs of arthritis or Raynaud's phenomenon. The eyelids, lashes, and eyelid margins should be examined for evidence of meibomian gland dysfunction (MGD), blepharitis, and *Demodex*. Careful attention should also be paid to any lid malpositioning such as lagophthalmos, trichiasis, symblepharon, and punctal occlusion.

A full ocular surface exam should then be performed. This includes careful examination of the cornea and conjunctiva looking for conditions such as conjunctivochalasis, superior limbic keratoconjunctivitis (SLK), and any corneal pathology including anterior basement membrane dystrophy or corneal scars. The order in which each test is performed is important. Topical anesthetic should not be administered prior to the ocular surface exam as this can affect test results by causing false-positive ocular surface staining. Instead, preservative-free sterile saline should be used to moisten fluorescein or lissamine green strips. Alternatively, preservative-free ocular staining drops are available through compounding pharmacies.

Thirty seconds after one drop of fluorescein is administered to the eye, the tear break-up time (TBUT) should be assessed using slit lamp biomicroscopy and a cobalt blue filter. Fluorescein staining of the cornea should be evaluated next, followed by lissamine green staining of the conjunctiva. It is important to examine both the superior and inferior bulbar conjunctival surfaces in addition to the interpalpebral areas. Finally, unanesthetized Schirmer testing should be performed. It is important that the Schirmer testing be done without anesthesia as this is part of the ocular portion of the current SS classification criteria (see Tables 5.1 and 5.3).

While many ophthalmologists commonly use fluorescein staining of the cornea in their ocular surface evaluation, few routinely assess staining of the conjunctiva, with only 5–10% of eye care professionals routinely performing this procedure [9, 10].

Table 5.1 American European Consensus Group (AECG) Sjögren's syndrome classification criteria [14]: Classification of SS[a] requires either: (1) Four out of the six following criteria (with at least one being autoantibodies (V) or histopathology (VI)) (2) Three of the four objective criteria (II, IV, V, or VI)

I. Subjective dry eye[b]
II. Objective dry eye (Schirmer's without anesthesia $\leq$5 mm at 5 min or vital dye staining of ocular surface $\geq$4 according to van Bijsterveld's scoring)
III. Subjective dry mouth[c]
IV. Objective dry mouth (unstimulated whole salivary flow $\leq$1.5 ml in 15 min or parotid sialography showing diffuse sialectasias without obstruction of major ducts; salivary scintigraphy showing delayed uptake, reduced concentration and/or delayed excretion of tracer)
V. Positive SSA and/or SSB
VI. Minor labial salivary gland biopsy

[a]*Exclusion criteria:* past head and neck radiation treatment, hepatitis C infection, acquired immunodeficiency syndrome (AIDS), pre-existing lymphoma, sarcoidosis, graft-versus-host disease, current use of anticholinergic drugs

[b]*Subjective dry eye* defined as positive response to at least one of the following questions: (1) Have you had daily, persistent, troublesome dry eyes for more than 3 months? (2) Do you have a recurrent sensation of sand or gravel in the eyes? (3) Do you use tear substitutes more than three times a day?

[c]*Subjective dry mouth* defined as positive response to at least one of the following questions: (1) Have you had a daily feeling of dry mouth for more than 3 months? (2) Have you had recurrently or persistently swollen salivary glands as an adult? (3) Do you frequently drink liquids to aid in swallowing dry food?

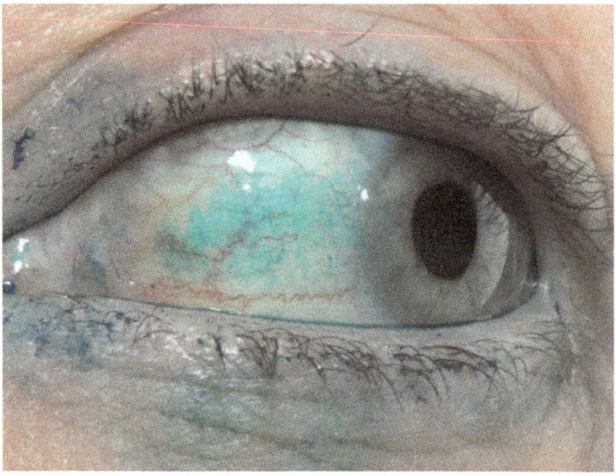

Fig. 5.1 (Case 1) External photograph showing 3+ lissamine green staining of nasal conjunctiva of left eye

It is crucial to include conjunctival staining with lissamine green in the ocular surface evaluation, as this is needed to assess the ocular criteria for SS and can also reveal ocular surface changes that will not be detected through the use of fluorescein staining alone. The current underutilization of conjunctival staining may contribute to the under-referral of dry eye patients for SS workups and delays in diagnosis.

On exam, she has evidence of 2+ meibomian gland dysfunction (MGD) (scale 0–3) with a tear break-up time (TBUT) of 4 s (normal >10 s) in both eyes. Her right eye has 1+ scattered punctate staining (scale 0–3) of her cornea with fluorescein, but no central staining, confluence, or corneal filaments. Her left cornea does not stain with fluorescein. After lissamine green administration, she has 1+ nasal conjunctival staining in her right eye (scale 0–3) and 3+ staining nasally in her left eye (Fig. 5.1). Unanesthetized Schirmer testing measured her tear production to be 5 mm/5 min in the right eye and 6 mm/5 min in the left eye (normal > 10 mm/5 min).

What Is Your Assessment? What Is the Ocular Staining Score (OSS) and How Is It Interpreted?

This patient has evidence of evaporative dry eye in addition to some signs of aqueous deficiency. This patient has an ocular staining score (OSS) of 2 in her right eye and 3 in her left eye. The OSS is a scoring system used as part of the American College of Rheumatology (ACR)-Sjögren's International Clinical Collaborative Alliance (SICCA) criteria for SS. Whitcher and colleagues described the OSS scoring system in detail and proposed a cutoff for abnormal OSS of 3 or more [11]. Briefly, the OSS score is a sum of corneal staining with fluorescein (score of 0–3) and conjunctival staining with lissamine green (score of 0–3 for each area—nasal and temporal). An additional point is given for corneal staining for any of the following: (1) patches of confluent staining, (2) staining in the central cornea or pupillary area, and (3) the presence of one or more filaments. It is important to use the OSS (score 0–12) when evaluating a dry eye patient for possible SS.

In addition, the patient has evidence of aqueous tear deficiency with a low Schirmer score in the right eye and a borderline score in the left eye. Although this patient did not demonstrate any filaments, the presence of filaments should always raise the suspicion for SS.

How Would You Manage the Patient at This Point?

We would recommend immediately stopping all bottled tears and switching to frequent preservative-free artificial tears. It is important to treat both the aqueous deficient and evaporative components of her ocular surface disease. Patients with low or borderline low Schirmer scores (i.e., Schirmer $\leq$5 mm/5 min) typically will not have any excess tearing after punctal occlusion, and we have a low threshold for punctal occlusion in these patients (typically after controlling ocular surface inflammation). To address her MGD, we would also recommend starting warm compresses twice daily, lid hygiene, oral omega-3 fatty acid supplements, and/or oral doxycycline or azithromycin.

The patient returns for a follow-up visit 4 months later and feels that her symptoms are about the same. Her ocular exam remains unchanged except that her TBUT has increased slightly to 6 s in each eye. However, she is now experiencing dry mouth symptoms and some fatigue.

What Is Your Assessment and What Are Your Next Steps?

At this point, we would refer the patient to a rheumatologist for a workup. She has evidence of both aqueous tear deficiency and evaporative dry eye. In addition, she has extraocular symptoms that are suspicious for possible SS, and she has not had any significant improvement after 4 months of treatment. In general, a referral to a rheumatologist should be considered when a patient has any of the following: (1) signs of severe ocular surface disease, (2) positive OSS (OSS > 3 in either eye) or unanesthetized Schirmer $\leq$5 mm/5 min in either eye and positive ROS, or (3) positive OSS or unanesthetized Schirmer $\leq$5 mm/5 min in either eye and is refractory to treatment. The length of time when a patient is considered refractory to treatment varies by each individual, but in general, we would consider someone refractory after 4–6 months of appropriate therapy.

What Are Your Next Management Steps?

We would start topical cyclosporine or lifitegrast twice daily. To treat her MGD, we would consider oral doxycycline or azithromycin (if not started previously) and/or topical erythromycin ointment at bedtime. At this point, one could also consider a short course of topical steroids such as loteprednol drops or tobramycin/dexamethasone ointment with careful monitoring for side effects such as increased intraocular pressure. The patient should then return in about 3–4 months to assess for any improvement (sooner if topical steroids are started).

The patient was evaluated by her rheumatologist and has negative bloodwork for SSA, SSB, rheumatoid factor (RF), and antinuclear antibody (ANA). She then undergoes a labial salivary gland biopsy that comes back positive. The biopsy showed focal lymphocytic sialadenitis with a focus score of 1.7/4 mm^2, which was above the required diagnostic threshold of $\geq$1/4 mm^2.

Can You Have SS with Negative Bloodwork?

Negative bloodwork for the traditional SS antibodies (SSA, SSB, RF, and ANA) does not rule out this diagnosis since about 40% of patients with SS lack immunologic markers in the serum. This "seronegative" subset of SS patients may have a lower rate of extraglandular manifestations [12].

The Sjo kit (Bausch & Lomb) allows for in-office testing of an expanded set of blood tests, which includes three novel antibodies that were described in a mouse model for SS [13]. In that study, the authors found that these novel antibodies appeared earlier than traditional SS antibodies in their mouse model. However, understanding the significance of these antibodies in humans requires further clinical study.

In a seronegative patient whose signs and symptoms are suggestive of SS, a minor salivary gland biopsy is a reasonable next step in the workup. Other conditions which can lead to both dry eye and dry mouth should also be entertained. These include chronic sialadenitis, sialadenosis, complications of radiation therapy, sarcoidosis, HIV, IgG4-related disease, chronic hepatitis C, and medication side effects.

What Are the Current Classification Criteria for SS?

It is important to work with the patient's rheumatologist to apply published classification criteria that meet the case definition for SS. In the past decade, two sets of classification criteria have been most commonly used (Tables 5.1 and 5.2): (1) the American European Consensus Group (AECG) criteria [14] and (2) the American College of Rheumatology (ACR)/Sjögren's International Clinical Collaborative Alliance (SICCA) criteria [15]. Both criteria sets have strengths and weaknesses but greater than 90% sensitivity and specificity for classification of a patient as having SS [14, 15]. More recently, a new set of classification criteria

Table 5.2 American College of Rheumatology (ACR)/SICCA Sjögren's syndrome classification criteria [15]: Classification of SS applies to individuals[a] with signs or symptoms suggestive of SS requires two out of the three objective criteria

Keratoconjunctivitis sicca with ocular staining score (OSS) ≥3[b]
Positive serum anti-SSA/Ro and/or anti-SSB/La *or* (positive rheumatoid factor *and* ANA titer ≥1:320)
Labial salivary gland biopsy exhibiting focal lymphocytic sialadenitis with a focus score of ≥1 focus/4 mm^2

[a]*Exclusion criteria:* history of head and neck radiation treatment, hepatitis C infection, acquired immunodeficiency syndrome (AIDS), sarcoidosis, amyloidosis, graft-versus-host disease, IgG4-related disease
[b]Not currently using any daily eyedrops for glaucoma and has not had corneal surgery or cosmetic eyelid surgery within past 5 years

Table 5.3 American College of Rheumatology (ACR)/European League Against Rheumatism (EULAR) classification criteria for primary Sjögren's syndrome [16]

The classification of primary Sjögren's syndrome (SS) applies to any individual who meets the inclusion criteria[a], does not have any of the conditions listed as exclusion criteria[b], and has a score of ≥4 when the weights from the five criteria items below are summed	
	Weight/score
Labial salivary gland with focal lymphocytic sialadenitis and focus score of ≥1 foci/4 mm^2	3
Anti-SSA/Ro-positive	3
Ocular staining score ≥5 (or van Bijsterveld's score ≥4 in at least one eye)	1
Schirmer test ≤5 mm/5 min without anesthesia in at least one eye[c]	1
Unstimulated whole saliva flow rate ≤0.1 mL/min	1

[a]**INCLUSIONS:** These classification criteria are applicable to any patient with at least **one symptom of ocular or oral dryness**, defined as a positive response to at least one of the following questions: (1) Have you had daily, persistent, troublesome dry eyes for more than 3 months? (2) Do you have a recurrent sensation of sand or gravel in the eyes? (3) Do you use tear substitutes more than three times a day? (4) Have you had a daily feeling of dry mouth for more than 3 months? (5) Do you frequently drink liquids to aid in swallowing dry food? [14] Additionally, these criteria can be applied to any individual who presents with at least one extraglandular manifestation of SS as defined by the European League Against Rheumatism SS Disease Activity Index (ESSDAI) [37]
[b]**EXCLUSIONS**: Include a diagnosis of any of the following conditions, which would preclude a diagnosis of SS and participation in SS studies or therapeutic trials because of overlapping clinical features or interference with criteria tests: (1) history of head and neck radiation treatment, (2) active hepatitis C infection (with confirmation by PCR), (3) AIDS, (4) sarcoidosis, (5) amyloidosis, (6) graft-versus-host disease, (7) IgG4-related disease [14]
[c]Patients who are normally taking anticholinergic drugs should be evaluated for objective signs of salivary hypofunction and ocular dryness after a sufficient interval without these medications in order for these components to be a valid measure of oral and ocular dryness

(ACR/European League Against Rheumatism (EULAR)) has been developed in an attempt to reconcile differences between the AECG and ACR/SICCA criteria [16]. The 2016 ACR-EULAR criteria (Table 5.3) have now been endorsed by both the American College of Rheumatology and the European League Against Rheumatism and will likely be more widely utilized in the future than older criteria sets.

While all of the above classification criteria were originally developed to define homogeneous populations of patients for research studies including clinical trials, these criteria also provide a framework for diagnostic testing as well. Therefore, in clinical practice, any patient who fulfills any of the three aforementioned criteria sets can be considered to have SS.

What Is the Role of Punctal Occlusion in SS?

Because patients with SS often have low aqueous tear production, punctal occlusion plays an important role in the management of ocular surface disease in these patients. The decision of whether to perform total punctal occlusion (i.e., both the lower puncta and upper puncta) or to initially only occlude the lower puncta should be based on the severity of the aqueous tear deficiency at the time of evaluation. For SS patients with mild or moderate aqueous tear deficiency, punctal occlusion can be performed in a staged fashion with initial occlusion of the lower puncta followed at a later date by occlusion of the upper puncta if needed. In patients with severely diminished aqueous tear production, immediate total punctal occlusion is indicated as occlusion of the lower puncta alone is unlikely to have any meaningful effect on the patient's signs and symptoms. In these cases, the small amount of aqueous tears being produced is mostly lost to evaporation. If one is considering total punctal occlusion, it is best to first perform a trial with plugs (dissolvable or non-dissolvable) followed by punctal cauterization if there is a positive clinical response and no epiphora. In addition, the degree of aqueous tear deficiency should be reassessed after the initiation of any oral secretagogues for the treatment of dry mouth in order to avoid possible epiphora. Topical steroids are initiated prior to the insertion of punctal plugs in order to decrease the buildup of inflammatory factors that may be present in the tear film.

What Are Other Treatment Options for This Patient?

Other treatment options that could be considered in the future for this patient include:

- Autologous serum drops: We typically start with a 20% compounded preparation every 2 h. While we previously had concerns about the serum having an inflammatory effect on the ocular surface, this has not been the case as nearly all patients have a positive response to this treatment.
- Oral secretagogues (cevimeline 30 mg PO t.i.d. or pilocarpine 5 mg PO t.i.d. and qhs) are also effective in select SS patients.
- Scleral lenses including PROSE (prosthetic replacement of the ocular surface ecosystem) lens are highly effective for SS patients. The patient must be able to learn how to handle the lenses (not a very good choice for elderly patients). Fitting these lenses requires special expertise.
- Intense pulsed light (IPL) and Lipiflow® Thermal Pulsation System may be considered, but the effects are generally temporary, and, since MGD is not a primary problem in these patients, we don't recommend it very often.

- We would also work closely with her rheumatologist who might choose to start systemic immunosuppressive therapy. In a patient who is very symptomatic with significant signs of inflammation (injection), a course of oral prednisone (alongside their topical therapy) can help suppress the inflammation more rapidly and give the patient more immediate relief.

Case 2

A 66-year-old Caucasian woman with a history of SS presents with decreased vision and glare in her right eye greater than her left eye, which has gradually worsened over the past year. She has a moderate cataract in the right eye with 2+ nuclear and 1+ cortical lens changes. She elects to have cataract surgery in the right eye to improve visual acuity and symptoms of glare.

What Are Important Preoperative Considerations When Planning Cataract Surgery for Patients with Sjögren's Syndrome?

It is important to evaluate a patient's preoperative dry eye regimen and to assess how well it is working. As with all SS patients, we recommend performing a full ocular surface exam as outlined above. Surgery should be delayed until the ocular surface is optimized as much as possible. Ideally, there should be no or minimal corneal/conjunctival staining, the lid margin and lashes should be clean, and topography and keratometry measurements should remain stable over two visits. Keratometry and A scan measurements should be performed *prior* to the instillation of any eye drops, particularly topical anesthetic agents.

Visual quality has been shown to be worse in dry eye disease, and outcomes after cataract surgery in patients with SS have been shown to be less favorable as compared to patients with dry eye who do not have connective tissue disease [17]. Thus, the threshold to proceed with surgery in patients with SS should be higher, and the patient should be well informed about possible complications and a potentially difficult postoperative period.

What Role Do In-office Tests Such as MMP-9 Testing and Tear Osmolarity Play in Preoperative Surgical Planning for SS Patients?

Matrix metalloproteinase-9 (MMP-9) is an inflammatory marker that has been found to be elevated in the tears of patients with dry eye. Rapid in-office testing is both sensitive and specific for identifying inflammatory dry eye and ocular surface disease [18]. This has been postulated to help with earlier diagnosis of dry eye and may allow for more targeted perioperative therapeutic management, which is expected to reduce complications from surgery [19, 20]. However, further studies are needed to clarify the role of MMP-9 testing in patients with ocular surface disease.

In addition, studies have shown that patients with dry eye have tear film instability and increased tear osmolarity secondary to reduced tear secretion and/or increased evaporation [21–23]. One important consideration for SS patients undergoing surgery is that tear film instability can affect keratometry (K) readings and preoperative measurements. In one study, there was significantly more variability in the average K readings and anterior corneal astigmatism in patients with higher tear osmolarity (>316 mOsm/L in at least one eye) compared to patients with normal tear osmolarity (<308 mOsm/L in both eyes) with significant resultant differences in IOL power calculations [24].

In our experience, we have found a high amount of variability in repeated measurements of tear osmolarity in patients with SS compared to patients without dry eye disease, which makes clinical interpretation of measurements unclear [25]. Thus, we do not routinely check osmolarity in our patients. However, MMP-9 and tear osmolarity testing are sometimes used in general ophthalmology offices for screening patients preoperatively for undiagnosed dry eye disease that could affect preoperative measurements.

The patient currently uses preservative-free artificial tears several times per day in both eyes and underwent lower lid punctal occlusion with silicone plugs several years before. She complains of a gritty sensation in both eyes. Her eyelid exam is significant for moderate MGD, with a few collarettes. The lower lids have punctal plugs in place. There is 2+ staining of the cornea with fluorescein (Fig. 5.2) in each eye with involvement of the pupillary area, the presence of confluent PEK, but no filaments. In addition there is 1+ staining of

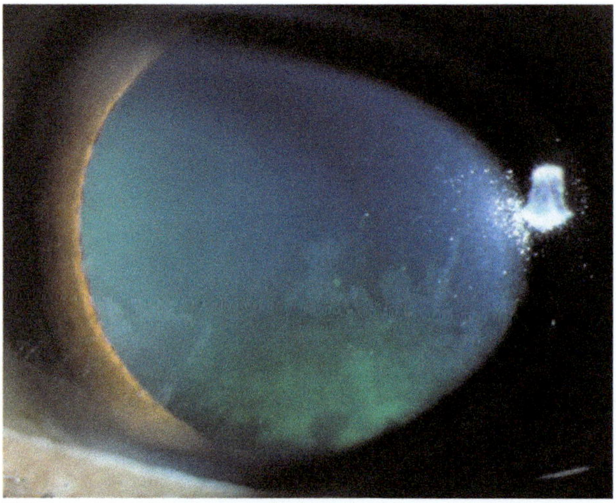

Fig. 5.2 (Case 2) Slit lamp photograph showing mild nuclear sclerosis, cortical changes, and 2+ punctate epithelial keratopathy

the temporal conjunctiva with lissamine green in both eyes. Therefore, the patient's OSS score is 6 in each eye. Schirmer testing without anesthesia is 7 mm/5 min in the right eye and 5 mm/5 min in the left eye.

How Would You Change her Treatment Regimen Prior to Cataract Surgery Based on These Findings?

To optimize patients for surgery and improve the health of the ocular surface, it is important to address both the aqueous deficient and evaporative components of ocular surface disease. SS patients are classically thought of as having aqueous tear deficiency, but there is increasing evidence in the literature that they also commonly have significant MGD [26, 27].

In any patient with moderate-to-severe ocular surface disease, it is important to treat them aggressively preoperatively and postpone surgery until the ocular surface has been optimized.

We recommend early punctal occlusion, starting with the lower puncta, followed by the upper puncta at a later date if more effect is required, and the continued use of preservative-free artificial tears. In addition, to address the patient's MGD, we would recommend starting warm compresses and eyelid hygiene twice daily. Eyelid hygiene can be performed with either dilute baby shampoo or any over the counter eyelid scrub. In patients who continue to have signs and symptoms of dry eye despite these measures, we would consider the addition of oral omega-3 fatty acid supplements, oral doxycycline or azithromycin, and/or erythromycin ointment [28]. Other options would be to start topical cyclosporine drops or autologous serum drops at least 6–8 weeks prior to surgery.

Additional appointments prior to the planned cataract surgery date to ensure improvement in the ocular surface can be helpful.

The surgery was uneventful with a sutureless clear corneal incision and phacoemulsification, with a one-piece IOL being placed within the capsular bag.

How Do You Manage Postoperative Cataract Patients with Severe Dry Eye and/or SS?

If possible, the typical postoperative eye drops should be ordered in non-preserved formulations to avoid additional corneal toxicity, which may exacerbate ocular surface issues (we generally recommend the use of non-preserved drops obtained through a compounding pharmacy in order to minimize ocular surface toxicity). Preservative-free prednisolone acetate 1% drops are available from compounding pharmacies. Nonsteroidal anti-inflammatory drops have been linked to corneal melts, and patients with dry eyes are potentially more prone to this complication [29]. As such, we recommend not using nonsteroidal anti-inflammatory drops postoperatively in patients with SS, but if they must be used, the preservative-free form should be chosen. Fluoroquinolone antibiotic drops are used three or four times a day starting 3 days before surgery and continued for 1 week after surgery. Patients should also continue their dry eye treatment regimens postoperatively.

It is important to follow patients closely after cataract surgery. We recommend reexamining these patients every 1–2 weeks postoperatively and monitoring their ocular surface closely. We have seen cases of corneal and scleral melting in otherwise routine cataract surgery in patients with moderate-to-severe dry eye with or without rheumatologic diseases.

Case 3 [30]

A 79-year-old Caucasian man presents to you with a 5-day history of right eye pain, with no history of dry eye or dry mouth symptoms. His past medical history is significant for hypertension, coronary artery disease, and osteoarthritis of the hip. His current medications are oral diclofenac, nifedipine, and nadolol.

On examination, visual acuity is count fingers in the right eye and 20/30 in the left eye. Evaluation of the periocular skin shows no evidence of rash or other lesions. There is no trichiasis, significant lid laxity, or lagophthalmos. There is significant anterior and posterior blepharitis in both eyes with a rapid TBUT of 3 s. His conjunctiva is moderately injected in the right eye with a large paracentral corneal ulcer with stromal melting and perforation in the inferior limbal area. The iris has plugged the wound inferiorly, and it is Seidel negative (Fig. 5.3a). Fluorescein staining shows severe dryness with multiple epithelial defects in both eyes.

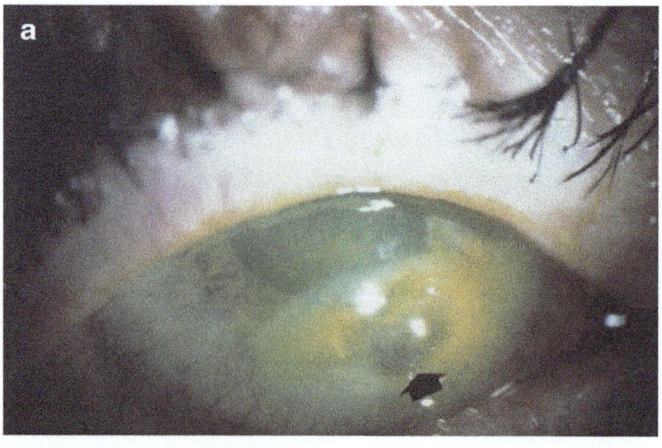

Fig. 5.3 (Case 3) (**a**) Slit lamp photograph showing marked inferior corneal thinning and ulceration of the right eye with iris plugging corneal perforation (*arrow*). (**b**) Slit lamp photograph of right eye showing patch corneal transplant (Printed with permission [30])

Fig. 5.3 (continued)

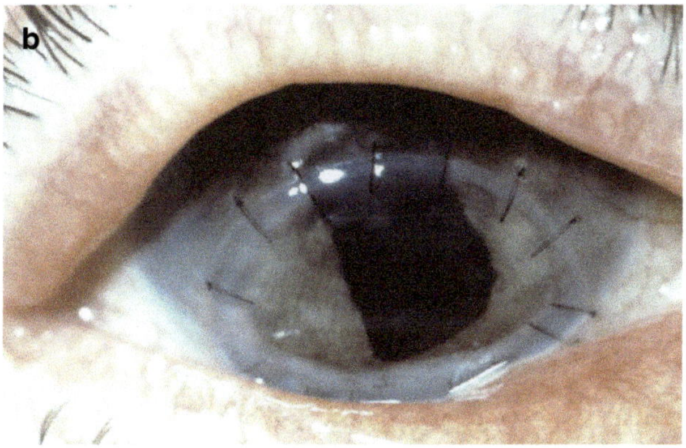

What Is the Initial Approach to This Patient? What Diagnosis Do These Findings Suggest?

When an underlying connective tissue disorder (CTD) has not yet been diagnosed, infection must always be excluded by culturing the ulcer for possible pathogens and treating with empiric prophylactic topical antibiotics. Nonbacterial infections, traumatic or surgical injuries, granulomatous disease, vasculitis, and neurologic and primary skin disorders should also be considered. Patients with evidence of severe ocular surface disease and epithelial defects should be evaluated for an underlying CTD. In addition, patients with CTD can develop bacterial superinfections, which should always be considered as a possible complication.

Testing reveals a positive fluorescent antinuclear antibody test at a titer of 1:640 with a speckled pattern, as well as a positive SS-A (Ro) antibody. The remaining laboratory results are normal. The patient also complains of dry eye and dry mouth symptoms.

What Are Your Next Diagnostic Steps?

The presence of dry eyes and dry mouth, objective signs of keratoconjunctivitis sicca, and anti-SSA positivity are suggestive of a diagnosis of SS (see Tables 5.1 and 5.2). In this patient, a salivary scintigraphic scan, measurement of whole mouth unstimulated salivary flow, and a lip biopsy were performed to confirm the diagnosis.

While the workup is still underway, and only 2 days after the patient's initial presentation, the ulcer has progressed with further stromal thinning and leakage of aqueous humor.

The patient undergoes repair of his right corneal perforation with a therapeutic contact lens applied over a corneal tissue adhesive. A Tc-99m

pertechnetate salivary scintigraphic scan and measurement of whole mouth unstimulated salivary flow (0.375 ml/min) are both normal. However, a labial minor salivary gland biopsy confirms the diagnosis of primary SS and reveals focal lymphocytic sialadenitis and fibrosis with a focus score of 7/4 mm^2.

Unfortunately, 3 weeks after contact lens placement, the patient returns, and the contact lens has fallen off. The cornea has melted further in the same area as the original ulceration with even more stromal loss than before the gluing.

What Is the Pathophysiology of Corneal Melts in SS Patients?

Sterile corneal melts in SS patients classically present in the paracentral cornea and most likely begin with a breakdown in the epithelium due to severe dryness. While a breakdown in the epithelium may not lead to rapid stromal melting in non-SS patients, there are several factors that contribute to rapid stromal degradation in patients with SS. There is likely an excess of matrix metalloproteinases (due to inflammation) on the ocular surface. In addition, persistent epithelial defects stimulate the infiltration of the stroma by inflammatory cells, causing lysosomal enzymatic degradation of collagen and ground substance by collagenase and other proteases. Stimulation of collagenase production by corneal fibroblasts or stromal keratocytes may further contribute to stromal degradation. It is important to remember that corneal melting can occur at any time in a patient's clinical course and does not always correlate with the activity of the underlying connective tissue disease.

As noted in case 2, a common offending agent that can precipitate such melts in SS patients is topical nonsteroidal anti-inflammatory drugs (NSAIDs), which are not only toxic to the epithelium but also inhibit tissue repair. Since dryness and local inflammation play a central role, treatment is aimed at local control of inflammation (topical cyclosporine/tacrolimus), inhibition of matrix metalloproteinases (doxycycline/minocycline), protecting the cornea (bandage contact lens, tarsorrhaphy), and improving the tear film (copious non-preserved tears and later punctal occlusion). Systemic anti-inflammatory therapy with oral corticosteroids is also helpful acutely since topical steroids are contraindicated in such settings. Recurrent or refractory corneal melts may require the use of systemic immunosuppression. These paracentral melts should be distinguished from another classic corneal melting condition known as peripheral ulcerative keratitis (PUK). PUK, which can occur in the setting of conditions such as rheumatoid arthritis or granulomatosis and polyangiitis (GPA) (formerly known as Wegener's), indicates active systemic inflammation and requires intense systemic therapy (high-dose systemic steroids, TNF inhibitors) in order to be controlled.

What Is the Approach to Corneal Ulcerations with Corneal Perforation or Threatened Corneal Perforation in SS Patients?

Controversy exists regarding the optimal treatment of sterile corneal ulceration in patients with SS. Therapy often consists of a combination of local treatments to decrease corneal melting in addition to systemic medications aimed at treating the underlying disease. After excluding infection, the goal is to close the epithelial defect, limit further ulceration, and provide tectonic support of any stromal melting. Topical steroids are generally contraindicated in SS patients with an epithelial defect and corneal thinning. They are postulated to inhibit corneal repair by reducing fibroblast synthetic activity or by stimulating collagenase production [31, 32].

The initial approach to a patient with sterile corneal melt without perforation would consist of the following:

1. Stopping topical steroids and/or NSAIDs
2. Frequent use of preservative-free artificial tears
3. Prophylactic antibiotic ointment and drops
4. Topical 1–2% cyclosporine (or 0.01–0.03% compounded tacrolimus) qid
5. Systemic doxycycline 100 mg bid
6. Bandage contact lens
7. Punctal occlusion

The use of amniotic membrane overlays may be considered if there is no improvement with the above measures in order to promote epithelialization and to resist further stromalysis. AmbioDisk™ Amniotic Membrane (IOP Ophthalmics) with an accompanying bandage lens is a convenient device which allows for application of the membrane over the cornea without the need for any suturing or operating room procedure. It can easily be applied in the clinic.

If there is significant corneal stromal thinning (>50%), then the approach needs to be even more aggressive. A sterile corneal melt with impending perforation in patients with SS (or presumed SS) should be treated aggressively with either cyanoacrylate glue and bandage contact lens placement or with a temporary complete tarsorrhaphy, while therapy is initiated. The application of corneal tissue adhesive can usually be performed in the examination lane with the patient supine under topical anesthesia. Amniotic membrane overlays with a bandage contact lens (AmbioDisk or Prokera) can also be applied in the clinic setting.

Once a corneal perforation has occurred, if small (<1 mm), treatment may consist of applying corneal adhesive or stacking small segments of amniotic membrane layers within the melting area. If the perforation is >1 mm, usually tissue adhesive is not effective and may enter the anterior chamber and bridge the iris or lens to the cornea. In these cases of contact lens failure or larger perforations, lamellar patch grafting or penetrating keratoplasty can be used along with one or more of the other modalities mentioned above including tarsorrhaphy, punctal occlusion, amniotic membrane overlays, and copious lubrication [32]. In addition, topical cyclosporine/tacrolimus may be helpful in treating patients with recurrent corneal ulcerations [33, 34]. Ocular surface moisture can also be maintained through either temporary or permanent tarsorrhaphy to decrease tear evaporation, as well as punctal occlusion [35]. Increasing the oral intake of vitamin C and the use of tetracycline formulations may also be of benefit to promote stromal healing and retard further stromal melting.

Concomitant systemic immunosuppressant treatment is very important, as lamellar or penetrating grafts are susceptible to further melting if the underlying disease is not treated. Ideally it is preferable to delay corneal grafting until the acute inflammatory phase has stabilized.

Of note, a contact lens and corneal adhesive alone would not have been sufficient in this patient, and his course was complicated by further corneal melting requiring corneal graft surgery.

The patient undergoes an emergent corneal patch graft, tarsorrhaphy, and cautery punctal occlusion. Immunosuppressive therapy is begun with 100 mg prednisone daily. Within 2 weeks, the corneal patch graft melts. Histological examination reveals marked loss of stromal tissue with scattered acute and chronic inflammatory cells.

How Would Your Management Change at This Point?

As described above, definitive management of corneal melting generally cannot be achieved by local measures alone. Patients often require the institution of systemic treatment including immunosuppressive therapy. A combination of glucocorticosteroids and steroid-sparing immunosuppressive agents is generally the preferred approach to the treatment of severe autoimmune features in primary SS. Studies have shown the benefit of immunosuppressives with respect to graft survival [36]. However, there is no consensus on which immunosuppressive agent is best for these patients. Therapeutic success has been reported with the use of methotrexate, azathioprine, oral cyclosporine, cyclophosphamide, or combination therapy [30, 36]. We recommend involving a rheumatologist with experience in treating SS before initiating immunosuppressive treatment.

It is also important to remain vigilant and watch for signs of relapse. If relapse occurs, there should be a low threshold to increase or change immunosuppressive medications.

The patient is transitioned to azathioprine 50 mg daily, and a second patch corneal transplant finally succeeds (Fig. 5.3b). The prednisone dose is tapered over the course of 4 months, and the dose of azathioprine is slowly increased to 100 mg daily. Ocular symptoms improve. Visual acuity is now 20/60 in the right eye.

Over the next several months, the patient remains stable on maintenance azathioprine 75 mg daily and ocular lubricants.

Another useful adjunctive therapy for both acute management and long-term maintenance of sterile paracentral melts is topical 1–2% cyclosporine drops (compounded) or topical 0.01–0.03% tacrolimus drops (compounded). These can provide potent local immunosuppression as an alternative to topical steroids. The use of topical lifitegrast has not been studied in this setting but may be potentially helpful.

Acknowledgments *Financial Disclosure*: Dr. Vivino is a consultant and/or participant in clinical trials for Immco Diagnostics, Inc. *Conflict of Interest*: Dr. Vivino is a consultant and/or participant in clinical trials for Immco Diagnostics, Inc.

References

1. Segal B, Bowman SJ, Fox PC, et al. Primary Sjogrens Syndrome: health experiences and predictors of health quality among patients in the United States. Health Qual Life Outcomes. 2009;7:46.
2. Fox PC, Bowman SJ, Segal B, et al. Oral involvement in primary Sjogren syndrome. J Am Dent Assoc. 2008;139(12):1592–601.
3. Markusse HM, Oudkerk M, Vroom TM, Breedveld FC. Primary Sjogren's syndrome: clinical spectrum and mode of presentation based on an analysis of 50 patients selected from a department of rheumatology. Neth J Med. 1992;40(3-4):125–34.
4. Kassan SS, Moutsopoulos HM. Clinical manifestations and early diagnosis of Sjogren syndrome. Arch Intern Med. 2004;164(12):1275–84.
5. Kruszka P, O'Brian RJ. Diagnosis and management of Sjogren syndrome. Am Fam Physician. 2009;79(6):465–70.
6. Manthorpe R, Asmussen K, Oxholm P. Primary Sjogren's syndrome: diagnostic criteria, clinical features, and disease activity. J Rheumatol Suppl. 1997;50:8–11.
7. Zintzaras E, Voulgarelis M, Moutsopoulos HM. The risk of lymphoma development in autoimmune diseases: a meta-analysis. Arch Intern Med. 2005;165(20):2337–44.
8. Fox RI. Sjogren's syndrome. Lancet. 2005;366(9482):321–31.
9. Nichols KK, Nichols JJ, Zadnik K. Frequency of dry eye diagnostic test procedures used in various modes of ophthalmic practice. Cornea. 2000;19(4):477–82.
10. Korb DR. Survey of preferred tests for diagnosis of the tear film and dry eye. Cornea. 2000;19(4):483–6.
11. Whitcher JP, Shiboski CH, Shiboski SC, et al. A simplified quantitative method for assessing keratoconjunctivitis sicca from the Sjogren's syndrome international registry. Am J Ophthalmol. 2010;149(3):405–15.
12. Garcia-Carrasco M, Ramos-Casals M, Rosas J, et al. Primary Sjogren syndrome: clinical and immunologic disease patterns in a cohort of 400 patients. Medicine (Baltimore). 2002;81(4):270–80.
13. Shen L, Suresh L, Lindemann M, et al. Novel autoantibodies in Sjogren's syndrome. Clin Immunol. 2012;145(3):251–5.
14. Vitali C, Bombardieri S, Jonsson R, et al. Classification criteria for Sjogren's syndrome: a revised version of the European criteria proposed by the American-European Consensus Group. Ann Rheum Dis. 2002;61(6):554–8.
15. Shiboski SC, Shiboski CH, Criswell L, et al. American College of Rheumatology classification criteria for Sjogren's syndrome: a data-driven, expert consensus approach in the

Sjogren's International Collaborative Clinical Alliance cohort. Arthritis Care Res (Hoboken). 2012;64(4):475–87.
16. Shiboski CH, Shiboski SC, Seror R, Criswell LA, Labetoulle M, Lietman TM, Rasmussen A, Scofield H, Vitali C, Bowman SJ, Mariette X, International Sjögren's Syndrome Criteria Working Group 2013. American College of Rheumatology/European League against rheumatism classification criteria for primary Sjögren's syndrome: a consensus and data-driven methodology involving three international patient cohorts. Ann Rheum Dis. 2017;76(1):9–16.
17. Ram J, Sharma A, Pandav SS, Gupta A, Bambery P. Cataract surgery in patients with dry eyes. J Cataract Refract Surg. 1998;24(8):1119–24.
18. Sambursky R, Davitt WF III, Latkany R, et al. Sensitivity and specificity of a point-of-care matrix metalloproteinase 9 immunoassay for diagnosing inflammation related to dry eye. JAMA Ophthalmol. 2013;131(1):24–8.
19. Kaufman HE. The practical detection of mmp-9 diagnoses ocular surface disease and may help prevent its complications. Cornea. 2013;32(2):211–6.
20. Sambursky R, Davitt WF III, Friedberg M, Tauber S. Prospective, multicenter, clinical evaluation of point-of-care matrix metalloproteinase-9 test for confirming dry eye disease. Cornea. 2014;33(8):812–8.
21. Sullivan BD, Crews LA, Sonmez B, et al. Clinical utility of objective tests for dry eye disease: variability over time and implications for clinical trials and disease management. Cornea. 2012;31(9):1000–8.
22. Tomlinson A, Khanal S, Ramaesh K, Diaper C, McFadyen A. Tear film osmolarity: determination of a referent for dry eye diagnosis. Invest Ophthalmol Vis Sci. 2006;47(10):4309–15.
23. Versura P, Profazio V, Campos EC. Performance of tear osmolarity compared to previous diagnostic tests for dry eye diseases. Curr Eye Res. 2010;35(7):553–64.
24. Epitropoulos AT, Matossian C, Berdy GJ, Malhotra RP, Potvin R. Effect of tear osmolarity on repeatability of keratometry for cataract surgery planning. J Cataract Refract Surg. 2015;41(8):1672–7.
25. Bunya VY, Fuerst NM, Pistilli M, et al. Variability of tear osmolarity in patients with dry eye. JAMA Ophthalmol. 2015;133(6):662–7.
26. Menzies KL, Srinivasan S, Prokopich CL, Jones L. Infrared imaging of meibomian glands and evaluation of the lipid layer in Sjogren's syndrome patients and nondry eye controls. Invest Ophthalmol Vis Sci. 2015;56(2):836–41.
27. Villani E, Beretta S, De Capitani M, Galimberti D, Viola F, Ratiglia R. In vivo confocal microscopy of meibomian glands in Sjogren's syndrome. Invest Ophthalmol Vis Sci. 2011;52(2):933–9.
28. Kangari H, Eftekhari MH, Sardari S, et al. Short-term consumption of oral omega-3 and dry eye syndrome. Ophthalmology. 2013;120(11):2191–6.
29. Asai T, Nakagami T, Mochizuki M, Hata N, Tsuchiya T, Hotta Y. Three cases of corneal melting after instillation of a new nonsteroidal anti-inflammatory drug. Cornea. 2006;25(2):224–7.
30. Vivino FB, Minerva P, Huang CH, Orlin SE. Corneal melt as the initial presentation of primary Sjogren's syndrome. J Rheumatol. 2001;28(2):379–82.
31. Krachmer JH, Laibson PR. Corneal thinning and perforation in Sjogren's syndrome. Am J Ophthalmol. 1974;78(6):917–20.
32. Pfister RR, Murphy GE. Corneal ulceration and perforation associated with Sjogren's syndrome. Arch Ophthalmol. 1980;98(1):89–94.
33. Kervick GN, Pflugfelder SC, Haimovici R, Brown H, Tozman E, Yee R. Paracentral rheumatoid corneal ulceration. Clinical features and cyclosporine therapy. Ophthalmology. 1992;99(1):80–8.
34. Gottsch JD, Akpek EK. Topical cyclosporin stimulates neovascularization in resolving sterile rheumatoid central corneal ulcers. Trans Am Ophthalmol Soc. 2000;98:81–7. discussion 87–90
35. Colon LE, Enzenauer RJ. Corneal thinning as the sole manifestation of active undifferentiated connective tissue disease. South Med J. 1990;83(1):48–50.

36. Bernauer W, Ficker LA, Watson PG, Dart JK. The management of corneal perforations associated with rheumatoid arthritis. An analysis of 32 eyes. Ophthalmology. 1995;102(9):1325–37.
37. Seror R, Ravaud P, Bowman SJ, et al. EULAR Sjögren's Syndrome Disease Activity Index: development of a consensus systemic disease activity index for primary Sjögren's syndrome. Ann Rheum Dis. 2010;69:1103–9.

Chapter 6
Diagnosis and Management of Ocular Graft-Versus-Host Disease

Ketki Soin, Ali R. Djalilian, and Sandeep Jain

Case 1

VP is a 27-year-old male referred to our clinic for evaluation of ocular graft-versus-host disease (GVHD). His past medical history is significant for acute lymphocytic leukemia status post hematopoietic stem cell transplantation (HSCT) 6 months ago and Bell's palsy secondary to a brain lesion that has resolved. His medications include valacyclovir, folic acid, sulfamethoxazole and trimethoprim, calcium, lanoconazole, and dasatinib.

What Is Your Examination Approach to Ocular GVHD?

Ocular GVHD occurs in 38–50% patients after allogeneic HSCT. Therefore, it is important to perform a thorough ocular history and anterior segment exam. The Ocular Surface Disease Index (OSDI) is a valid and reliable 12-symptom analysis tool that can be used to assess dry eye disease severity and effect on vision-related function. The OSDI score is assessed on a scale of 0–100, with higher scores representing severe dry eye disease. The anterior segment exam includes close attention to the position of eyelids, direction of eyelashes, expressibility and keratinization of

K. Soin, MD • A.R. Djalilian, MD • S. Jain, MD (✉)
Department of Ophthalmology and Visual Sciences, Illinois Eye and Ear Infirmary,
University of Illinois at Chicago, Chicago, IL 60612, USA
e-mail: jains@uic.edu

A.R. Djalilian (ed.), *Ocular Surface Disease*,
https://doi.org/10.1007/978-3-319-15823-5_6

meibomian glands, vascularity of the eyelid margin, conjunctival injection, and corneal vascularization. Schirmer testing and fluorescein or rose bengal staining are all necessary.

He has no symptoms of ocular discomfort (OSDI = 0) and has no changes in his vision. On exam his visual acuity is 20/20 in both eyes. He has normal tear production in both eyes (Schirmer I >20 mm) and no ocular surface disease.

Is There a Diagnostic Criterion for Chronic Ocular GVHD?

The International Chronic Ocular Graft-vs-Host-Disease Consensus Group created a diagnosis criterion for chronic ocular GVHD. Parameters for diagnosis include (1) OSDI score, (2) Schirmer's test score without anesthesia, (3) corneal fluorescein staining, and (4) conjunctival injection. Each parameter is given a score, and the aggregate score determines the disease severity as none, mild/moderate, and severe (Table 6.1). A diagnosis of ocular GVHD is made as none, probable GVHD, and definitive GVHD based on the aggregate score and the presence or absence of systemic GVHD (Table 6.2) [1].

Given his exam findings and absence of systemic GVHD, he scores zero in both eyes and does not have ocular GVHD.

Table 6.1 Severity scale in chronic ocular GVHD

Severity scores (points)	Schirmer's test (mm)	Corneal fluorescein staining	OSDI	Conjunctival injection
0	>15	0	<13	None
1	11–15	<2	13–22	Mild/moderate
2	6–10	2–3	23–32	Severe
3	≤5	≥4	≥33	

From: With permission from International Chronic Ocular Graft-vs-Host-Disease (GVHD) Consensus Group: Proposed Diagnostic Criteria for Chronic GVHD [1]

OSDI ocular surface disease index. Total score (points); (Schirmer's test score + corneal fluorescein staining score + OSDI score + conjunctival injection score) = 0–4 (none); 5–8 (mild/moderate); 9–11 (severe)

Table 6.2 Diagnosis of chronic ocular GVHD

	None (points)	Probable GVHD (points)	Definite GVHD (points)
Systemic GVHD (−)	0–5	6–7	≥8
Systemic GVHD (+)	0–3	4–5	≥6

From: With permission from International Chronic Ocular Graft-vs-Host-Disease (GVHD) Consensus Group: Proposed Diagnostic Criteria for Chronic GVHD [1]

Can You Perform Any Other Tests to Determine If He Has Any Signs of Ocular Inflammation?

Several laboratory tests can be performed to assess for early signs and markers of dry eye disease and ocular inflammation. Tear fluid osmolarity and noninvasive Keratograph tear break-up time (NIKBUT) are two tests that can aid in the diagnosis of dry eye disease. Tear fluid osmolarity test measures the osmolarity of human tears. The lower the water content of tears, the higher the osmolarity of tears and the more severe the dry eye. Normal tear osmolarity ranges from 280 to 295 mOsm/L, which is equivalent to normal blood osmolarity (citation 5 from tear lab cards). Measurements >300 mOsm/L or an inter-eye difference >8 mOsm/L demonstrates loss of homeostatic osmolarity regulation. NIKBUT measures tear film stability by measuring the first and mean break-up times without the need for fluorescein.

The ocular redness score using Keratograph, and tear matrix metalloproteinase-9 (MMP-9) level, can suggest early ocular surface inflammation if positive. The oculus Keratograph scans the exposed bulbar conjunctiva and generates a bulbar redness (BR) score. The BR score range between 0.0 and 4.0. MMP-9 are proteolytic enzymes that play a role in wound healing and inflammation. They have been shown to be higher in tears of individuals with dry eye disease. The InflammaDry test is used to detect MMP-9 levels in the tear film. A positive result indicates the presence of MMP-9 ≥ 40 ng/ml.

We performed NIKBUT, which was reduced in both eyes (3.70 s in the right eye and 2.68 s in the left eye) which indicates rapid breakup of the tear film and is suggestive of early dry eye disease. The tear fluid osmolarity was high in both eyes (330 in the right eye and 315 in the left eye) suggestive of dry eye disease. The ocular redness score using Keratograph was 1.1 in the right eye and 0.8 in the left eye, which is also high normal and may suggest early ocular surface inflammation. MMP-9 was positive in both eyes suggestive of ocular surface inflammation.

How Do These Laboratory Tests Help You in Counseling and Treating This Patient?

Taken together, despite the clinical signs pointing to "none" ocular GVDH, the laboratory tests suggest that early dry eye disease and ocular surface inflammation may be present. Therefore it would be reasonable to initiate mild anti-inflammatory therapy to hopefully prevent development of overt signs and symptoms.

We suggested he perform warm compresses, start cyclosporine eye drops twice a day, and use artificial tears as needed. The patient needs to be followed up every 3 months to check for signs of ocular GVHD.

Case 2

CL is a 65-year-old female with history of chronic GVHD and dry eyes, referred for evaluation of ocular GVHD. She was diagnosed with multiple myeloma 2 years ago and underwent HSCT 4 and 10 months following her diagnosis. She was diagnosed with chronic GVHD because she had clinical signs of her skin, mouth, and eyes.

She experiences dry eyes in both eyes; however her right eye is worse than her left eye. She has eye discomfort, soreness, irritation, and redness. Her symptoms are worse in the morning and evenings. She uses lubricating drops at bedtime and wears contact lenses in both eyes during the day.

Her best corrected visual acuity is 20/20 in both eyes. She has minimal symptoms of ocular discomfort (OSDI = 2.08), severe tear deficiency in the right eye (Schirmer I = 0 mm), and borderline tear deficiency in the left eye (Schirmer I = 8 mm). Her corneal fluorescein staining showed moderate ocular surface disease (5 points OD, 2 points OS). She had extensive conjunctival staining of the right eye as well. Given these findings her disease severity is mild/moderate in both eyes (total points: 6 OD, 4 OS). In the presence of systemic chronic GVHD, these scores lead to a diagnosis of "definite" ocular GVHD in the right eye and "probable" ocular GVHD in the left eye.

We performed laboratory tests to see if she had other markers of dry eye disease and ocular inflammation. NIKBUT was reduced in both eyes (5.93 s OD and 2.48 s OS), which indicates rapid breakup of the tear film. The tear fluid osmolarity was high in both eyes (347 OD and 308 OS). Both of these tests are suggestive of dry eyes. The MMP-9 test was positive in both eyes, and the ocular redness score using Keratograph was 1.2 OD and 1.4 OS, which is also high—these tests are suggestive of ocular surface inflammation.

Why Are Her Ocular Symptoms Asymmetric?

Even though ocular GVHD is a systemic disease, patients can present with asymmetric symptoms and clinical signs. Both eyes are usually affected; however one eye can be more symptomatic and show more clinical signs. Studies have shown some patients with asymmetric disease have differences in their corneal nerve fiber density between both eyes. The morphological changes in corneal nerves also may explain the lack of correlation between signs and symptoms in dry eye patients [2].

Despite having less symptoms, a greater Schirmer I test, and decreased corneal staining in the left eye, her other laboratory tests suggested she had ocular inflammation in the left eye. Given the laboratory tests were very similar between the two eyes, her contact lenses could have been masking her symptoms in the left eye greater than the right eye. Soft contact lenses have been shown to decrease dry eye symptoms and improve visual acuity without significantly affecting the Schirmer test, tear break-up time, or corneal staining, in patients with ocular GVHD [3].

How Do You Treat This Patient, Given She Has Minimal Symptoms (OSDI = 2.08)?

A symptom sign disconnect in dry eye is very well known. She has definite ocular GVHD in the right eye and probable GVHD in the left eye, and laboratory tests suggest inflammation in both eyes. Therefore, aggressive control of inflammation is warranted in both eyes despite her mild symptoms.

Treatment options for ocular GVHD are based on four main principles: lubrication and tear preservation, reduction of inflammation, prevention of tear evaporation, and epithelial support [4].

Topical lubrication with non-preserved artificial tears is used for patients with aqueous-deficient dry eye to provide lubrication and dilution of inflammatory mediators present at the ocular surface. Punctal plugs can also be used to maintain lubrication; however if ocular inflammation is present, the inflammation should be treated prior to placement of punctal plugs. It should be noted that in patients with moderate to severe GVHD (with very low Schirmer values), total punctal occlusion (both upper and lower puncta) is needed for a meaningful clinical response. In other words, occluding a single punctum is unlikely to have any value. Given the permanent nature of the disease, cauterization of both upper and lower puncta is a more definitive therapy compared to plugs which likely need to be replaced from time to time.

Ocular inflammation can be reduced with topical cyclosporine and steroid drops. Cyclosporine inhibits T-cell activation and downregulates inflammatory cytokines in the conjunctiva. Topical cyclosporine also increases conjunctival goblet cell density and decreases epithelial cell turnover. Topical cyclosporine has been shown to decrease dry eye symptoms and corneal fluorescein staining in patients with ocular GVHD [5]. Topical cyclosporine can be used long term without causing side effects. Topical steroids are also be used for their anti-inflammatory properties; however low-dose steroids used for a short-time period are preferred given their side effect profile. Topical tacrolimus may be even more effective that cyclosporine but is only available as a compounded medication at this time.

Meibomian gland dysfunction can lead to an unstable tear film, resulting in tear evaporation. Warm compresses applied twice a day for 5–10 min combined with lubricating ointments over the lid margin can treat meibomian gland disease. Oral tetracycline antibiotics such as doxycycline and minocycline are also indicated. They are used for their anti-inflammatory properties as they inhibit MMP and interleukin-1 activity [4]. Patients with chronic GVHD typically have progressive meibomian gland dropout, and in long-standing disease, most of the glands may be lost (Fig. 6.1).

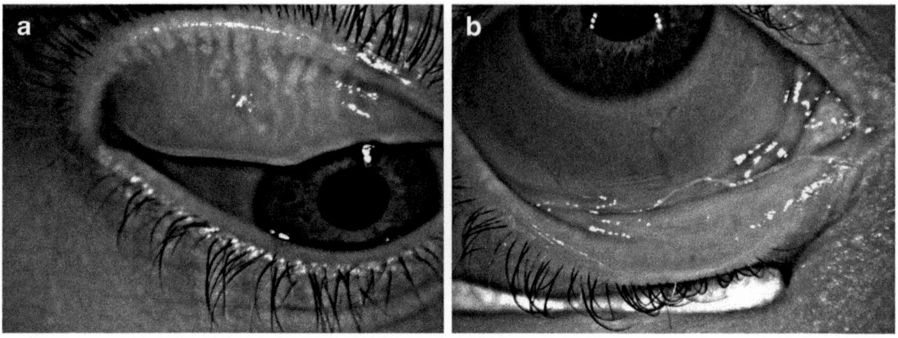

Fig. 6.1 Loss of meibomian glands in the upper (**a**) and lower lid (**b**) of a patient with chronic ocular GVHD

Bandage soft contact lenses or scleral lenses can provide epithelial support by hydrating the corneal surface, stabilizing the tear film, promoting corneal healing, and restoring normal cell turnover. As mentioned earlier bandage soft contact lenses with high oxygen diffusion capacities and scleral lenses have been shown to improve subjective dry eye symptoms and visual acuity in patients with ocular graft-versus-host disease [3, 6–8].

She was started on compounded methylprednisolone eye drops four times a day, doxycycline 50 mg daily, and erythromycin ointment at bedtime in both eyes. In addition she was advised to perform warm compress twice a day. She was referred to the contact lens clinic for either soft daily disposable bandage contact lens fitting or regular scleral lens or prosthetic replacement of the ocular surface ecosystem (PROSE) treatment.

What Is the Role of Autologous Serum Tears in the Management of Chronic Ocular GVHD?

Serum tears are invaluable in the management of ocular GVHD. We offer this treatment to all patients, typically starting with 20% concentration applied every 2–3 h. It is considered prior to contact lenses or in patients who are unable to handle contact lenses. Previously, we had theoretical concerns about circulating immune factors exacerbating the inflammation on the surface, however clinically that has not been a problem, perhaps because patients are also frequently receiving anti-inflammatory treatment. In our experience, GVHD patients universally like serum tears, improving both their signs and symptoms of ocular disease. Patients are encouraged to remain on serum tears for at least 6–12 months and, if possible, indefinitely. Patient can continue to use serum tears even if they end up using contacts/scleral lenses. Some patients use the serum tears to partially fill the scleral lens before placing it on the eye.

Case 3

BI is a 53-year-old male with history of non-Hodgkin's lymphoma status post bone marrow transplant 15 years ago resulting in chronic systemic and ocular GVHD, presented for a second opinion for dry eyes. His ocular symptoms began 14 years ago. His past ocular history included cataract extraction and intraocular lens placement in both eyes 5 years ago, cauterization of all four puncta 3 years ago, and herpes keratitis treated with valacyclovir a few years ago. His ocular medications include artificial tears every 15–60 min and lubricating ointment at bedtime in both eyes. He has tried cyclosporine drops, however is unable to use them due to burning. His systemic medications include CellCept, prednisone 2.5 mg, doxycycline 20 mg twice a day, Ambien, and amlodipine.

He experiences dryness, irritation, and photophobia everyday. His symptoms are worse in the morning and have become worse over the past 6 months.

His best corrected visual acuity is 20/25 OD and 20/30 OS. Anterior segment exam was significant for ectropion of the right and left lower eyelid, mild telangiectasia of the lid margins, cauterization of all four puncta, hyperemia of the conjunctiva OU, and punctate fluorescein staining of the superior cornea OS > OD. He had severe tear deficiency of both eyes (Schirmer I < 1 mm OU).

Why Did He Have Fluorescein Staining of the Superior Cornea?

Fine punctate staining of the superior cornea and conjunctiva is seen in superior limbic keratoconjunctivitis (SLK) [9]. SLK is thought to occur secondary to contact between the upper eyelid and superior bulbar conjunctiva while blinking. It is thought that localized tear deficiency in the upper conjunctiva can lead to loss of lubrication between the upper eyelid and superior conjunctiva and cornea. This can cause recurrent microtrauma to the superior conjunctiva and cornea [10]. This entity is often overlooked partly because the superior cornea/conjunctiva may not be routinely examined as it requires lifting the upper lid (Fig. 6.2). The staining pattern of the superior cornea can be mistakenly attributed to the dry eyes; however as seen in this example (Fig. 6.3), it is a distinct staining pattern.

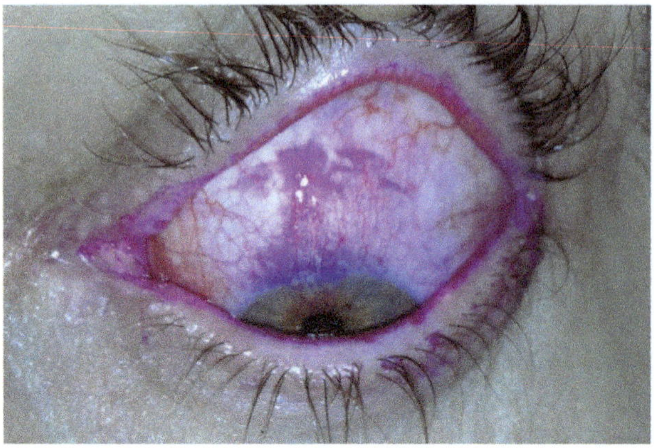

Fig. 6.2 Rose bengal staining of the superior conjunctiva in an ocular GVHD patient with SLK (with permission from [11])

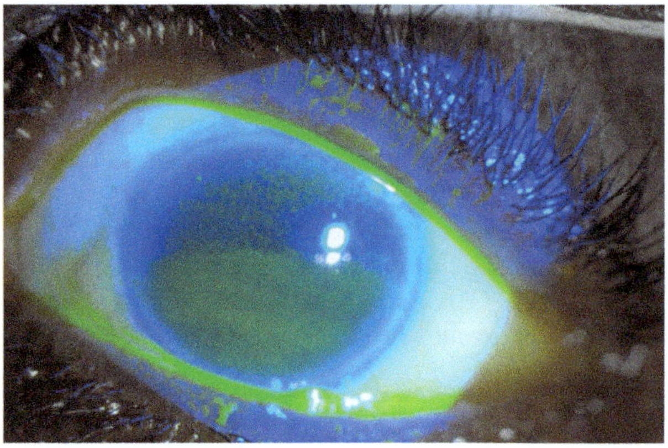

Fig. 6.3 Superior corneal epithelial staining (due to SLK) which is distinct from the inferior/interpalpebral staining due to dry eyes in a patient with chronic ocular GVHD

Is SLK Seen in Chronic Ocular GVHD?

Yes. There are no signs or symptoms specific to ocular GVHD. Ocular GVHD usually presents with signs and symptoms that mimic other immune-mediated ocular surface disorders [11]. Patients with ocular GVHD have dry eyes secondary to tear deficiency, and SLK can be seen in patients with tear deficiency. In particular, we hypothesize that the loss of goblet cells/mucin combined with the frequent forceful blinking leads to the development of SLK in these patients.

How Do You Treat SLK in Patients with Dry Eyes?

Improving the tear film with punctal occlusion and autologous serum tears are two options to treat SLK in patients with dry eyes. Punctal occlusion allows for more tears to accumulate on the ocular surface. However punctal occlusion should be used with caution in patients with ocular inflammation because punctal occlusion can cause decrease in clearance of inflammatory proteins. Alternate or adjunctive therapy to punctal occlusion is the use of autologous serum tears. Serum tears provide lubrication and many vitamins and growth factors that improve the health of the ocular surface.

His symptoms and exams were consistent with severe aqueous tear deficiency and SLK secondary to chronic ocular graft-versus-host disease. He was advised to start methylprednisolone drops four times a day, restart cyclosporine drops twice a day, and continue lubrication with preservative-free artificial tears and lubricating ointment. He was also referred to the contact lens clinic for scleral lens fitting.

The patient did not follow up with our practice for 3 years. He returned to see us because his vision and ocular symptoms were worsening. His left eye was more symptomatic compared to his right eye. He experienced constant dryness, redness, and photophobia. His medications at that visit included loteprednol four times a day, preservative-free artificial tears every 30 min, and lubricating ointment two times a day.

His best corrected visual acuity was 20/25 OD and 20/60 OS. Anterior segment exam was essentially stable in the right eye compared to 3 years ago. Anterior segment exam of the left eye was significant for 3+ injection of the conjunctiva, superior corneal vascularization, and conjunctivalization of the superior cornea. A whorl-like pattern of the superior corneal limbus was noted after instillation of fluorescein dye (Fig. 6.4).

His examination was consistent with limbal stem cell deficiency (LSCD) OS secondary to chronic superior limbic keratoconjunctivitis. He was advised to start using serum tears every hour and cyclosporine twice a day in both eyes. He was also referred to a contact lens clinic for scleral lenses to help treat his dry eyes and SLK.

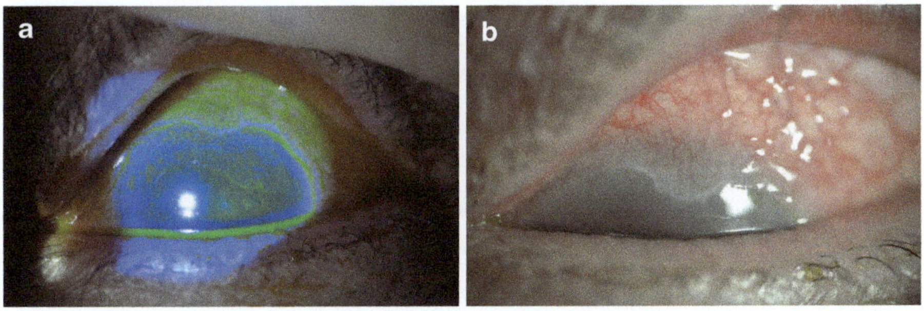

Fig. 6.4 Patient with untreated chronic SLK due to ocular GVHD which has now developed limbal stem cell deficiency as evident by whorl staining of the superior epithelium (**a**) and a peripheral corneal pannus and injection (**b**) (With permission from [11])

Why Does He Have LSCD in the Left Eye?

Since the patient did not follow up and was not adequately treated for SLK for 3 years, he developed secondary LSCD. The continuous microtrauma to the superior cornea and conjunctiva in SLK can destroy limbal stem cells. The left eye had worse SLK at initial examination and likely progressed to LSCD for that reason.

Two months later he returned for follow-up. His symptoms improved partially with serum tears. He saw contact lens clinic and was tried with soft bandage contact lenses; however he was unable to tolerate them. He was also unable to tolerate the cyclosporine drops because they caused burning.

On exam his vision improved to 20/25 OU. Anterior segment exam was stable except for mild subepithelial haze in the superior cornea of the right eye.

Patient was then referred back to contact lens where he was successfully fit with PROSE lenses. He continues to wear PROSE lenses everyday.

This case highlights the importance of recognizing and treating SLK in GVHD patients. We have seen other cases where long-standing SLK in a GVHD patient has led to permanent LSCD in both eyes. Examination of the superior cornea (with fluorescein staining) is a standard part of the exam for every ocular GVHD patient. The staining will often follow a more whorl-like pattern indicating "stress" to the limbus. Anti-inflammatory therapy (topical steroids followed by cyclosporine/tacrolimus) and serum tears are the first-line treatments for SLK. Scleral lenses are the most definitive therapy for persistent cases as it provides a physical barrier between the eyelid and the superior cornea and conjunctiva.

References

1. Ogawa Y, et al. International Chronic Ocular Graft-vs-Host-Disease (GVHD) Consensus Group: proposed diagnostic criteria for chronic GVHD (part I). Sci Rep. 2013;3:3419. PMC. Web. 29 2015
2. Dastjerdi MH, Hamrah P, Al-Arfaj K, Dana R. Disparate corneal nerve alterations between the two eyes in dry eye patients with asymmetric ocular surface manifestations: in vivo confocal microscopy Study. Invest Ophthalmol Vis Sci. 2008;49(13):5315.
3. Russo PA, Bouchard CS, Galasso JM. Extended-wear silicone hydrogel soft contact lenses in the management of moderate to severe dry eye signs and symptoms secondary to graft-versus-host disease. Eye Contact Lens. 2007;33:144–7.
4. Shikari H, Antin JH, Dana R. Ocular graft-versus-host disease: a review. Surv Ophthalmol. 2013;58(3):233–51.
5. Lelli GJ Jr, Musch DC, Gupta A, et al. Ophthalmic cyclosporine use in ocular GVHD. Cornea. 2006;25:635–8.
6. Pflugfelder SC. Management and therapy of dry eye disease: report of the Management and Therapy Subcommittee of the International Dry Eye WorkShop (2007). Ocul Surf. 2007;5(2):163–78.

7. Jacobs DS, Rosenthal P. Boston scleral lens prosthetic device for treatment of severe dry eye in chronic graft-versus-host disease. Cornea. 2007;26(10):1195–9.
8. DeLoss KS, et al. PROSE treatment for ocular chronic graft-versus-host disease as a clinical network expands. Eye Contact Lens. 2015;42(4):262–6.
9. Theodore FH, Ferry AP. Superior limbic keratoconjunctivitis: clinical and pathological correlations. Arch Ophthalmol. 1970;84:481–4.
10. Yang HY, Fujishima H, Toda I, et al. Lacrimal punctal occlusion for the treatment of superior limbic keratoconjunctivitis. Am J Ophthalmol. 1997;124:80–7.
11. Sivaraman KR, Jivrajka RV, Soin K, Bouchard CS, Movahedan A, Shorter E, Jain S, Jacobs DS, Djalilian AR. Superior limbic keratoconjunctivitis-like inflammation in patients with chronic graft-versus-host disease. Ocul Surf. 2016;14(3):393–400.

Chapter 7
Management of Ocular Surface Allergic Diseases

Jeanie Paik and Priti Batta

Case 1

A 5-year-old female presents in the spring with occasional tearing and frequent rubbing of her eyes for 5 weeks. She states her eyes feel itchy. The patient's mother states that the symptoms began at the start of the autumn season and were associated with rhinitis. She has not noticed any deviation of the eyes or difficulty with vision. On exam, the patient's vision is 20/20 in both eyes. She is orthotropic with full motility and gross stereoscopic vision.

What Is Seasonal Allergic Conjunctivitis, and How Does It Typically Present?

Seasonal allergic conjunctivitis is a markedly common allergic eye condition. It is usually a reaction to the presence of environmental allergens in the air, typically plant pollens during the spring and autumn months. Seasonal allergic conjunctivitis is distinguished from perennial allergic conjunctivitis in that the latter is present year-round, resulting in more chronic conjunctival inflammation. Allergic conjunctivitis is a type I immediate IgE-mediated hypersensitivity reaction in which mast cells play a major role. The degranulation of mast cells upon IgE-mediated activation causes the release of histamine, as well as the downstream production of leukotrienes and prostaglandins.

J. Paik, MD • P. Batta, MD (✉)
New York Eye and Ear Infirmary, New York, NY, USA
e-mail: pritibatta1@gmail.com

A.R. Djalilian (ed.), *Ocular Surface Disease*,
https://doi.org/10.1007/978-3-319-15823-5_7

The binding of histamine to H1 and H2 receptors leads to the classic and well-known symptoms of eye allergy: itching, tearing, redness, frequent blinking, conjunctival and eyelid swelling, and mucus production. The symptoms may be quite severe, especially the itching and resultant desire to rub the eyes; this should help to distinguish allergy from other ocular surface conditions such as dry eye syndrome and blepharitis, in which the itching and eye rubbing are usually mild and less frequent. The conjunctival chemosis can be very prominent, creating a "glassy" appearance to the eye, due to sudden severe influx of inflammatory cells into the conjunctiva. Patients with chronic ocular allergy often develop eyelid ptosis and wrinkling of the eyelid skin, sometimes with hyperpigmentation, due to repeated bouts of eyelid swelling as well as chronic eye rubbing. The condition is often associated with other manifestations of seasonal allergy such as rhinitis and cough.

Slit-lamp examination commonly reveals papillary changes in the upper and lower tarsus. These are closely packed, flat-topped nodules of the tarsal conjunctival surface, ranging in size and number. Histologic examination of these papillae reveals a central vascular core surrounded by eosinophils and other inflammatory cells.

On slit-lamp exam, the patient has 1+ conjunctival injection in both eyes with boggy conjunctival chemosis. There is no corneal staining. On lid eversion, diffuse, fine papillae are noted on the upper and lower tarsus of both eyes.

Is Any Further Diagnostic Testing Needed? How Would You Manage This Patient?

The diagnosis of seasonal allergic conjunctivitis can typically be made based on clinical history and examination findings. Diagnostic testing is rarely necessary but may be useful in cases that do not seem to respond to medical therapy. A conjunctival scraping may reveal eosinophils which are not normally present in the conjunctiva. However, this is not very sensitive in the diagnosis of allergy, as false negatives are common [1]. Similarly, levels of eosinophil-derived proteins, as well as IgE, are likely to be elevated in the tear film of patients with any form of ocular allergy [2, 3]. However, it does not appear that these levels correlate with disease activity. Serum IgE levels can also be elevated, and these typically correlate with tear film IgE levels [3].

Allergen testing, usually via skin prick testing, may be valuable in guiding treatment by reducing exposures to identifiable allergens. Reducing allergen exposure is often challenging, but when successful, it may be sufficient in controlling the condition. Topical antihistamine eye drops, such as azelastine and epinastine, are very effective in reducing acute allergic symptoms, though they may be inadequate in severe ocular allergy. Similarly, oral antihistamine medications can also be considered, especially if other forms of allergy are also present, such as rhinitis. Topical mast cell stabilizers, such as cromolyn sodium, prevent degranulation of mast cells and therefore reduce both histamine production and the downstream inflammatory mediators. Antihistamines are effective for acute allergy; however mast cell stabilizers are intended for prophylaxis and are appropriate for more chronic cases of ocular allergy. Newer agents have multiple mechanisms of action with both antihistamine and mast cell-stabilizing effects; these include olopatadine, alcaftadine, and ketotifen.

For more severe cases or acute exacerbations, topical corticosteroids may need to be employed. Due to their broader anti-inflammatory activity, they are often highly effective against seasonal allergy, but the significant side effects of cataract and increased intraocular pressure must be considered. The use of topical corticosteroids in ocular allergy should be brief and with the lowest concentration and dosing necessary to achieve control. When possible, milder topical steroids such as loteprednol should be favored over the more potent steroids such as prednisolone acetate. While nonsteroidal anti-inflammatory medications have been used in the management of allergic disease, we generally do not use these agents and prefer to use more targeted therapies.

In this case, the patient was treated with a combined mast cell stabilizer and antihistamine drop (olopatadine) which effectively controlled her symptoms. If the patient had more allergic rhinitis, then preference would have been given to an oral antihistamine (e.g., loratadine 5–10 mg/day). If the patient was experiencing an acute exacerbation, a short course of loteprednol 0.5% may also be considered at the same time, while the other agent(s) starts to work.

Case 2

A 13-year-old male presents with itching of both eyes for several weeks. He also reports light sensitivity with moderate eye pain in his left eye and states that he wakes up with his eyes "stuck together" due to mucus accumulation. He states that for approximately the last 4 years, he has had similar symptoms every year during spring. He is from West Africa and is currently visiting the United States. His family denies any other medical history.

What Is the Typical Clinical History of VKC? How Can the History Help to Differentiate Between VKC and Other Forms of Allergic Eye Disease, Specifically AKC?

VKC is a bilateral chronic allergic conjunctivitis characterized by itching, foreign body sensation, conjunctival injection and chemosis, photophobia, and filamentous "ropy" mucous discharge [4–6]. The presenting complaints are therefore very similar to AKC, with which it shares many common immunologic mechanisms, and are generally much more severe than seasonal or perennial allergic conjunctivitis.

The disease is termed "vernal" due to its usual presentation during the spring season; however the term is a bit misleading, as some patients with VKC present with year-round symptoms. VKC peaks in the first decade of life and is more commonly seen in boys than girls. It is also more common in hot, dry climates, such as

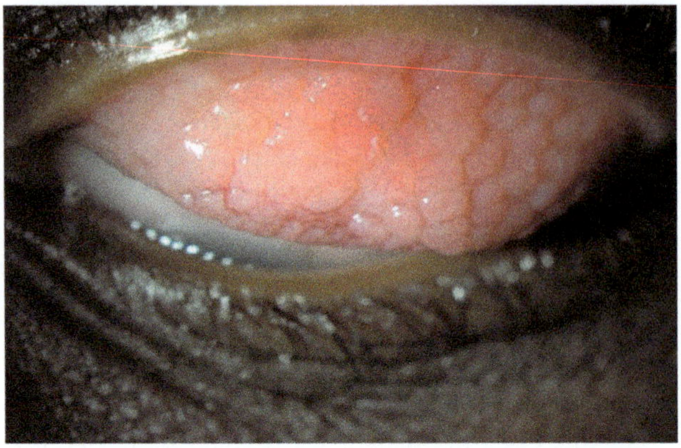

Fig. 7.1 Giant Papillae in a patient with VKC

in West Africa or the Middle East [5]. About half of VKC patients have a personal or family history of atopy. In milder cases, VKC is generally a self-limited condition, as it typically resolves by the late teens. However, in some patients, the disease may be more persistent. Importantly, even if the disease becomes quiescent, the long-term sequelae can be lifelong.

In contrast, AKC presents in an older patient population, peaking in the second to fifth decades of life [7]. It has less seasonal variation and geographic specificity than VKC. AKC is much more likely to have a chronic indolent course with greater potential for ocular surface and corneal scarring. AKC patients are more likely to have atopy and have dermatologic disease requiring chronic therapy.

Upon examination, the patient's visual acuity was 20/20 in the right eye and 20/50 in the left. Pupils were equal, round, and reactive. Intraocular pressure was 12 mmHg in both eyes. With lid eversion, giant cobblestone papillae were observed in both upper eyelids (Fig. 7.1).

What Are Common Examination Findings in VKC? What Are the Long-Term Sequelae of VKC?

AKC and VKC have similar clinical presentations, with conjunctival hyperemia, papillary reaction, corneal epitheliopathy, and ulceration as common features of each. A trademark feature of VKC is giant "cobblestone" papillae of the upper tarsus; these are less common in AKC. These giant papillae are greater than 1 mm in diameter. A thick ropy discharge frequently accumulates in the septa in between the giant papillae. Limbal papillae may also be seen and are typically large, gelatinous, and confluent. Frequently, either tarsal papillae or limbal papillae predominate, leading to two broad categories of VKC: palpebral vernal and limbal vernal. In the limbal papillae, Horner-Trantas dots may develop, another classic feature of VKC. These are collections of degenerated epithelial debris and eosinophils that form small white dots at the limbus [5, 6].

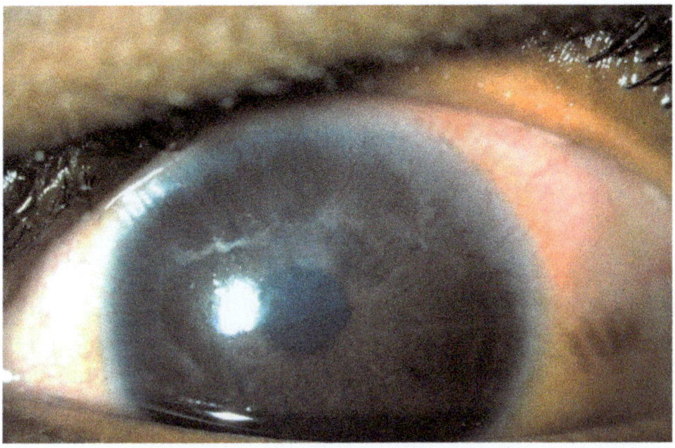

Fig. 7.2 Superior limbal stem cell deficiency in a patient with chronic VKC

Patients with VKC almost always have quiet, uninflamed eyelids and periorbital skin, in contrast to the nearly universal presence of periorbital atopic dermatitis seen in AKC patients. Subepithelial fibrosis of the palpebral conjunctiva and symblepharon formation are also much less common in VKC compared to AKC [8]. The mechanical rubbing of giant papillae against the cornea, along with release of inflammatory mediators, contributes to punctate epithelial erosions and sometimes macroerosions. Long-term sequelae of VKC can lead to corneal neovascularization and scarring. A pseudogerontoxon may be seen; this is a linear corneal scar, resembling a partial arcus senilis (gerontoxon). Chronic inflammation may result in severe stromal thinning and even corneal perforation. These findings are not common, and the long-term prognosis for mild VKC is generally good. However, 6% of patients will go on to develop visual impairment secondary to cataract, glaucoma, or corneal damage [4].

Slit-lamp exam revealed a white and quiet right eye and 1+ conjunctival injection in his left eye. His right cornea was clear. His left cornea showed a superior pannus and superficial neovascularization with diffuse, confluent punctate epithelial erosions (Fig. 7.2). The anterior chamber was deep and quiet in both eyes.

Based on the clinical history and presentation, the patient was diagnosed with VKC.

What Is the Pathophysiology of VKC? What Is Appropriate Medical Management for These Patients?

The pathogenesis of VKC is complex and not entirely understood; a thorough discussion of the immune mechanisms involved is beyond the scope of this chapter. In brief, as with allergic conjunctivitis, eosinophils and mast cells play an important role in VKC, and on cytopathologic examination these cells are seen in the conjunctiva of these patients. However, other inflammatory cells, such as lymphocytes, neutrophils, plasma cells, and macrophages, are clearly involved in VKC, as these are also found in large numbers in the conjunctiva [6]. In particular, T-helper lymphocyte cells (i.e., Th2 cells) are responsible for the production of specific interleukins, such as IL-4 and IL-5, which mediate several of the immune responses in VKC [6]. The production of interleukins and chemokines leads to recruitment of leukocytes, as well as increased production of IgE. Interleukins also promote the proliferation of fibroblasts.

Initial management for VKC is similar to that of other forms of allergic conjunctivitis and should include topical antihistamines and lubrication with artificial tears. Nonsteroidal anti-inflammatory drops may also provide some benefit in symptomatic relief. Mast cell stabilizers and preferably dual-acting agents can be useful for chronic maintenance.

Because of the numerous inflammatory mechanisms involved, these measures are usually inadequate. Topical steroids may be used for exacerbations in moderate to severe VKC and should be used judiciously with close monitoring for side effects. Topical cyclosporine eye drops are highly effective as an adjunctive therapy to decrease chronic inflammation. Cyclosporine has been shown to block T-lymphocyte proliferation, conjunctival fibroblast proliferation, and histamine release from mast cells. The commercially available concentration of 0.05% cyclosporine (Restasis, Allergan) can be used up to four times a day, though higher concentrations of 1–2% (compounded) may yield better results. Our standard treatment for these patients is to use topical cyclosporine and a dual-acting antihistamine on a long-term continuous basis. Topical steroids are used for exacerbations and at the lowest effective dose. Topical tacrolimus drops (if available) may be used as an alternative to cyclosporine and likely is more effective given that tacrolimus is 10–100 times more potent than cyclosporine.

Systemic treatment is rarely needed in VKC; however montelukast (Singulair, Merck) has been shown to be effective in reducing symptoms in VKC [9, 10]. Oral antihistamines may have minimal efficacy on VKC but may reduce systemic hyperreactivity. Systemic corticosteroids are rarely necessary but may need to be considered in vision-threatening cases. In cases where systemic steroids are needed, oral tacrolimus is a highly effective steroid-sparing agent which can be used for at least 6–12 months. Comanagement with a pediatric allergist or immunologist is highly recommended in such cases.

Case 3

A 12-year-old male is referred to you by a pediatric ophthalmologist for a chronic corneal ulcer. The child describes severe pain, tearing, and lid swelling of his left eye for approximately 1 month. The parents report that the child has had intermittent itching, tearing, and redness in both eyes for several years. He has been prescribed several different eye drops over the years, with varying

effectiveness. The referral note states that the child had a small corneal ulcer in the same eye approximately 2 years ago, which resolved with topical antibiotics and steroids.

Is There Any Further History You Would Like to Elicit from the child's family? What Is the Differential Diagnosis of a Chronic Corneal Ulcer in This Patient?

The initial evaluation of a corneal ulcer should differentiate between infectious and noninfectious etiologies. Chronic or recurrent corneal ulceration, along with long-standing symptoms of ocular surface irritation and redness, as in this child's case, points toward an inflammatory cause as the underlying pathology. The differential diagnosis for chronic or recurring corneal ulcer in the pediatric patient includes the following common conditions: atopic and vernal keratoconjunctivitis, staphylococcal blepharitis, ocular rosacea, and herpetic viral keratitis. Pertinent history may include prior episodes of red eye, a history of allergies and/or systemic atopic disease such as eczema and asthma, frequent chalazia or hordeola, history of eyelid blisters or cold sores that may suggest a herpetic etiology, and contact lens wear. It is also important to realize that chronic ocular surface inflammation predisposes the eye to microbial superinfection, and corneal cultures should be considered in all cases of chronic corneal ulceration.

His past medical history is significant only for asthma and allergies, including a severe peanut allergy. He takes oral montelukast and uses an albuterol inhaler as needed for his asthma. He is not currently on any topical medications.

Upon exam, his vision is 20/25 in both eyes. His external lid exam shows moderate swelling of his left upper lid with secondary ptosis (Fig. 7.3).

Upon lid eversion of his left upper lid revealed giant papillae (Fig. 7.4).

His corneal exam showed a 2.5 mm × 1 mm corneal "shield" ulcer with a plaque deposit; fluorescein staining revealed extensive filamentary and punctate keratopathy (Fig. 7.5a, b).

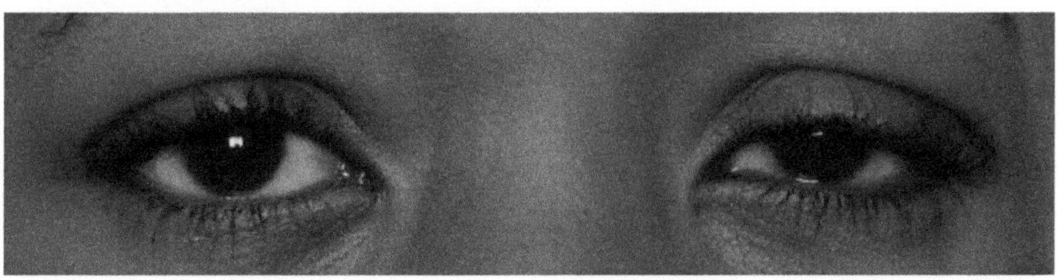

Fig. 7.3 Moderate swelling of the left upper lid with secondary ptosis in a patient with VKC

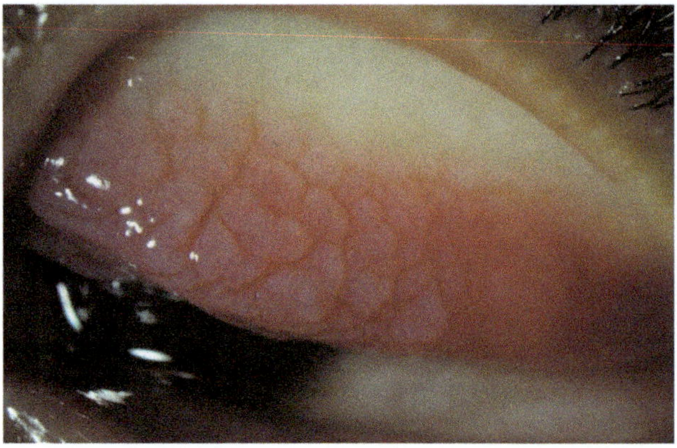

Fig. 7.4 Giant Papillae in a patient with VKC

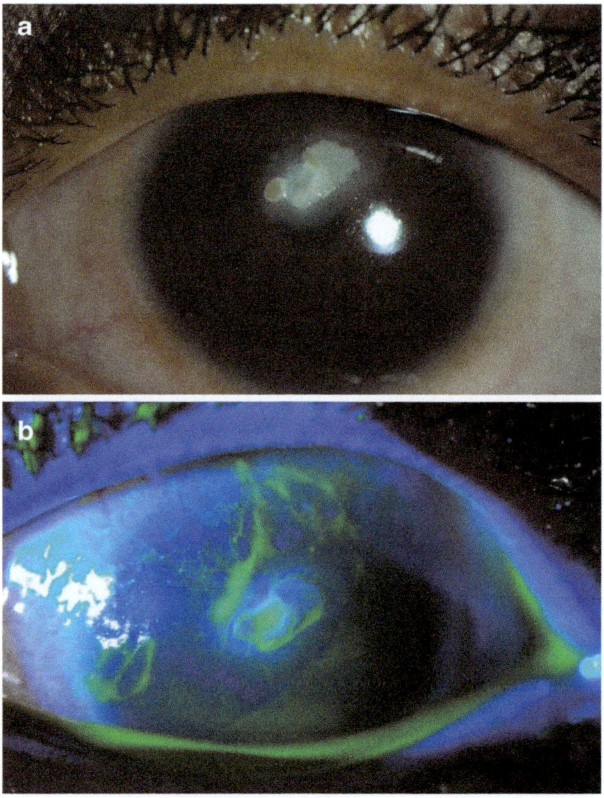

Fig. 7.5 Typical central shield ulcer with a plaque in a p atient with VKC (**a** and **b**)

What Is the Pathogenesis of a Shield Ulcer?

Shield ulcers of the cornea may develop secondarily from the mechanical injury from giant papillae, as well as chronic inflammation. Initially, a punctate epithelial keratitis develops which may lead to a frank erosion. Eventually a "vernal" plaque at the level of Bowman's membrane may deposit in these erosions, referred to as a shield ulcer due to its appearance. These are adherent mucus plaques consisting of degraded epithelial cells, eosinophils, and inflammatory cells. The incidence of shield ulcers in VKC has been reported from 3 to 11% [4, 6, 11]. They are typically localized to the superior half of the cornea, which underlies the tarsal papillae. The plaque impedes epithelial healing, and chronic shield ulcers may result in corneal scarring, neovascularization, and stromal thinning.

The patient was diagnosed with VKC and the edges of the shield ulcer were cultured. The patient was started on moxifloxacin four times a day in the left eye and olopatadine 0.1% in both eyes two times a day. The culture had no growth at follow-up. The patient was then started on loteprednol (Lotemax, Bausch & Lomb) four times a day in the left eye.

How Should Shield Ulcers Initially Be Managed?

Shield ulcers can often be difficult to treat and may follow a chronic or relapsing course. Topical steroids should be employed to reduce surface inflammation contributing to plaque deposition, and topical antibiotics should be administered for prophylaxis. After the eye drop regimen has been optimized, debridement of the shield ulcer manually or with the use of phototherapeutic keratectomy can be attempted to stimulate re-epithelization [12, 13]. If the epithelial defect persists, surface treatments such as a bandage contact lens and amniotic membrane transplant can be considered.

The shield ulcer and papillae remained unchanged on topical therapy at the patient's next follow-up 2 weeks later, though his symptoms of itching and pain were improved. Debridement of the plaque was performed with eventual recurrence of his shield ulcer on further follow-up.

What Are Some Other Treatment Options for Recalcitrant Shield Ulcers?

The size of the giant papillae has been directly correlated with the persistence or worsening of symptoms [4]. In retrospect, loteprednol was likely inadequate, and more potent steroids (e.g., prednisolone acetate 1% every 2 h) may have been more effective at reducing the inflammation for our patient. Alternatively, a supratarsal injection of steroids can be considered in cases of shield ulcer unresponsive to medical therapy, both to reduce the size of the giant papillae (thereby relieving the mechanical corneal irritation) and to decrease the number of inflammatory mediators on the ocular surface [14, 15]. Multiple injections may be needed. The patient should also be treated with topical cyclosporine on a long-term basis.

Case 4

A 27-year-old male presents with decreased vision in both eyes for 5 years. He also reports a chronically itchy rash around his eyes. His medical history is significant for eczema, asthma, and allergies since childhood.

His visual acuity at presentation was 20/200 and 20/40, respectively. The external lid exam revealed an excoriated, scaly periorbital dermatitis (Fig. 7.6). and inspissated meibomian glands with thickened lid margins. Upon lid eversion, diffuse micropapillae were noted on the upper and lower tarsus.

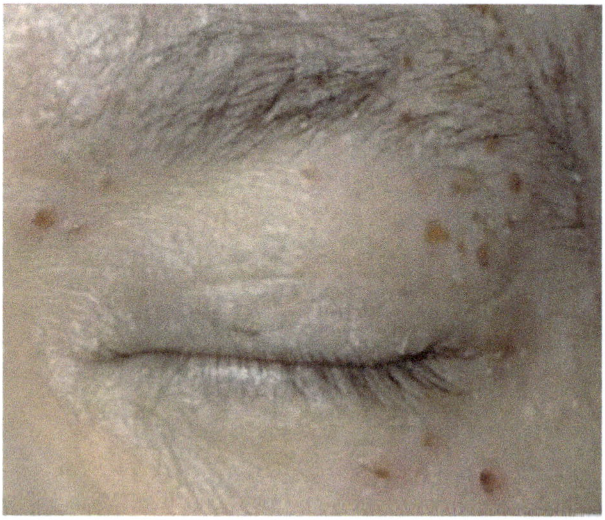

Fig. 7.6 Skin changes in a patient with AKC

What Is the Typical Clinical History of Patients with AKC? What Are Common Skin and Eyelid Findings in AKC?

Of the diseases in the allergic spectrum, AKC has the most severe, chronic course marked by significant ocular morbidity from corneal and conjunctival scarring. A thorough medical history should be obtained. Of AKC patients, 95% have concurrent eczematous dermatitis [8, 16, 17]. Other common associations include asthma and allergies, seen in up to 65–87% of patients [8, 16, 18]. AKC patients commonly present in the third to fifth decades [7]. Unlike VKC, AKC often persists, and patients may need lifelong treatment.

Clinically, AKC presents with chronic, erythematous itchy eyes with tearing [19, 20]. Pain is rarely reported; however the patient may have ocular irritation with photophobia. The external eyelid exam often reveals wrinkled, flaky, excoriated periorbital skin classic for eczematous dermatitis. Other signs include Dennie-Morgan folds, which are additional linear creases of the lower lids secondary to edema and eyelid thickening, and de Hertoghe sign, referring to the loss of hairs in the outer third of the brow [21]. Vertical corrugations near the medial canthus of the upper and lower lids may be seen. With progression of eczema, fissuring of the skin can be seen, and in long-standing AKC, ectropion, ptosis, lagophthalmos, and madarosis may result.

The patient's slit-lamp exam was significant for boggy chemotic conjunctiva and 1+ injection in both eyes. He had diffuse punctate epithelial erosions, central corneal steepening with apical scarring, and a positive Munson's sign in his right eye. The anterior chamber was deep and quiet in both eyes.

How Does AKC Affect the Conjunctiva and Cornea? What Are Other Ocular Associations Seen in AKC?

As in VKC, papillary hypertrophy is prominent, though the conjunctival papillae in AKC preferentially involve the lower tarsus and are smaller than those seen in VKC. The conjunctiva is inflamed and chemotic, though limbal papillae and Horner-Trantas dots are less common. Punctate epithelial erosions and corneal hypoesthesia in the setting of a poor ocular surface may lead to macroerosions. As in VKC, shield ulcers with plaque formation can develop.

Of all the allergic eye diseases, AKC is the most chronic and difficult to control, and patients often exhibit the usual complications of persistent ocular surface inflammation. Subepithelial fibrosis may occur with long-term disease, and end-stage cicatricial changes include symblepharon formation and fornix foreshortening [22]. Mechanical surface irritation and chronic inflammation can result in limbal stem cell deficiency. Late-stage corneal involvement including limbal stem cell deficiency, neovascularization, pseudopterygium, subepithelial haze, and stromal scarring and thinning can be seen in 60–70% of patients, leading to visual debilitation and even blindness [18, 22]. Approximately 30–50% of these patients require penetrating keratoplasty for visual rehabilitation or tectonic support [18].

Cataract develops early in these patients and usually presents as anterior subcapsular changes in a stellate or shield-like pattern. Posterior subcapsular cataracts can develop secondarily from chronic steroid use. HSV keratitis is more common in these patients due to underlying immune dysfunction and may manifest as a bilateral keratitis. There is a known association of AKC with keratoconus and pellucid marginal degeneration, which may be partly related to excessive eye rubbing [23, 24]. In this particular patient, the keratoconus was more advanced in his right eye which correlated with the side of his hand dominance [25]. There is also a higher observed rate of retinal detachment in AKC patients which may be due to vitreous degeneration from eye rubbing [26]. These patients also appear to be at higher risk for developing glaucoma which may be exacerbated by the chronic use of topical steroids.

The patient was prescribed topical tacrolimus ointment for the eyelid skin and olopatadine eye drops in both eyes twice daily. Lid hygiene and warm compresses were suggested, as well as frequent lubrication with artificial tears. The patient was also referred to an allergist.

What Is the Treatment Approach to AKC?

Treatment goals include controlling ocular inflammation and preventing visual debilitation while using the lowest dose and safest medications possible. A multidisciplinary team is needed including allergists and dermatologists. Improving atopic dermatitis lid disease can secondarily improve the ocular surface in AKC. Daily lid hygiene with warm compresses and lid scrubs should be initiated to control any meibomian gland dysfunction and staphylococcal colonization which can exacerbate surface inflammation. Periocular eczema can be controlled with topical emollients and, as needed, mild topical steroid ointments and emollients [27]. If steroid side effects are a concern, steroid-sparing ointments can be considered. Tacrolimus (Protopic, Astellas) is a calcineurin inhibitor that, like cyclosporine, leads to decreased T-cell production, inhibiting the release of interleukin-2. Compared to cyclosporine, tacrolimus is a more potent immunosuppressant and inhibitor of IgE-mediated enzyme release [21, 28]. Tacrolimus is available as a 0.03% and 0.1% topical ointment and has been shown to be effective in treating atopic lid disease as a steroid-sparing immunosuppressive. An ophthalmic preparation of tacrolimus is not available (except by compounding), but studies have reported symptomatic improvement with off-label ophthalmic use of the ointment in the conjunctival sac and topical use on the external lids with presumed ocular spillover [28, 29].

For conjunctival symptoms, we prefer to start with a combination of mast cell stabilizer and H1 receptor inhibitor (olopatadine, ketotifen, azelastine) to help reduce itch symptoms and overall decrease eye rubbing. As with VKC, cyclosporine may be effective in controlling T-cell-mediated inflammation. Cyclosporine 0.05% (Restasis, Allergan) has been studied in a small number of AKC patients in two randomized controlled trials; a 2004 study showed improvement of signs and symptoms of AKC [30], and a more recent study showed no statistical difference with placebo in steroid-dependent AKC [31]. Cyclosporine 0.05% (Restasis) or compounded 1–2% is recommended in all AKC patients. Clinical experience has shown topical T-cell inhibitors (cyclosporine or tacrolimus) to be extremely effective in all patients with chronic allergic eye disease and are recommended as a long-term treatment in every case. More severe AKC will require topical steroids such as prednisolone acetate 1% or difluprednate 0.05% with gradual tapering to more mild topical steroids (loteprednol or fluorometholone) as ocular inflammation is controlled. Prudent short-term use of steroids should be utilized to reduce long-term effects of cataract and glaucoma. It is well known that patients with AKC are at higher risk of developing herpetic keratitis, and AKC is a frequent cause of bilateral HSV keratitis. Thus, patients on chronic steroids are monitored for reactivation of HSV. Finally, in our experience, patients with AKC tend to be more sensitive to BAK; therefore, preservative-free or non-BAK preserved drops may be preferred whenever possible.

Systemic antihistamine may be used in addition to topical therapy and may provide additional anti-inflammatory effect. However, for severe refractory AKC, we prefer to use systemic immunosuppression with oral agents particularly cyclosporine or preferably tacrolimus. These agents have been found to be extremely effective and should be considered in all patients with ongoing inflammation and vision-threatening disease despite topical therapy [27, 32]. More recently, the use of anti-IgE (omalizumab) has been reported for the treatment of AKC, but experience is very limited [33].

At a follow-up visit 3 weeks later, the patient had mild improvement of his symptoms; however his clinical exam was unchanged. Cyclosporine 0.05% (Restasis, Allergan) four times a day in both eyes and tobramycin/dexamethasone ointment (TobraDex, Alcon) to the lid margin three times a day in both eyes were added to his regimen with the plan to transition to topical tacrolimus ointment (0.03%). An extensive discussion with the patient stressed the need for optimization of the ocular surface and his disease prior to keratoplasty for his keratoconus.

What Are Some Considerations When Planning Penetrating Keratoplasty in AKC Patients?

Penetrating keratoplasty in AKC patients is associated with higher rates of graft failure. The risk of graft rejection is relatively high, not only because of ocular surface inflammation and corneal neovascularization but also due to the underlying systemic immune dysregulation in atopic patients. Reports suggest that patients with higher serum IgE levels have increased risk of corneal graft rejection [25]. Penetrating keratoplasty in AKC may also stimulate further ocular surface inflammation, worsening the atopic disease. This is known as post-keratoplasty atopic keratitis [34]. A persistent epithelial defect is more likely to occur, due to limbal stem cell deficiency and irregular corneal epithelium.

It is important to optimize the ocular surface and minimize inflammation prior to keratoplasty. Ideally a keratoplasty should only be considered when the ocular surface inflammation is under control. If keratoplasty cannot be avoided in a patient with severely active AKC, then systemic immune suppression should be strongly considered, starting several weeks to months before surgery. The quality of the tear film should be optimized with appropriate agents recommended to treat blepharitis, meibomian gland dysfunction, and tear deficiency. Amniotic membrane transplantation can be considered at the time of keratoplasty to reduce the chances of persistent epithelial defect in patients. Additionally, atopies tend to be eye rubbers, and the importance of refraining from this after keratoplasty should be clearly conveyed to patients. Finally, limbal stem cell deficiency is a long-term complication of AKC (and VKC), and therefore management of LSCD (e.g., through limbal transplantation) may be indicated prior to keratoplasty (Fig. 7.7).

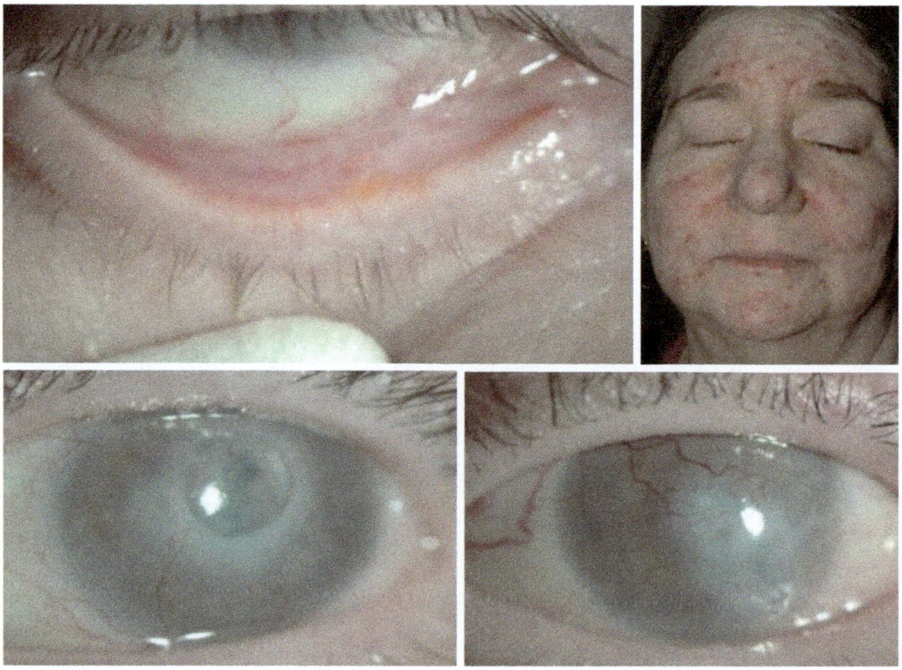

Fig. 7.7 Patient with chronic AKC leading to conjunctival scarring and bilateral limbal stem cell deficiency. Patient had a history of recurrent epithelial defects and corneal perforation requiring patch grafting. The patient later underwent limbal stem cell transplantation and penetrating keratoplasty

Summary

Allergic eye disease includes several conditions that vary in clinical presentation and severity. Common among all allergic eye diseases is a type I hypersensitivity reaction to antigens, mediated by IgE, which leads to mast cell degranulation and histamine release. In vernal and atopic keratoconjunctivitis, T-cell activation plays a prominent role. In all forms of ocular allergy, topical antihistamines/mast cell stabilizers are a mainstay of treatment, with topical steroids reserved for exacerbations. The topical T-cell inhibitors, cyclosporine and tacrolimus, are very effective and are recommended for all patients requiring long-term therapy. Chronic allergic eye disease can lead to conjunctival and corneal scarring, resulting in significant visual impairment. In addition to corneal complications such as shield ulcers, patients with long-standing disease often develop limbal stem cell deficiency and corneal scarring from chronic AKC suggesting that earlier intervention with T-cell inhibitors (cyclosporine or tacrolimus) topically and perhaps systemically (for the most severe cases) could have prevented these devastating long-term complications (Fig.7.7).

References

1. Tsubota K, Takamura E, Hasegawa T, Kobayashi T. Detection by brush cytology of mast cells and eosinophils in allergic and vernal conjunctivitis. Cornea. 1991;10(6):525–31.
2. Montan PG, van Hage-Hamsten M. Eosinophil cationic protein in tears in allergic conjunctivitis. Br J Ophthalmol. 1996;80(6):556–60.
3. Inada N, Shoji J, Kato H, Kiely S, Mulyanto SM. Clinical evaluation of total IgE in tears of patients with allergic conjunctivitis disease using a novel application of the immunochromatography method. Allergol Int. 2009;58(4):585–9. doi:10.2332/allergolint.09-OA-0101.
4. Bonini S, Bonini S, Lambiase A, et al. Vernal keratoconjunctivitis revisited: a case series of 195 patients with long-term follow up. Ophthalmology. 2000;107(6):1157–63. doi: S0161-6420(00)00092-0 [pii]
5. Pattnaik L, Acharya LA. comprehensive review on vernal keratoconjunctivitis with emphasis on proteomics. Life Sci. 2015;128:47–54. doi:10.1016/j.lfs.2015.01.040.
6. Bonini S, Lambiase A, Sgrulletta R, Bonini S. Allergic chronic inflammation of the ocular surface in vernal keratoconjunctivitis. Curr Opin Allergy Clin Immunol. 2003;3(5):381–7. doi:10.1097/01.all.0000092610.76804.8a.
7. Donshik PC. Allergic conjunctivitis. Int Ophthalmol Clin. 1988;28(4):294–302.
8. Tuft SJ, Kemeny DM, Dart JK, Buckley RJ. Clinical features of atopic keratoconjunctivitis. Ophthalmology. 1991;98(2):150–8.
9. Lambiase A, Bonini S, Rasi G, Coassin M, Bruscolini A, Bonini S. Montelukast, a leukotriene receptor antagonist, in vernal keratoconjunctivitis associated with asthma. Arch Ophthalmol. 2003;121(5):615–20. doi:10.1001/archopht.121.5.615.
10. Gane J, Buckley R. Leukotriene receptor antagonists in allergic eye disease: a systematic review and meta-analysis. J Allergy Clin Immunol Pract. 2013;1(1):65–74. doi:10.1016/j.jaip.2012.07.001.
11. Neumann E, Gutmann MJ, Blumenkrantz N, Michaelson IC. A review of four hundred cases of vernal conjunctivitis. Am J Ophthalmol. 1959;47(2):166–72.
12. Cameron JA. Shield ulcers and plaques of the cornea in vernal keratoconjunctivitis. Ophthalmology. 1995;102(6):985–93.

13. Cameron JA, Antonios SR, Badr IA. Excimer laser phototherapeutic keratectomy for shield ulcers and corneal plaques in vernal keratoconjunctivitis. J Refract Surg. 1995;11(1):31–5.
14. Holsclaw DS, Whitcher JP, Wong IG, Margolis TP. Supratarsal injection of corticosteroid in the treatment of refractory vernal keratoconjunctivitis. Am J Ophthalmol. 1996;121(3):243–9.
15. Saini JS, Gupta A, Pandey SK, Gupta V, Gupta P. Efficacy of supratarsal dexamethasone versus triamcinolone injection in recalcitrant vernal keratoconjunctivitis. Acta Ophthalmol Scand. 1999;77(5):515–8.
16. Bielory B, Bielory L. Atopic dermatitis and keratoconjunctivitis. Immunol Allergy Clin North Am. 2010;30(3):323–36. doi:10.1016/j.iac.2010.06.004.
17. Bremond-Gignac D, Nischal KK, Mortemousque B, Gajdosova E, Granet DB, Chiambaretta F. Atopic keratoconjunctivitis in children: clinical features and diagnosis. Ophthalmology. 2015;123(2):435–7. doi: S0161-6420(15)00703-4 [pii]
18. Power WJ, Tugal-Tutkun I, Foster CS. Long-term follow-up of patients with atopic keratoconjunctivitis. Ophthalmology. 1998;105(4):637–42. doi: S0161-6420(98)94017-9 [pii]
19. Hogan MJ. Atopic keratoconjunctivitis. Am J Ophthalmol. 1953;36(7 1):937–47.
20. Guglielmetti S, Dart JK, Calder V. Atopic keratoconjunctivitis and atopic dermatitis. Curr Opin Allergy Clin Immunol. 2010;10(5):478–85. doi:10.1097/ACI.0b013e32833e16e4.
21. Chen JJ, Applebaum DS, Sun GS, Pflugfelder SC. Atopic keratoconjunctivitis: a review. J Am Acad Dermatol. 2014;70(3):569–75. doi:10.1016/j.jaad.2013.10.036.
22. Foster CS, Calonge M. Atopic keratoconjunctivitis. Ophthalmology. 1990;97(8):992–1000.
23. Bawazeer AM, Hodge WG, Lorimer B. Atopy and keratoconus: a multivariate analysis. Br J Ophthalmol. 2000;84(8):834–6.
24. Rahi A, Davies P, Ruben M, Lobascher D, Menon J. Keratoconus and coexisting atopic disease. Br J Ophthalmol. 1977;61(12):761–4.
25. Harrison RJ, Klouda PT, Easty DL, Manku M, Charles J, Stewart CM. Association between keratoconus and atopy. Br J Ophthalmol. 1989;73(10):816–22.
26. Yoneda K, Okamoto H, Wada Y, et al. Atopic retinal detachment. Report of four cases and a review of the literature. Br J Dermatol. 1995;133(4):586–91.
27. Darsow U, Wollenberg A, Simon D, et al. ETFAD/EADV eczema task force 2009 position paper on diagnosis and treatment of atopic dermatitis. J Eur Acad Dermatol Venereol. 2010;24(3):317–28. doi:10.1111/j.1468-3083.2009.03415.x.
28. Attas-Fox L, Barkana Y, Iskhakov V, et al. Topical tacrolimus 0.03% ointment for intractable allergic conjunctivitis: an open-label pilot study. Curr Eye Res. 2008;33(7):545–9. doi:10.1080/02713680802149115.
29. Rikkers SM, Holland GN, Drayton GE, Michel FK, Torres MF, Takahashi S. Topical tacrolimus treatment of atopic eyelid disease. Am J Ophthalmol. 2003;135(3):297–302. doi: S0002939402019827 [pii]
30. Akpek EK, Dart JK, Watson S, et al. A randomized trial of topical cyclosporin 0.05% in topical steroid-resistant atopic keratoconjunctivitis. Ophthalmology. 2004;111(3):476–82. doi:10.1016/j.ophtha.2003.05.035.
31. Daniell M, Constantinou M, Vu HT, Taylor HR. Randomised controlled trial of topical ciclosporin A in steroid dependent allergic conjunctivitis. Br J Ophthalmol. 2006;90(4):461–4. doi: 90/4/461 [pii]
32. Friedlaender MH. Ocular allergy. Curr Opin Allergy Clin Immunol. 2011;11(5):477–82. doi:10.1097/ACI.0b013e32834a9652.
33. Taille C, Doan S, Neukirch C, Aubier M. Omalizumab for severe atopic keratoconjunctivitis. BMJ Case Rep. 2010;2010:pii: bcr0420102919. doi:10.1136/bcr.04.2010.2919.
34. Daniell MD, Dart JK, Lightman S. Use of cyclosporin in the treatment of steroid resistant post-keratoplasty atopic sclerokeratitis. Br J Ophthalmol. 2001;85(1):91–2.

Chapter 8
Neuropathic Corneal Pain

Sunali Goyal, Alessandro Abbouda, Nicholas Pondelis, and Pedram Hamrah

Case 1: Corneal Neuropathy and Light Sensitivity (Photoallodynia)

OG, a 53-year-old female, was referred to our center with a diagnosis of dry eye disease. Her past medical history included significant migraines and photophobia, which began about 6 years ago. The patient had a recent MRI that was normal. No physical reasons were found to explain her symptoms. Several systemic medications were prescribed to control the alleged depressive state. She was on duloxetine 30 mg twice daily, quetiapine fumarate 150 mg per day, tizanidine 2 mg every 6 hours, gabapentin 300 mg three times a day, dextroamphetamine saccharate 5 mg once a day, and a sumatriptan injection at the onset of each episode of migraine. The patient displayed hypothyroidism and was being treated with daily levothyroxine 25 mcg. Approximately 9 months ago, she was seen by her ophthalmologist, who did not note any clinical signs associated with her ocular symptoms of photophobia. Artificial tears were prescribed to give her some relief. For the next several months, her symptoms were refractory to artificial tears.

S. Goyal, MD
Department of Ophthalmology, University of Arkansas for Medical Sciences, Little Rock, AR, USA

A. Abbouda, MD • P. Hamrah, MD, FRCS (✉)
Cornea Service, New England Eye Center, Boston, MA, USA

Department of Ophthalmology, Center for Translational Ocular Immunology, Tufts Medical Center, Tufts University School of Medicine, Boston, MA 02111, USA
e-mail: PHamrah@tuftsmedicalcenter.org

N. Pondelis, BA
Department of Ophthalmology, Center for Translational Ocular Immunology, Tufts Medical Center, Tufts University School of Medicine, Boston, MA 02111, USA

A.R. Djalilian (ed.), *Ocular Surface Disease*,
https://doi.org/10.1007/978-3-319-15823-5_8

At her first visit to our center, the patient complained of severe photoallodynia (perception of pain on exposure to light). She wore sunglasses throughout the day. She was referred for a decrease in vision and a "strained" feeling in both eyes. Her corrected visual acuity was 20/30 in both eyes. Near corrected vision was J1+ in both eyes. Evaluation of the periocular skin showed no evidence of a rash or other lesions. There was no trichiasis, lagophthalmos, or significant lid laxity. The meibomian glands and the eyelid margin appeared normal. Her conjunctiva was normal. Slit-lamp examination revealed minimal superficial punctate keratopathy. Intraocular pressure and fundus examination were normal.

What Is Causing Her Pain? Given the Normal Eye Exam, Could the Patient Be Malingering?

Unfortunately, many of these patients are misdiagnosed as malingering. Neuropathic pain was recently redefined as "pain caused by a lesion or disease of the somatosensory system." [4]. Nociceptors are sensory receptors, which result in the perception of pain. Long-term deregulation in the peripheral nociceptive (pain) input can cause pain signal pathways to not function properly and this in turn leads to central pain pathways to become more autonomous. Nociceptors may respond to various environmental stimuli, which can be mechanical, thermal, or chemical in nature [5]. Some nociceptors are polymodal and can react to more than one of these modalities. Polymodal receptors are activated by near noxious or noxious mechanical, thermal, and to a large variety of endogenous chemical stimuli. Once activated, tissue injury and inflammation can cause these polymodal receptors to cause irregular firing at even lower thresholds. These receptors are connected centrally to higher-order pain pathways and sensitization to these results in allodynia (pain due to innocuous stimuli), hyperalgesia (enhanced pain perception), and spontaneous pain [6, 7]. Worthwhile to mention here is that there are two different types of nociceptor axons—myelinated Aδ fibers with an action potential travel rate of about 20 m/s and the more slowly conducting unmyelinated C fiber axons that have a speed of around 2 m/s [7]. As a result of the different fiber types, pain has an early phase facilitated by the fast-conducting Aδ fibers that can be extremely sharp and a later segment carried out by the polymodal C fibers that is more prolonged and somewhat dull in nature.

The cornea is the most densely innervated tissue in the body, which comes with a price of making it a powerful pain generator. Corneal nerves relay sensations of touch, chemical, pain, and temperature signals to the brain. They also induce reflex tear production, blinking, and release trophic factors, which help maintain the important structural and functional integrity of the ocular surface [8–11]. Due to this dense innervation, the non-keratinized epithelium of cornea has the ability to detect minute magnitude nociceptive insults of unparalleled sensitivity and generate defense reflexes, crucial for protection of the ocular surface. Over-sensitization of these receptors can cause neuropathic eye pain which can be perceived as itch, irritation, dryness, grittiness, burning, aching, and light sensitivity, which are integrated at higher brain centers and are patient specific [12, 13]. Hyperalgesia and allodynia draw a parallel in the cornea. Hyperalgesia can be perceived as hypersensitivity to moving air, minimal noxious stimuli, and to normal light (photoallodynia). Corneal allodynia can be manifested as burning sensation generated by normal non-noxious stimuli, such as wetting drops or even by patient's own tears.

How Do We Approach This Patient?

Any clinic visit should start with a detailed ocular exam including inspection of the lid anatomy, cornea and conjunctival surface, and a complete fundus exam. There are various direct and indirect methods to assess the function of corneal nerves. Indirect measures include slit-lamp examination with various vital dyes, such as fluorescein and lissamine green, and reveal the general health of the ocular surface. Direct measures use various esthesiometers, such as the Cochet-Bonnet contact esthesiometer, which can detect mechanical nociceptor responses, thereby quantifying Aδ fibers function. The non-contact Belmonte esthesiometer is capable of detecting polymodal functionality of both Aδ and C fibers and may be more informative, albeit not commonly available [14].

What Is the Difference Between Peripheral vs. Central Neuropathic Pain? What Is the Proparacaine (Anesthetic) Challenge Test?

It is important to ascertain whether the pain perception thought to be originating from the ocular surface has its inception in the cornea (peripheral) or is it more located centrally and only perceived as coming from the ocular surface. This is important as it can aid in proper management. Some basic tests may aid in distinguishing between peripheral and central pain, although many patients may suffer from a combination of both. The proparacaine challenge with instillation of a drop topical anesthesia of 0.5% proparacaine hydrochloride (Alcaine, Alcon) on the ocular surface will attenuate peripheral but not central pain. Measures, such as the use of soft contact lenses and moisture goggles, may also help to neutralize the evaporative component of the tears and will decrease peripheral but not central pain. Patients with no relief from any of the above measures likely suffer, at least in part, from central neuropathic pain. Likewise those who have some relief with the proparacaine challenge likely suffer from combined peripheral and central neuropathic pain.

What Can Aid in Definitive Diagnosis?

In vivo confocal microscopy (IVCM) has proven to be an extremely useful tool in the modern cornea practice. IVCM is a noninvasive procedure that allows the study of corneal cells, nerves, and the immune cells and their various interactions in ocular and systemic diseases [15–17]. IVCM has been utilized to study nerve changes in various conditions including normal eyes, keratoconus, dry eye disease [18], contact lens wear, neurotrophic keratopathy [19], infectious keratitis [20], and post-refractive surgery, among others [15–17, 21]. Moreover, IVCM has enabled us to study the regenerative changes of the corneal nerves and correlation with corneal sensation [8, 17, 22]. Studies in different corneal pathologies have shown varying degrees of reduced nerve fiber density, increased subbasal nerve tortuosity, increase in nerve fiber beading, branching, reflectivity, neuromas, and nerve sprouting [23–25]. A baseline IVCM in patients with neuropathic pain can help assess and confirm nerve abnormalities like microneuromas (highly specific), increased nerve tortuosity, increased beading, decreased density of nerve fibers, and variable increase in dendritic cells, which can be subsequently followed by posttreatment IVCM to monitor for changes and reversal of baseline findings [3].

IVCM examination was performed on this patient. The test revealed severe nerve tortuosity, beading, and large microneuromas (Fig. 8.1a). These findings led to a diagnosis of corneal neuropathy. No relief was obtained with the instillation of proparacaine drops, so a strong component of central pain was considered.

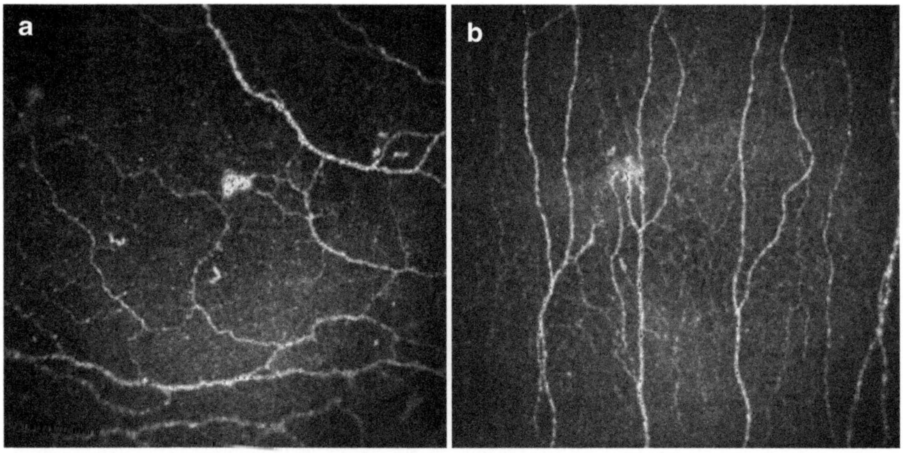

Fig. 8.1 IVCM examination of a patient with corneal neuropathy and light sensitivity. At the beginning of the follow-up, IVCM showed an abnormal subbasal nerve plexus with a large neuroma, nerve tortuosity, and bleeding. Some dendritic cells are visible (**a**). At 9 months, IVCM showed an increase in the nerve density and persistence of bleeding and neuroma (**b**)

Nortriptyline 10 mg once a day at night was prescribed with a gradual increase to 50 mg, along with eight drops of autologous serum tears 20% a day, and loteprednol etabonate 0.5% drops four times a day for a week tapering to a drop each week. In addition, twice-a-week acupuncture and an increase in cardiovascular exercise were suggested to the patient. IVCM at 9 months showed a reduction of number of neuromas compared to the first visit, as well as an increase in nerve density (Fig. 8.1b). Serum tears were maintained whereas nortriptyline was stopped according to the improvement of patient's symptoms.

Case 2: Corneal Neuropathy After LASIK Surgery (Post-LASIK Neuralgia)

TB, a 35-year-old healthy male, was referred to our center for ocular pain and dry eye symptoms in both eyes. He had no past significant medical history. The ocular history was significant for LASIK surgery in both eyes performed 10 years ago. Two years post-LASIK, he started noticing ocular pain. He had been to several different ophthalmologists. A diagnosis of dry eye disease was made, and he was given artificial tears and steroid eye drops, both of which provided no relief. A different ophthalmologist diagnosed scleritis. He took prednisone 60 mg per day for 1 week, which reduced the pain. He then switched to naprosyn 250 mg twice daily, and the pain returned. An MRI of the brain and orbits was performed which was normal.

At the first visit to our clinic, the patient complained of an increase in pain duration and intensity over the past few months. He was on prednisolone acetate drops, vitamin C tablets, Omega-3, B complex vitamins, and calcium. His visual acuity was 20/20 in the both eyes. Slit-lamp examination revealed mild blepharitis, normal LASIK flaps, and no corneal staining. The rest of the ocular exam was also normal.

Which Patients Are Susceptible to Corneal Pain?

Various inflammatory diseases, neurological diseases, or surgical interventions can be the underlying cause of corneal neuropathic pain (Table 8.1). Some of them include refractive surgery [26], dry eye disease [27, 28], Sjögren's syndrome [29, 30], neuralgia associated with herpes virus [31], benzalkonium chloride (BAK) preserved eye drops, accutane, chemotherapy, and radiotherapy to mention a few [3]. In addition to refractive surgery, particularly LASIK, we have also observed cataract surgery—clear cornea incision—to also trigger neuropathic corneal pain.

Table 8.1 Causes of corneal neuropathic pain

1.	Dry eye disease
2.	Infectious keratitis
3.	Herpetic keratitis
4.	Recurrent erosions
5.	Postsurgical (cataracts, refractive surgery, corneal transplantation)
6.	Chemical burns
7.	Toxic keratopathy
8.	Radiation keratopathy
9.	Miscellaneous: ocular surface neoplasia, trauma, post-blepharoplasty, iatrogenic trigeminal neuralgia, chronic corneal pain with blepharospasm, fibromyalgia, small fiber neuropathy

What Is the Social Impact of Corneal Pain?

Corneal nerve damage may be associated with symptoms of pain, light sensitivity, irritation, and sometimes a vague sensation of pressure. As a physician, one must understand that pain does not affect the patient alone, but it affects the entire social structure of the patient. Eye pain decreases work performance and can have huge impact on aspects of physical, social, and psychological functioning [32, 33]. Crucial daily activities like reading, driving, and computer work are affected giving a sense of handicap [33]. Severe cases with photoallodynia may require dark glasses indoors affecting social quality of life. Many patients are unable to work and go on disability. Unfortunately, we have witnessed many patients with severe form of pain where anxiety and depression have forced them to contemplate and even seek ending their own life.

What Should We Do Next for This Patient?

As outlined earlier, after a complete ocular exam, IVCM should be done. In this patient, IVCM examination revealed an increase in the presence of dendritic cells, neuromas, and nerve tortuosity, while also revealing a reduction in nerve density (Fig. 8.2a). A diagnosis of corneal neuropathy was made. The pain was significantly reduced with proparacaine drops, confirming the theory of peripheral corneal neuropathy following LASIK surgery.

The patient was prescribed autologous serum tears (20%) eight times a day and loteprednol etabonate 0.5% drops four times a day for a week, tapering to a drop each week. After 6 months, the patient reported significant resolution of his symptoms and occasional flare-ups. Ocular examination was normal, and IVCM revealed no neuromas but persistent inflammation with a maintained reduction of nerve density (Fig. 8.2b). The previous treatment was maintained.

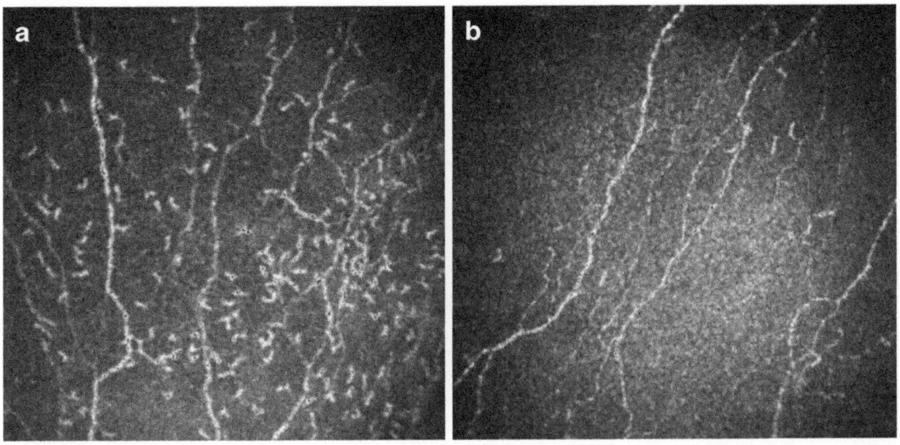

Fig. 8.2 IVCM examination of a patient with corneal neuropathy and inflammation. At the beginning of the follow-up, IVCM showed a marked increase in dendritic cell density and a significant reduction in the nerve density (**a**). At 6 months, IVCM revealed a substantial decrease in dendritic cells and a moderate increase in the nerve density (**b**)

Case 3: Ocular Pain and Centralized Pain

A 70-year-old female was referred to our center with a diagnosis of filamentary keratitis and photophobia. She was followed for 2 years elsewhere with partial response to removal of filaments with forceps and the use of bandage contact lenses. She had received punctal plugs and topical steroids with limited improvement.

At her first examination, she was taking cyclosporine 0.05% drops four times daily and non-preserved artificial tears on a very regular basis (more in her left eye than right eye). She was complaining of photophobia and ocular pain. The pain interfered with driving, watching TV, and sleeping. Her initial visual acuity was 20/40 in the right eye and 20/20 in the left eye. She had a tender posterior lid margin and telangiectasia, with trace fine vessel injection on her conjunctiva. She had mild blepharitis, with partial occlusion of meibomian gland ducts. The central cornea showed punctate epithelial keratitis and few central debris filaments. Tear breakup time was abnormally rapid, and tear meniscus was reduced. She was pseudophakic in both eyes with no signs of intraocular inflammation. Fundus examination was normal.

IVCM showed neuromas in both eyes, high corneal nerve tortuosity, and a reduction of corneal nerve density (Fig. 8.3a). Proparacaine drops did not provide relief from pain. A diagnosis of corneal neuropathy associated with central pain was made.

The patient was started on autologous serum tears 20% eight drops a day, loteprednol etabonate 0.5% drops four drops a day for a week, tapering to a drop each week, and carbamazepine 400 mg orally twice daily. After 6 months

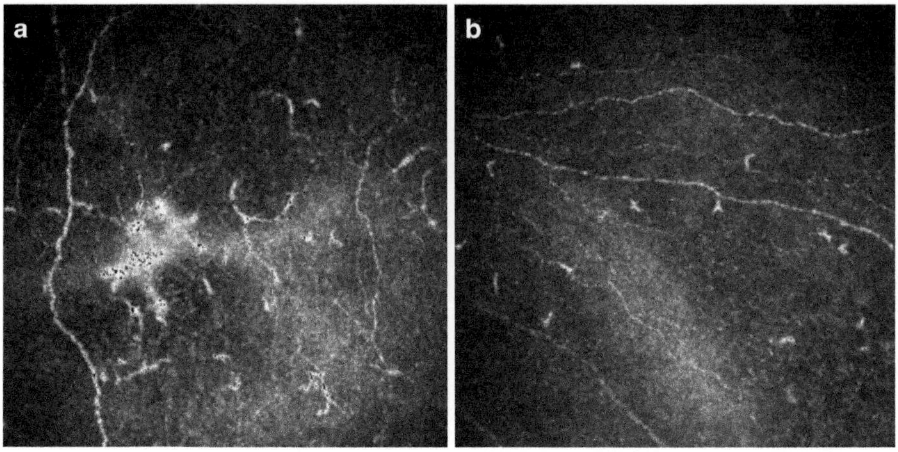

Fig. 8.3 IVCM examination of a patient with ocular pain after LASIK surgery performed 10 years ago. IVCM examination at the beginning of the follow-up showed a large neuroma, dendritic cells with long dendrites, and a reduction in the nerve density (**a**). After 6 months, IVCM displayed reduced dendritic cells in number and size. Nerve density was still low (**b**)

of the treatment, the patient reported a substantial improvement of his symptoms, with only occasional discomfort. His visual acuity was stable. Slit-lamp examination was normal. IVCM at 6 months showed a reduction of dendritic cells compared to the first visit, as well as an increase in nerve density (Fig. 8.3b). Serum tears were maintained. An additional month of loteprednol etabonate 0.5 % drops was suggested, followed by one drop twice a week for 4 weeks.

Case 4: Corneal Neuropathy and Inflammation

RO, a 21-year-old male, was referred to our center with a diagnosis of systemic neuralgia, progressive ocular pain, and photophobia. He was undergoing treatment with high-dose duloxetine, 120 mg per day, but noticed worsening photophobia. The patient decided to reduce the treatment without any improvement in his ocular symptoms. He was not able to wear contact lenses but wore special sunglasses constantly. The patient denied having any other significant disease. His medical family history was negative for significant disease.

His corrected visual acuity was 20/25 in both eyes. Eyelid and slit-lamp examination, intraocular pressure, and fundus examination were all normal. The Schirmer's test was normal (>10 mm in both eyes), and tear breakup time was >7 s. After the instillation of proparacaine drops, the patient reported an important reduction of the symptoms. The central component of the pain was minimal. IVCM revealed a significant increase of dendritic cells in the subbasal layer, associated with a clinically important reduction of the nerve density in both eyes (Fig. 8.4a).

Nortriptyline was prescribed (10 mg once a day at night) associated with autologous serum tears 20 % eight drops a day, and fluorometholone 0.1 % one

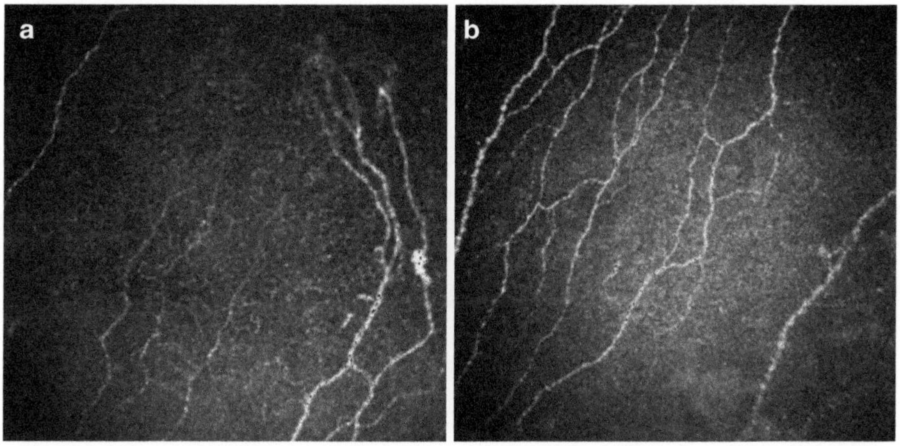

Fig. 8.4 IVCM examination of a patient with ocular pain with a central component. At the first visit, IVCM showed reduced nerve density and neuromas. After 6 months, a substantial improvement was observed with significant increase in nerve regeneration

drop a day for 4 weeks, and cyclosporine 0.05% drops. Doxycycline 100 mg two times per day was prescribed to improve meibomian gland disease. After 6 months, the patient reported an improvement of her symptoms. Her visual acuity was 20/20 in both eyes. Slit-lamp examination showed superficial punctate epitheliopathy. IVCM showed severe focal areas of inflammation but a reduction of neuromas with significant increase in nerve regeneration (Fig. 8.4b). The patient was instructed to follow the same treatment and to consider acupuncture two times per week. An increase in cardiovascular exercise was also suggested to the patient.

Summary of the Management of Neuropathic Corneal Pain

Nerve injury results in the release of inflammatory cytokines from both the injured and healthy nerves [16, 29]. We always begin treatment with palliative care regardless of the underlying pathology of dry eyes or neuralgia. Lubricating the surface with modest frequency of non-preserved artificial tears or emulsion-based tears is our initial step. We have seen that adding punctal plugs to maintain a more generous tear lake benefits patients. The authors discourage placing punctal plugs in eyes with active allergies and inflammation, as this may increase the contact time of the allergens on the surface. Treating any concomitant posterior blepharitis and meibomian gland dysfunction with hot compresses and lid massage or medical therapy is always beneficial. For MGD cases refractory to medical management, procedures such as intraductal meibomian gland probing, thermal pulsation devices (Lipiflow), and intense pulse-lighted therapy may aid in the treatment of meibomian gland dysfunction and subsequent increase of TBUT [34].

Anti-inflammatory Agents

In our experience, patients with corneal neuropathic pain typically require chronic use of anti-inflammatory agents (Table 8.2) to prevent recurrent episodes. Steroids are the main stay of treatment, especially for initial rapid relief. The authors prefer loteprednol 0.5% at an initial qid dose with biweekly taper to once or twice a week over a 6–8 week period. For severe refractory cases, we might add Anakinra (Kineret) human IL-1 receptor antagonist 2.5% at TID dosing for 3–6 months or Tacrolimus (calcineurin inhibitor) 0.03% at bid dosing for 3–6 months as they tend to be efficacious in reducing

Table 8.2 Evidence-based treatment of neuropathic corneal pain

A. Treatment of ocular surface disease 1. Increase tear production – Use PFATs 2. Increase tear retention – Punctal plugs, contact lenses, and moisture goggles 3. Treatment of lids and ocular surface disease – Treat blepharitis with lid hygiene and warm compresses – Refractory cases: meibomian gland probing, Lipiflow, intense pulse-lighted therapy 4. Managing comorbid conditions – Treat allergies, conjunctival chalasis, lagophthalmos, and nocturnal exposure
B. Anti-inflammatory agents 1. Topical corticosteroids 2. Azithromycin ointment and oral doxycycline 3. Cyclosporine 4. Tacrolimus 5. Anakinra
C. Regenerative therapy 1. Autologous serum eye drops (20–100%) 2. Nerve growth factor 3. Platelet rich plasma 4. Umbilical cord serum eye drops
D. Protect ocular surface when required 1. Bandage contact lenses 2. Scleral contact lenses 3. Special scleral lenses like PROSE
E. Systemic pharmacotherapy for pain 1. TCAs like nortriptyline and amitriptyline 2. GABAergic drugs (gabapentin, pregabalin) 3. SNRI like duloxetine and venlafaxine 4. Opioids like oxycodone, methadone, morphine, and levorphanol
F. Complementary and alternative measures 1. Acupuncture 2. Transcranial magnetic stimulation 3. Scrambler therapy 4. Cardio exercise 5. Omega-3-rich diet

PFAT's preservative free artificial tears, *PROSE* Prosthetic Replacement of the Ocular Surface Ecosystem; *TCAs* tricyclic anti-depressants, *SNRI* serotonin- norepinephrine reuptake inhibitors corneal surface inflammation and epitheliopathy [35, 36]. In addition, topical azithromycin 1% application at bedtime is a very effective and well-tolerated therapy of lid margin disease and meibomian gland dysfunction [37, 38]. It is both an anti-inflammatory, inhibiting pro-inflammatory cytokines, and an effective antibacterial agent. Likewise, oral doxycycline is an antimicrobial that also inhibits matrix metalloproteinases that degrade connective tissue [39]. We use oral doxycycline at a dose of 100 mg once or twice a day for 2–3 months followed by daily dosing for another 3 months.

Neuro-regenerative Therapy

Autologous serum tears (ASTs) are the mainstay of therapy for these patients. They contain a variety of pro-epithelial and pro-neural factors like epidermal growth factor (EGF), NGF, insulin-like growth factor (IGF-1), etc. [3, 40]. Concentrations from 20 to 100% have been shown to encourage epithelial healing, increase nerve density, and decrease nerve tortuosity [3]. IVCM has demonstrated significantly improved nerve parameters including total length, number, reflectivity, and also reduction of beading and neuromas in patients treated with ASTs [3]. Recent studies with the help of IVCM have shown a substantial correlation between the increase in dendritic cell numbers and decreased subbasal corneal nerves signifying a possible interaction between the immune and nervous system in the cornea [16]. In our experience, the combination of steroids with ASTs is extremely synergistic as steroids decrease the initial inflammation on the ocular surface, providing an environment conducive to neuronal regeneration with the help of ASTs.

Protective Contact Lenses

In patients with strong peripheral pain component (as revealed by the proparacaine challenge test), shielding the sensitized corneal receptors from the triggering environmental stimulus by using protective bandage lenses may be advantageous. The most effective lens in maintaining the pre-corneal nociceptive barrier is the liquid corneal bandage created by the fluid-filled scleral lenses like PROSE (prosthetic replacement of the ocular surface ecosystem, Boston Foundation for Sight) [41, 42]. It is felt that treating corneal epitheliopathy early in the disease process may help to reverse chronic pain. However, once established, the corneal bandage by itself is usually not adequate.

More recently, we have begun to use a self-retaining amniotic membrane device (Prokera, Bio-Tissue) for acute management of patients with corneal neuropathic pain. It is mainly used as a short-term strategy to give some relief to the patient, while the other long-term treatments begin to work. We typically use the device in one eye at a time and use the specific device that has a hole in the center—which allows the patient to see.

Systemic Pharmacotherapy for Pain

Data on the use of systemic pharmacotherapy for corneal neuropathic pain is scarce. The authors have borrowed this from pain literature elsewhere in the body and have had rewarding results with these patients. Various options are available that include anticonvulsants (e.g., carbamazepine), tricyclic antidepressants (e.g. Nortriptyline), serotonin uptake inhibitors, opioids, etc. Gamma aminobutyric acid (GABA) is the key inhibitory neurotransmitter of the central nervous system [43]. Drugs like gabapentin (Neurontin) and pregabalin (Lyrica) that were first developed and used as anticonvulsants are now endorsed as first-line agents for the treatment of neuropathic pain arising from diabetic neuropathy, post-herpetic neuralgia, and central neuropathic pain [44]. These drugs bind to the α-2-delta subunit of voltage-dependent calcium channels, causing decrease in the inflow of calcium into the neurons thus stabilizing them throughout the central nervous system [45]. We initiate gabapentin on day 1 as a single 600 mg dose, on day 2 as 1200 mg/day, and on day 3 as 1800 mg/day. Patients are instructed to subsequently titrate the dose up as needed for pain relief to a maximum dose of 3600 mg/day (900 mg four times a day). We warn the patients of the most common dose-limiting side effects which can include sedation, somnolence, and dizziness which can often be judicially dealt by a slow titration of the dose.

Tricyclic antidepressants (TCAs) exert effect by inhibiting presynaptic reuptake of serotonin and norepinephrine and by blocking cholinergic, adrenergic, histaminergic, and sodium channels. Drugs like amitriptyline, nortriptyline, desipramine, and imipramine are classified as TCAs. We initiate therapy with nortriptyline at a dose of 10–25 mg nightly. Depending on the response and tolerance, this can be titrated by 10–25 mg every 3–7 days up to a maximum of 150 mg nightly. Anticholinergic side effects like dry mouth and eyes, excess sedation, urinary retention, constipation, orthostatic hypotension, and blurry vision need to be discussed upfront. Serotonin-norepinephrine inhibitors like duloxetine (Cymbalta) and venlafaxine (Effexor) have also been studied for the treatment of neuropathic pain [44, 46]. While we recommend that one agent at a time be tried in patient with corneal neuropathic pain, combination therapy is often required in refractory cases.

Carbamazepine, an antiepileptic drug typically used for trigeminal neuralgia, may be tried in some of these patients. The usual effective dose for corneal neuralgia ranges from 800 to 1600 mg divided in two to four doses per day. Once response has been achieved, it can be tapered to a minimal effective dose. Opioids, such as tramadol, bind to the μ-opioid receptor and inhibit the reuptake of serotonin and norepinephrine. They can be tried in moderate to severe acute neuropathic pain when immediate and short-term relief of pain is desired [44, 46]. Side effects such as nausea, vomiting, constipation, sedation, and dependence limit their use to second-line medications, when the first-line medications fail to achieve a satisfactory response. In crunch situations, mexiletine can serve as an alternative second line therapy [47]. Mexiletine (225–675 mg/day) is an orally active local anesthetic agent, which is structurally related to lidocaine and has been used to alleviate neuropathic pain of various origins [47]. Side effects like nausea, sleep disturbance, headache, shakiness, dizziness, and tiredness may however limit its prolonged use.

Complementary and Alternative Medical Approaches

Despite the use of all the above measures in various combinations, adequate pain relief may not be achieved. The authors have found that use of adjunctive therapies, such as acupuncture [48] and vigorous exercise, may provide temporary relief and/or decrease the need for pharmacotherapy in many patients. Many of our patients report getting the extra relief ranging between a few hours to a few days that was not achieved by the above algorithm. We now have started referring refractory patients for a trial of Transcranial Magnetic Stimulation (TMS) or Scrambler therapy. TMS is a noninvasive method to cause depolarization or hyperpolarization in the neurons of the brain. High-frequency repetitive TMS (rTMS) of those brain regions which parallel the body parts in pain may be effective in controlling refractory cases [49]. Another useful therapy used to control chronic neuropathic pain is Scrambler therapy. The Scrambler therapy works on the principle of interfering with pain signal transmission, by mixing a non-pain information with the pain signal into the nerve fibers and thus confusing the nervous system ability to sense pain [50]. Another intervention, neuromodulation, involves stimulation or administration of medications directly to the body's nervous system for therapeutic purposes. It involves implantable as well as non-implantable devices that deliver electrical, chemical, or other agents to reversibly modify brain and nerve cell activity. Neuromodulation therapies allow focused delivery of modifying agents—e.g., electrical, optical, or chemical signals—to targeted areas of the nervous system in order to improve neural function [51].

Evidence suggests that cardio exercise may alter the perception of pain experience centrally. We recommend that our patients be involved in some kind of cardio exercise for about 30–45 min at least 3–5 times a week. Nutritional intervention strategies like increasing the ratio of omega-3 to omega-6 fatty acids can be exploited to decrease inflammation and pain in the body [52]. Foods like flaxseed oil, fish oil, walnuts, and soybeans are rich in omega-3 fatty acids. We recommend that our patients be on 1000 mg bid to tid daily dosing of either fish oil or flaxseed oil. Presence of allergies and conditions like conjunctival chalasis, lagophthalmos, and nocturnal exposure should be carefully assessed and addressed appropriately medically or surgically when needed. Interestingly, gluten sensitivity may be etiologically linked to a substantial number of idiopathic axonal neuropathies [53]. Gluten seems to cause and support neuronal inflammation, and in our experience, change to gluten-free diet has resulted in variable decrease in neuropathic corneal pain. We recommend our patients to be tested for gluten sensitivity and, if tested positive, abstain from gluten products.

References

1. Belmonte C. Eye dryness sensations after refractive surgery: impaired tear secretion or "phantom" cornea? J Refract Surg. 2007;23(6):598–602.
2. Rosenthal P, Borsook D. The corneal pain system. Part I: the missing piece of the dry eye puzzle. Ocul Surf. 2012;10(1):2–14.
3. Aggarwal S, Kheirkhah A, Cavalcanti BM, et al. Autologous serum tears for treatment of photoallodynia in patients with corneal neuropathy: efficacy and evaluation with in vivo confocal microscopy. Ocul Surf. 2015;13(3):520–62. pii: S1542-0124(15)00009-9
4. Jensen TS, Baron R, Haanpää M, et al. A new definition of neuropathic pain. Pain. 2011;152(10):2204–5.
5. Lee Y, Lee CH, Oh U. Painful channels in sensory neurons. Mol Cells. 2005;20(3):315–24.
6. Brooks J, Tracey I. From nociception to pain perception: imaging the spinal and supraspinal pathways. J Anat. 2005;207(1):19–33.
7. Reichling DB, Levine JD. Critical role of nociceptor plasticity in chronic pain. Trends Neurosci. 2009;32(12):611–8.
8. Beuerman RW, Schimmelpfennig B. Sensory denervation of the rabbit cornea affects epithelial properties. Exp Neurol. 1980;69(1):196–201.
9. Toivanen M, Tervo T, Partanen M, et al. Histochemical demonstration of adrenergic nerves in the stroma of human cornea. Invest Ophthalmol Vis Sci. 1987;28(2):398–400.
10. Nishida T. Neurotrophic mediators and corneal wound healing. Ocul Surf. 2005;3(4):194–202.
11. Müller LJ, Marfurt CF, Kruse F, Tervo TM. Corneal nerves: structure, contents and function. Exp Eye Res. 2003;76(5):521–42.
12. Feng Y, Simpson TL. Nociceptive sensation and sensitivity evoked from human cornea and conjunctiva stimulated by CO_2. Invest Ophthalmol Vis Sci. 2003;44(2):529–32.
13. Feng Y, Simpson TL. Characteristics of human corneal psychophysical channels. Invest Ophthalmol Vis Sci. 2004;45(9):3005–10.
14. Murphy PJ, Patel S, Kong N, et al. Noninvasive assessment of corneal sensitivity in young and elderly diabetic and nondiabetic subjects. Invest Ophthalmol Vis Sci. 2004;45(6):1737–42.
15. Cruzat A, Pavan-Langston D, Hamrah P. In vivo confocal microscopy of corneal nerves: analysis and clinical correlation. Semin Ophthalmol. 2010;25(5-6):171–7.
16. Cruzat A, Witkin D, Baniasadi N, et al. Inflammation and the nervous system: the connection in the cornea in patients with infectious keratitis. Invest Ophthalmol Vis Sci. 2011;52(8):5136–43.
17. Mantopoulos D, Cruzat A, Hamrah P. In vivo imaging of corneal inflammation: new tools for clinical practice and research. Semin Ophthalmol. 2010;25(5-6):178–85.
18. Alhatem A, Cavalcanti B, Hamrah P. In vivo confocal microscopy in dry eye disease and related conditions. Semin Ophthalmol. 2012;27(5-6):138–48.
19. Hamrah P, Cruzat A, Dastjerdi MH, et al. Unilateral herpes zoster ophthalmicus results in bilateral corneal nerve alteration: an in vivo confocal microscopy study. Ophthalmology. 2013;120(1):40–7.
20. Hamrah P, Cruzat A, Dastjerdi MH, et al. Corneal sensation and subbasal nerve alterations in patients with herpes simplex keratitis: an in vivo confocal microscopy study. Ophthalmology. 2010;117(10):1930–6.
21. Hamrah P, Sahin A, Dastjerdi MH, et al. Cellular changes of the corneal epithelium and stroma in herpes simplex keratitis: an in vivo confocal microscopy study. Ophthalmology. 2012;119(9):1791–7.
22. Patel DV, McGhee CN. In vivo confocal microscopy of human corneal nerves in health, in ocular and systemic disease, and following corneal surgery: a review. Br J Ophthalmol. 2009;93(7):853–60.
23. Tervo TM, Moilanen JA, Rosenberg ME, et al. In vivo confocal microscopy for studying corneal diseases and conditions associated with corneal nerve damage. Adv Exp Med Biol. 2002;506(Pt A):657–65.

24. Rosenberg ME, Tervo TM, Müller LJ, et al. In vivo confocal microscopy after herpes keratitis. Cornea. 2002;21(3):265–9.
25. Labbé A, Alalwani H, Van Went C, et al. The relationship between subbasal nerve morphology and corneal sensation in ocular surface disease. Invest Ophthalmol Vis Sci. 2012;53(8):4926–31.
26. Toda I, Asano-Kato N, Komai-Hori Y, Tsubota K. Dry eye after laser in situ keratomileusis. Am J Ophthalmol. 2001;132(1):1–7.
27. Stern ME, Beuerman RW, Fox RI, et al. The pathology of dry eye: the interaction between the ocular surface and lacrimal glands. Cornea. 1998;17(6):584–9.
28. Solomon A, Dursun D, Liu Z, et al. Pro- and anti-inflammatory forms of interleukin-1 in the tear fluid and conjunctiva of patients with dry-eye disease. Invest Ophthalmol Vis Sci. 2001;42(10):2283–92.
29. Gøransson LG, Herigstad A, Tjensvoll AB, et al. Peripheral neuropathy in primary sjogren syndrome: a population-based study. Arch Neurol. 2006;63(11):1612–5.
30. Barendregt PJ, van den Bent MJ, van Raaij-van den Aarssen VJ, et al. Involvement of the peripheral nervous system in primary Sjögren's syndrome. Ann Rheum Dis. 2001;60(9):876–81.
31. Liesegang TJ. Herpes zoster ophthalmicus natural history, risk factors, clinical presentation, and morbidity. Ophthalmology. 2008;115(2 Suppl):S3–12.
32. Friedman NJ. Impact of dry eye disease and treatment on quality of life. Curr Opin Ophthalmol. 2010;21(4):310–6.
33. Miljanović B, Dana R, Sullivan DA, Schaumberg DA. Impact of dry eye syndrome on vision-related quality of life. Am J Ophthalmol. 2007;143(3):409–15.
34. Qiao J, Yan X. Emerging treatment options for meibomian gland dysfunction. Clin Ophthalmol. 2013;7:1797–803.
35. Amparo F, Dastjerdi MH, Okanobo A, et al. Topical interleukin 1 receptor antagonist for treatment of dry eye disease: a randomized clinical trial. JAMA Ophthalmol. 2013;131(6):715–23.
36. Moscovici BK, Holzchuh R, Sakassegawa-Naves FE, et al. Treatment of Sjögren's syndrome dry eye using 0.03% tacrolimus eye drop: Prospective double-blind randomized study. Cont Lens Anterior Eye. 2015;38(5):373–8. pii: S1367-0484(15)00058-2
37. John T, Shah AA. Use of azithromycin ophthalmic solution in the treatment of chronic mixed anterior blepharitis. Ann Ophthalmol (Skokie). 2008;40:68–74.
38. Foulks GN, Borchman D, Yappert M, Kakar S. Topical azithromycin and oral doxycycline therapy of meibomian gland dysfunction: a comparative clinical and spectroscopic pilot study. Cornea. 2013;32(1):44–53.
39. Golub LM, Lee HM, Ryan ME, et al. Tetracyclines inhibit connective tissue breakdown by multiple non-antimicrobial mechanisms. Adv Dent Res. 1998;12:12–26.
40. Yoon KC, Heo H, Im SK, et al. Comparison of autologous serum and umbilical cord serum eye drops for dry eye syndrome. Am J Ophthalmol. 2007;144(1):86–92.
41. Stason WB, Razavi M, Jacobs DS, et al. Clinical benefits of the boston ocular surface prosthesis. Am J Ophthalmol. 2010;149(1):54–61.
42. Jacobs DS, Rosenthal P. Boston scleral lens prosthetic device for treatment of severe dry eye in chronic graft-versus-host disease. Cornea. 2007;26(10):1195–9.
43. Hirata H, Okamoto K, Bereiter DA. GABA (A) receptor activation modulates corneal unit activity in rostral and caudal portions of trigeminal subnucleus caudalis. J Neurophysiol. 2003;90(5):2837–49.
44. Attal N, Cruccu G, Baron R, et al. European Federation of Neurological Societies. EFNS guidelines on the pharmacological treatment of neuropathic pain: 2010 revision. Eur J Neurol. 2010;17(9):1113-e88.
45. Jensen TS, Madsen CS, Finnerup NB. Pharmacology and treatment of neuropathic pains. Curr Opin Neurol. 2009;22(5):467–74.
46. Dworkin RH, O'Connor AB, Kent J, et al. International Association for the Study of Pain Neuropathic Pain Special Interest Group. Interventional management of neuropathic pain: NeuPSIG recommendations. Pain. 2013;154(11):2249–61.

47. Carroll IR, Kaplan KM, Mackey SC. Mexiletine therapy for chronic pain: survival analysis identifies factors predicting clinical success. J Pain Symptom Manage. 2008;35(3):321–6.
48. Kaptchuk TJ. Acupuncture: theory, efficacy, and practice. Ann Intern Med. 2002;136(5):374–83.
49. Lefaucheur JP, André-Obadia N, Antal A, et al. Evidence-based guidelines on the therapeutic use of repetitive transcranial magnetic stimulation (rTMS). Clin Neurophysiol. 2014;125(11):2150–206. pii: S1388-2457(14)00296-X
50. Sabato AF, Marineo G, Gatti A. Scrambler therapy. Minerva Anestesiol. 2005;71(7-8):479–82.
51. Deer TR, Mekhail N, Provenzano D, et al. Neuromodulation Appropriateness Consensus Committee. The appropriate use of neurostimulation of the spinal cord and peripheral nervous system for the treatment of chronic pain and ischemic diseases: the Neuromodulation Appropriateness Consensus Committee. Neuromodulation. 2014;17(6):515–50. discussion 550
52. Raphael W, Sordillo LM. Dietary polyunsaturated fatty acids and inflammation: the role of phospholipid biosynthesis. Int J Mol Sci. 2013;14(10):21167–88.
53. Hadjivassiliou M, Grünewald RA, Kandler RH, et al. Neuropathy associated with gluten sensitivity. J Neurol Neurosurg Psychiatry. 2006;77(11):1262–6.

Chapter 9
Management of Glaucoma in Patients with Ocular Surface Disease

Elham Ghahari, Ali R. Djalilian, and Ahmad A. Aref

Case 1: Ocular Surface Toxicity/Allergy from Glaucoma Medications

The patient is a 55-year-old female who was referred to our institution for diagnosis and management of an opaque epithelial sheet in the superior cornea of both eyes. She reports a long history of ocular surface disease with chronic red irritated eyes for the last 2 years. Her past ocular medications included tobramycin-dexamethasone, doxycycline, olopatadine, epinastine, cyclosporine, prednisolone, and multiple antibiotics drops. Most recently she was started on loteprednol 0.5% three times a day, which she did not find to be helpful. She has a history of glaucoma for 10+ years which in the past has been treated with timolol-dorzolamide. Her current medication was timolol 0.5% once a day and loteprednol 0.5% twice a day in both eyes. Her vision was 20/50 in the right eye and 20/40 in the left eye. IOP was 21 and 23 in the right and left, respectively.

On examination, the patient demonstrated significant erythema and skin changes around the lids. She had significant meibomian gland plugging and lid margin telangiectasia. His puncta were stenotic due to cautery punctal occlusion ion the past. Both corneas demonstrated inferior punctate staining and an opaque epithelial sheet extending from limbus superiorly extending into the visual axis. The epithelial sheet stained late with fluorescein in a whorl pattern (Figs. 9.1 and 9.2).

E. Ghahari, MD • A.R. Djalilian, MD • A.A. Aref, MD (✉)
Department of Ophthalmology and Visual Sciences, Illinois Eye and Ear Infirmary,
University of Illinois at Chicago, Chicago, IL, USA
e-mail: aaref@uic.edu

A.R. Djalilian (ed.), *Ocular Surface Disease*,
https://doi.org/10.1007/978-3-319-15823-5_9

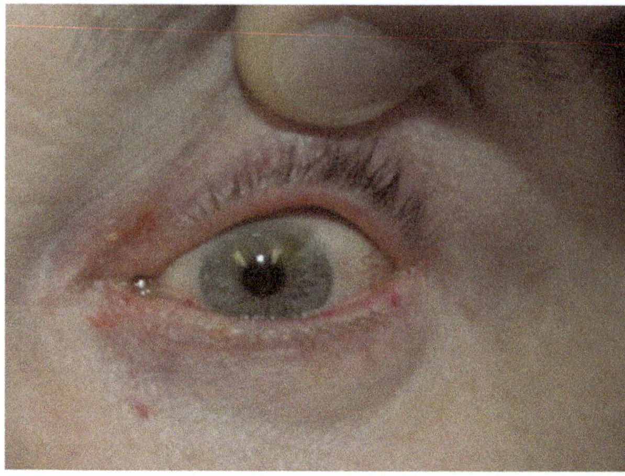

Fig. 9.1 External photograph demonstrating ocular adnexal erythema and edema as a result of chronic topical medications (in this case due to BAK allergy)

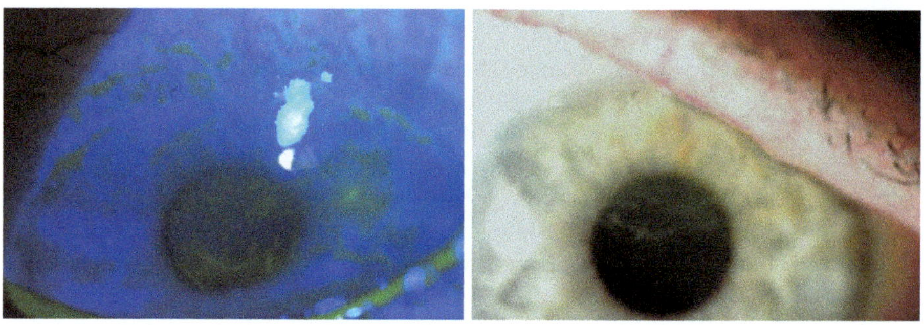

Fig. 9.2 Slit-lamp photograph demonstrating abnormal epithelial sheet extending from limbus superiorly and late staining with fluorescein. This sheet of epithelium regressed completely when BAK was eliminated and the patient was treated with preservative-free steroids and topical vitamin A ointment

What Diagnosis Do These Findings Suggest?

We have encountered a patient with ocular surface disease in the setting of chronic topical medication use. The patient has a chronic conjunctivitis along with periorbital skin changes suggestive of allergy. The late staining opaque epithelium extending into the visual axis from the superior limbus represents conjunctival-type epithelium and is consistent with the diagnosis of limbal stem cell deficiency (LSCD). The etiology of the LSCD was not quite clear at this initial visit. Given the superior location, the differential included superior limbal keratoconjunctivitis and contact lens-induced LSCD. There was no redundancy/staining of the conjunctiva superiorly, but upon questioning the patient did report a past history of soft contact lens wear for a number of years; however she had not worn lenses for over 10 years. The patient's dry eyes and meibomian gland disease also contribute to her surface disease and inflammation. The other important contributing factor to her ocular surface disease is her history of glaucoma medication use.

What Is the Basic Pathophysiology of the Ocular Surface Disease in the Setting of Glaucoma?

Ocular surface disease and dry eye syndrome (DES) are present in 15% of the elderly population and have been reported in up to 60% of glaucoma patients using topical therapy [1, 2]. OSD in glaucoma patients is often overlooked since the focus of management is typically on the possibility of glaucomatous progression.

Symptoms such as redness, stinging, burning, irritation, and dryness are common presentations of ocular surface disease related to IOP-lowering therapy. Examination findings often include superficial punctate keratitis of the cornea and conjunctiva, tear-film instability, and allergic reactions [3]. Long-term use of topical glaucoma medications may cause conjunctival inflammation and subconjunctival fibrosis (illustrated by the next case).

All classes of glaucoma medications have been reported as a cause of allergic reaction, and each drug class can manifest different allergic and/or toxic reactions. For example, beta blockers cause contact dermatitis in 11–13% of patients, and prostaglandin analogs can manifest as a mild allergic conjunctivitis in 1.5% [4]. Brimonidine-induced ocular allergies have been reported 9–11.5% [5].

Epithelial toxicity has been of particular interest in glaucoma therapy, most commonly associated with topical beta blockers and prostaglandin analogs [4].

Topical glaucoma medications can cause disruption of tear-film integrity. It is reported that tear-film breakup time and Schirmer values are abnormal in over 60% of glaucoma patients in addition to significant tear-film hyperosmolarity and meibomian gland loss [6, 7]. Laser scanning confocal microscopy and impression cytology documented glaucoma therapy-induced morphologic alterations of limbus, which may play a role in the glaucoma related ocular surface disease [8].

Glaucoma medication-induced allergic reaction can present as conjunctival hyperemia, eyelid erythema, and/or eczema. A type IV hypersensitivity reaction typically manifests as chronic eyelid inflammation and contact dermatitis. As this reaction may occur months after exposure, it may be difficult to distinguish this entity from a chronic blepharitis or a low-grade ocular toxicity secondary to preservative exposure. Follicular conjunctival reactions, a combination of type I and IV reactions, have been reported in the literature as common presentations of allergic reactions to glaucoma medications [9].

Differentiation between ocular surface allergy and toxicity is difficult in daily practice as they are usually coexistent. Allergic reaction presentation can vary from a typical periorbital dermatitis and papillary conjunctivitis to more subtle allergic blepharitis [3].

Ocular surface disease occurs due to both active compounds and preservatives, and differences are seen among the various classes of therapy [3, 9]. Most of the time, a trial-and-error approach may be necessary in order to reach to the diagnosis. After distinguishing allergy from toxicity, it is critical to discriminate whether the allergy is secondary to the active ingredient versus the preservative. Currently published data are inconclusive, but some studies have found a significant difference in the degree of SPK in patients maintained on preserved versus non-preserved topical glaucoma medications [5].

Benzalkonium chloride (BAK) is one of the first ophthalmic preservatives introduced and the most commonly used today. It is a cell wall and cytoplasmic membrane detergent and prevents microbial contamination in multi-dose containers. Its cationic quaternary ammonium structure allows it to promote drug transmission into the anterior chamber. BAK has toxic effects on ocular tissues [10]. Polyquarternium-1 is another quaternary ammonium preservative considered to be less toxic to the ocular surface based on studies examining toxicity to corneal and conjunctival epithelial cells; however it has also been shown to cause dendritic keratopathy. A newer generation preservative, SofZia (Alcon, Fort Worth, Texas, USA), functions as a microbicidal agent through oxidative properties and converts to non-toxic by-products after contact with the ocular surface.

In the presented case, multiple factors can contribute to the clinical picture. She has suffered at least two "hits" to her limbus, one is her history of contact lens wear and the other is her glaucoma medication usage. Other factors such as dry eye and inflammation clearly exacerbate the picture. Another common cause of superior LSCD in glaucoma patients is previous glaucoma surgeries like trabeculectomy with or without mitomycin C (Fig. 9.3). These factors tend to have additive effects and ultimately lead to surface failure focally (or globally).

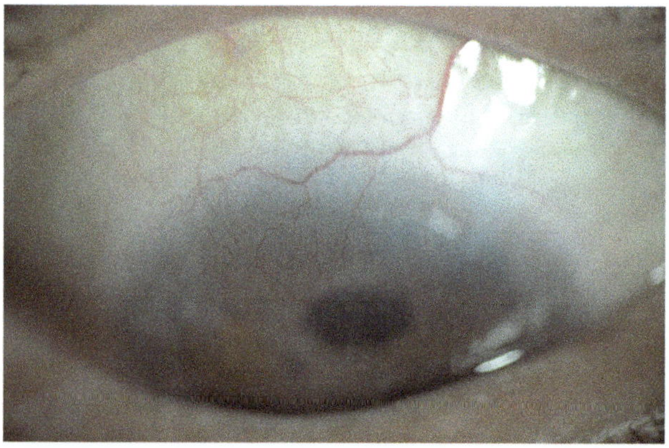

Fig. 9.3 Patient with history of extracapsular cataract extraction and long history of using glaucoma drops presents with superior limbal stem cell deficiency (i.e., iatrogenic LSCD). The patient had a partial response to stopping topical medications and using acetazolamide along with serum tears. He ultimately required a conjunctival limbal autograft from the other eye (which was no-light perception due to end-stage glaucoma)

What Is the Next Step in the Management of This Patient?

In a glaucoma patient with non-visually significant surface disease (mainly bothered by symptoms), the first step is to look for signs of allergy (skin changes, follicles) and discontinue suspected agent (e.g., brimonidine). The next step for a non-visually significant ocular surface disease is to change all drops to preservative-free. In a glaucoma patient with visually significant ocular surface disease, one should be more aggressive, and the first step is usually to hold all topical medications and temporarily use an oral agent (methazolamide or acetazolamide) to control the IOP. Short-term use of corticosteroid drops should also be considered, although one must be alert to the possibility of a steroid-induced elevation in IOP (Table 9.1).

In this case, all topical medications including the loteprednol and timolol were discontinued. IOP-lowering therapy with oral acetazolamide was initiated. To help with ocular surface inflammation, preservative-free topical steroid (compounded methylprednisolone 1%) was started at a frequency of every 6 h in each eye. Preservative-free artificial lubricating drops were continued. Oral doxycycline along with lid hygiene/massage was also recommended for her MGD. Finally, to help the LSCD, the patient was also prescribed topical vitamin A 0.01% qhs; however the patient did not get this until a few weeks later.

After 3 weeks, the patient had experienced remarkable improvement with significant reduction in her presenting symptoms. Patient reported that her eyes had not felt this good in years. We concluded that she *definitely was allergic to BAK.*

Once the surface disease has improved, a trial of a topical medication from a different class of active compound should be implemented but the possibility for cross-reaction should be noted. In cases where recurrent allergy is identified in association with multiple agents of differing drug classes, a BAK allergy must be suspected and a trial of BAK-free or preservative-free medication may be tried.

The concern for ocular surface damage from preservatives, especially BAK, has prompted the shift toward entirely preservative-free medications in single-unit dose vials.

Table 9.1 Stepwise management of OSD in glaucoma patients

• Begin with standard management of OSD (i.e., non-preserved artificial lubricants, aggressive treatment of MGD). If definite signs of allergy to topical medications (periocular skin changes, follicular reaction) stop or switch the offending agent (particularly brimonidine)
• If patient is still symptomatic, switch all glaucoma drops to preservative-free agents
• In more severe disease (e.g., visually significant limbal stem cell deficiency or active cicatricial disease), consider stopping all topical medications and temporarily using only oral agents
• A short trial of topical steroids (preferably preservative-free)—if positive response may add topical cyclosporine or lifitegrast for long-term maintenance
• May reintroduce topical glaucoma therapy (one at a time) using preservative-free or non-BAK preserved medications
• Consider SLT/ALT or minimally invasive procedures (e.g., iStent if undergoing cataract surgery) to eliminate or reduce the need for topical medications

Preservative-free timolol has been available for several years in the USA and Europe. Preservative-free prostaglandin analog, tafluprost (Zioptan; Merck, Whitehouse Station, New Jersey, USA), and preservative-free dorzolamide/timolol combination (Cosopt PF; Merck, Whitehouse Station, New Jersey, USA) have been released in the USA as well.

Several studies have reported improved ocular surface symptoms with preservative-free agents [5], but the results from alternative preservative formulations, particularly with the prostaglandin travoprost-Z (SofZia; Alcon), have been inconsistent [11]. Though efficacious in decreasing ocular surface disease and allergy, the higher cost of these medications largely limits their widespread application.

Three recent trials have studied the two preservative-free therapies approved in the USA, preservative-free tafluprost and dorzolamide/timolol. Significant decreases in subjective symptoms and tear-film abnormalities were found with both agents [12]. *Our own clinical experience with these agents confirms that, in glaucoma patients with dry eye symptoms, switching to preservative-free medications help reduce the symptom burden (not eliminate it).*

Finally, a patient with multiple allergies or severe ocular surface disease may not be able to tolerate any topical medication. For these patients, laser treatments such as argon laser trabeculoplasty, selective laser trabeculoplasty, or laser cyclophotocoagulation may be considered prior to proceeding with surgical interventions. It has been shown that a longer duration of glaucomatous disease is significantly correlated with worsening of OSD symptoms. In one study, patients with glaucoma diagnoses of less than 6 years had a significantly lower mean Ocular Surface Disease Index score relative to patients with glaucoma diagnoses of 6 years or more [13].

What About the Long-Term Management of This Patient's Glaucoma and OSD?

Moderate to severe OSD frequently requires a change of glaucoma medications. Switching to a different topical medication or systemic therapy with carbonic anhydrase inhibitor or performing laser trabeculoplasty or other surgery along with adding treatment to alleviate ocular surface symptoms is possible. Modification of glaucoma therapy due to OSD is practiced in approximately 40% of patients [14].

In a study of rabbit eyes, the beneficial effects of topical cyclosporine have been demonstrated to reverse adverse ocular surface changes produced by long-term glaucoma medical therapy [15]. It has been shown that glaucoma patients with significant ocular surface changes after topical glaucoma medication usage have altered morphology of subbasal nerve fibers. One study highlights that topical cyclosporine therapy seems to have beneficial effects in dry eye disease due to long-term topical hypotensive medications with improvement in ocular surface changes and central corneal subbasal nerve fiber density. Therefore, topical cyclosporine 0.05% (or perhaps lifitegrast) may be considered in eyes with dry eye disease due to long-term topical glaucoma therapy [16].

In this case, the patient was started on Zioptan while her acetazolamide was discontinued. Her IOP has remained well controlled. She was started on

Restasis in order to help get her off the steroids; however she required a very prolonged taper and continues to require very low dose (one drop every few days) to help control her inflammation and symptoms. Her topical vitamin A was discontinued after 3–4 months but did require repeat treatment later in her course for mild recurrence of the LSCD. At last follow-up, her visual acuity was 20/20 OU with well-controlled IOPs on preservative-free prostaglandin drops.

Case 2: Glaucoma Patient with Chronic Conjunctivitis and Scarring

The patient is a 57-year-old male with complaints of red eyes, foreign body sensation, light sensitivity, and tearing. He has been followed more than 15 years for an underlying diagnosis of primary open angle glaucoma for which has been treated with multiple topical IOP-lowering agents. His symptoms began about 3 years ago and were diagnosed as dry eyes and meibomian gland disease. In addition, he has had recurrent trichiasis of the lower and upper lids which has required multiple epilations. He denies any history of chemical injury or exposure. He works as an employee in an electrical engineering company and does not report any occupational exposure. His current IOP-lowering medical regimen includes fixed-combination dorzolamide/timolol twice daily in both eyes. His past treatments have included tobramycin-dexamethasone, olopatadine, Restasis, and doxycycline.

On presentation, visual acuity was 20/70 OD and 20/50 OS. IOP was 13 OU. Slit-lamp examination of the eyelids revealed bilateral mild inward rotation of the lower lids. The lid margin itself had prominent telangiectasia and severe meibomian gland dysfunction as well as lid margin keratinization extending onto the palpebral surface. The conjunctiva was 2+ injected, and there was subepithelial fibrosis, foreshortening of the inferior fornix (Fig. 9.4). The cornea has moderate diffuse punctuate epithelial erosion bilaterally.

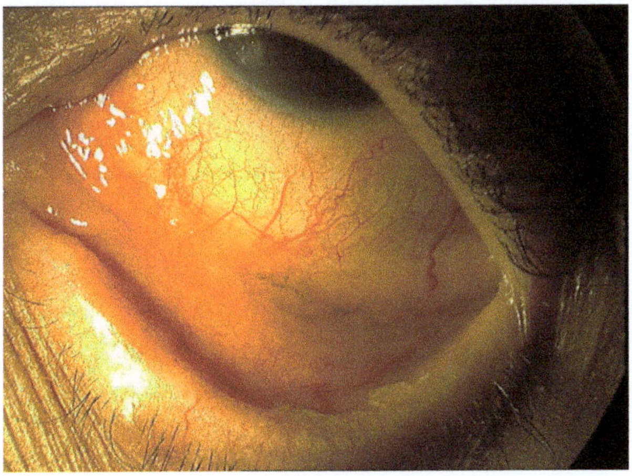

Fig. 9.4 Slit-lamp photograph demonstrating conjunctival hyperemia with forniceal foreshortening and lid margin keratinization (Photo courtesy of Mohammad Pakravan, M.D., Labbafinejad Medical Center, Iran)

What Is Your Diagnosis? What Else Do You Recommend?

This patient is presenting with chronic conjunctivitis and mild cicatricial changes. One important diagnosis that should be considered is mucous membrane pemphigoid, also known as ocular cicatricial pemphigoid (OCP). However, in this case, given the long history of glaucoma medication use, the diagnosis may in fact be "drug-induced" cicatricial conjunctivitis. We prefer this term over other terms such as "pseudo-pemphigoid" since the term "pseudo" can sometimes be misleading and leave the impression that the disease is not real and hence not serious. Ocular rosacea and atopic keratoconjunctivitis are two other causes so querying the patient with regard to any history of allergy and atopy [17]. The patient is questioned about skin and other mucous membrane involvement which he denies.

Topical and systemic drugs have been associated with the development of cicatricial conjunctivitis. In a study performed by Thorne and colleagues, the most common topical medical association with drug induced pemphigoid was topical IOP-lowering medications, which accounted for 28.3% of all cases. They reported beta blockers in 87.8%, epinephrine and alpha agonists in 61.0%, and miotics in 53.6% of patients with "pseudopemphigoid" [17]. In fact, any chronic topical medication can potentially lead to cicatricial changes. The preservative BAK has particularly been implicated.

OCP has an autoimmune etiology, with characteristic autoantibodies directed at the basement membrane zone (BMZ) of the epithelial-subepithelial junction of mucous membranes and/or skin. In contrast, patients with drug-induced "OCP" have a negative biopsy (no specific BMZ immune deposits detected) and presence of another cause of cicatrization [17].

Conjunctival biopsy is necessary to reach a definite diagnosis before considering specific systemic immunosuppressive therapy. It is noteworthy to mention that drug-induced cicatricial conjunctivitis caused by topical glaucoma drugs is almost identical to other causes in clinical presentation except for unilaterality in the eye receiving the medication and cessation of disease progression on discontinuation of the medication.

Systemic examination revealed no skin or mucous membrane abnormalities. The patient has no history of allergy, atopy, or recent infection. In this case, considering history of glaucoma, it is most likely that the glaucoma medication is the responsible agent causing ocular surface cicatrization and keratinization mimicking ocular pemphigoid. Nonetheless, a conjunctival biopsy was recommended to rule out an underlying cicatrizing disease.

How Was This Patient Managed?

The most immediate step in the management of this patient is to withdraw all topical glaucoma medications and use anti-inflammatory therapy to reduce the inflammation. The patient was started on oral prednisone 60 mg per day and topical preservative-free methylprednisolone every 4 h. He was also started on oral doxycycline 100 mg twice a day. Acetazolamide 125 mg every 12 h was started for IOP control after discontinuation of topical glaucoma medication.

In general, identification and removal of all aggravating factors that contribute to inflammation (trichiasis, meibomian gland dysfunction, dry eyes, colonization with bacterial pathogens, smoking) is critical [18]. Any causes of inflammation can lead to progression of cicatrizing conjunctivitis.

Trichiasis can lead to corneal abrasions, punctuate epitheliopathy, and may increase likelihood of bacterial keratitis. Epilation is recommended as treatment for this condition; however, regrowth of eyelashes makes this treatment a short-term option, and once inflammation is under control, surgical management may be considered. In the meantime, we frequently use bandage contact lenses to protect the cornea and ocular surface from the lashes.

It is important to emphasize that systemic immunosuppressive therapy should be offered only to patients with active, progressive disease. The decision to use chemotherapy requires careful consideration and close collaboration between the ophthalmologist and hematologist/oncologist.

After 3 weeks of these prescribed therapeutic measures, the patient reported marked improvement in ocular comfort. On examination, a significant improvement in conjunctival injection was noted. IOP measured 15 mmHg OU, which was acceptable given this patient's stage of glaucomatous optic neuropathy. Prednisolone and topical preservative-free methylprednisolone was slowly tapered over a course of 6 months while doxycycline was continued. Meanwhile, patient was using acetazolamide for IOP control. After this period, acetazolamide was replaced by topical preservative-free Cosopt twice a day which so far has been tolerated by the patient without recurrent inflammation.

In some patients, the inflammation may take a while to subside, and it may be necessary to use a secondary agent such as mycophenolate for several months after tapering the oral steroids. Many cases of drug-induced cicatricial conjunctivitis will eventually become quiet when the offending medications are eliminated. However, in some cases, the patient may actually have a true cicatricial process (e.g., pemphigoid) that could have preceded and become exacerbated by topical medications. In these cases, the inflammation will not subside even after medications are discontinued, and therefore prolonged immunosuppressive therapy will be necessary to prevent progression. The most important element on the exam is the level of conjunctival inflammation, which should be treated until it is completely under control.

Case 3: Glaucoma Surgery in the Limbal Transplant Patient

A 21-year-old Hispanic male is referred to your clinic for glaucoma evaluation. He has a history of severe chemical injury in both eyes at age 4 (due to a battery explosion). The right eye developed total LSCD and the left eye was only partially affected. He had previously undergone a penetrating keratoplasty in the

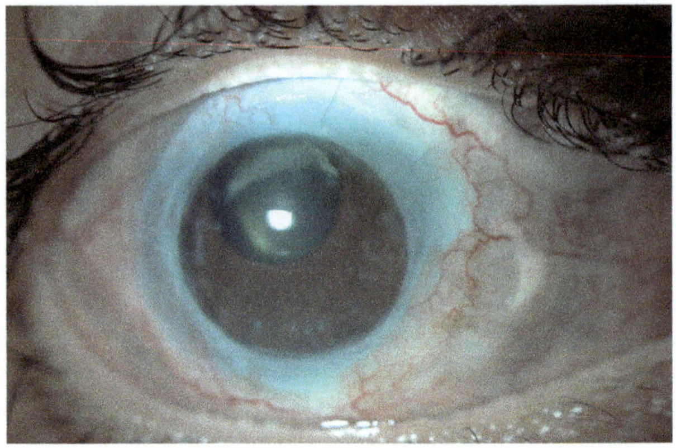

Fig. 9.5 Slit-lamp photograph demonstrating an intact 360-degree keratolimbal allograft

right eye at age 10 (at a different institution) which had failed due to recurrent surface disease. He successfully underwent combined keratolimbal allograft transplantation and penetrating keratoplasty in the right eye at age 17 with the use of systemic immunosuppression consisting of prednisone (4 months), tacrolimus, and mycophenolate. He also later underwent cataract extraction and lens implant in the same eye (Fig. 9.5). He was noted to have IOP elevation 1 year after original surgery in part due to the use of topical steroids.

Despite maximum medical therapy and two sessions of diode cyclophotocoagulation to the right eye, his IOP remained elevated at 27 mmHg 4 years after the keratolimbal allograft transplant. His uncorrected visual acuity at this time was 20/250 in the right eye with limited potential due to amblyopia. Examination of the left eye reveals vision achieving 20/20 with partial LSCD (total of 180° affected) not involving the visual axis. In the right eye, the limbal and corneal grafts were intact with minimal fluorescein staining. Dilated fundus examination reveals an optic nerve cup-disc ratio of 0.9 but otherwise unremarkable.

What Is the Pathophysiologic Basis for IOP Elevation in This Patient?

Glaucoma is frequently associated with severe OSD and is often exacerbated by ocular surface transplantation procedures [19]. The occurrence of progressive glaucomatous optic neuropathy may lead to irreversible visual field loss and a compromised visual outcome after otherwise successful ocular surface transplantation. The prevalence of concomitant glaucomatous disease in patients afflicted with severe OSD is relatively high. Tsai et al. reported an overall prevalence of 65.7%, ranging from 42.9% to 88.4% according to OSD subgroup, in 108 eyes [19]. Underlying mechanisms of glaucoma include congenital anomalies of the filtering angle associated with aniridia and inflammation/scarring of the ocular surface in patients with severe chemical and thermal injuries.

Although preexisting disease is an important contributor to glaucoma in this population, Tsai et al. also noted a 26% incidence of the disease after initial treatment with ocular surface transplantation and/or medical therapies [19]. Postoperative structural alterations to the ocular surface leading to decreased episcleral venous outflow as well as steroid-related IOP rise are thought to be the mechanisms by which this secondary glaucoma develops.

What Is the Treatment Plan for this Patient? What Are the Concerns When Proceeding to Treat Glaucoma in a Patient with History of Ocular Surface Transplantation?

The multiple complexities involved with glaucoma management in the setting of severe OSD and preexisting ocular surface transplantation require special consideration. Topical IOP-lowering therapies are effective in controlling glaucoma but may be toxic to a transplanted epithelial surface [20]. Diode laser transscleral cyclophotocoagulation has been found to be effective after ocular surface transplantation but is associated with increased postoperative inflammation requiring intensive immunosuppression. Standard trabeculectomy is often not possible because of conjunctival disease and may further traumatize the corneal limbus in the region of fistula creation and antifibrotic agents may lead to irreversible stem cell damage [21].

Glaucoma drainage implant (GDI) surgery is often the preferred for controlling IOP in eyes that have undergone prior ocular surgery. However, standard fornix-based GDI surgery (involving a limbal conjunctival incision) would lead to disruption of existing ocular surface transplant. Furthermore, a GDI tube placed in the anterior chamber increases the risk of future corneal transplant failure due to presumed direct endothelial cell contact and damage [22, 23].

This patient underwent GDI surgery utilizing a technique of limbal-based peritomy (i.e., where the incision is far away from the limbus) with ciliary sulcus tube placement. This technique helped to preserve the health of a preexisting ocular surface transplant while minimizing the risk of tube endothelium contact in order to maximize success of corneal transplant by decreasing mechanical endothelial cell damage.

While the two modifications noted above (placing the tube in the sulcus and using a limbal-based peritomy) can help preserve the limbal and corneal grafts both during and after GDI surgery, in general, we recommend placement of a GDI be performed prior to ocular surface transplant. Our current recommendation is that any patient requiring two or more IOP-lowering drops be considered for glaucoma surgery before undergoing limbal allograft transplantation. This would not only minimize the need for glaucoma medications, which can have detrimental effects on the limbal grafts but also reduce the likelihood of steroid-induced IOP spikes and avoid any induced inflammation from the glaucoma surgery.

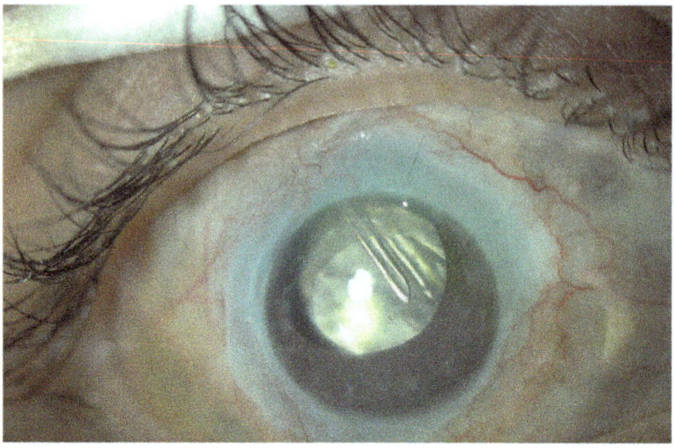

Fig. 9.6 Postoperative slit-lamp photograph corresponding to the case depicted in Fig. 9.5. The photo demonstrates a well-positioned glaucoma drainage implant tube in the ciliary sulcus with preservation of the preexisting keratolimbal allograft with a stable corneal epithelium

We prescribed topical prednisolone acetate 1% and topical gatifloxacin 0.5% solution. Six months after limbal-based GDI procedure with placement of the tube in the ciliary sulcus, IOP remained under excellent control at 8 mmHg in the right eye without the need for adjunctive topical or systemic ocular antihypertensive agents. The tube remained in good position in the ciliary sulcus. The limbal stem cell transplant also remained healthy, with no corneal fluorescein uptake, as of the last office visit (Fig. 9.6) with a postoperative uncorrected visual acuity of 20/500.

Previous studies have shown that GDI surgery with a tube placed in the anterior chamber may compromise the success of corneal transplantation procedures [22]. In a retrospective case-controlled study of 40 corneal grafts treated with GDI surgery, Alvarenga and colleagues identified GDI implantation as an independent risk factor for graft failure. In this series, the majority of GDI tubes were placed in the anterior chamber, with only a "low percentage" placed in the pars plana.

Summary

- OSD is extremely common in patients on topical glaucoma medications. When the OSD is not showing clinical improvement with standard measures, ocular allergy and/or toxicity from topical medications is considered as a contributing factor.
- In a glaucoma patient with symptoms and signs of OSD (non-visually significant) after initiating standard therapies (lubrication, lid hygiene), consideration should be given to switching to preservative-free medications.
- If the OSD is visually significant (e.g., limbal stem cell deficiency, cicatricial conjunctivitis), if possible, topical medications should be temporarily discontinued and patient should be treated with an oral carbonic anhydrase inhibitor with consideration given to short-term use of topical corticosteroids (preferably preservative-free) while closely watching the IOP.

- Once the OSD is better controlled, a trial of a different class of active compound and/or preservative free medications may be considered. Allergy to BAK should be suspected when there is documented intolerance to multiple medication classes, and, in these cases, a BAK-free or preservative-free medication may be prescribed.
- Some patients with severe OSD (cicatricial conjunctivitis) may not be able to tolerate any topical medication regardless of preservative until the inflammation is well controlled.
- Whenever possible, ALT/SLT should be considered in an effort to decrease dependency on medical therapy and hence exposure to toxic medications which can exacerbate the OSD.
- In a patient with drug-induced cicatricial conjunctivitis, conjunctival-based surgical treatments have a high failure rate particularly when there is active inflammation.
- In patients with severe OSD (e.g., limbal stem cell deficiency), glaucoma is very common. In patients using two or more topical glaucoma medications, a tube shunt (preferably placed in the sulcus) is recommended prior to any ocular surface transplantation.

Acknowledgments *Financial Disclosures*: None of the authors have any financial disclosures regarding the contents discussed in this manuscript. *Conflict of Interest*: None of the authors have any conflicts of interest with the contents discussed in this manuscript.

References

1. Leung EW, Medeiros FA, Weinreb RN. Prevalence of ocular surface disease in glaucoma patients. J Glaucoma. 2008;17(5):350–5.
2. Skalicky SE, Goldberg I, McCluskey P. Ocular surface disease and quality of life in patients with glaucoma. Am J Ophthalmol. 2012;153(1):1–9.
3. Baudouin C, Labbe A, Liang H, Pauly A, Brignole-Baudouin F. Preservatives in eye drops: the good, the bad and the ugly. Prog Retin Eye Res. 2010;29(4):312–34.
4. Servat JJ, Bernardino CR. Effects of common topical antiglaucoma medications on the ocular surface, eyelids and periorbital tissue. Drugs Aging. 2011;28(4):267–82.
5. Pisella PJ, Pouliquen P, Baudouin C. Prevalence of ocular symptoms and signs with preserved and preservative free glaucoma medication. Br J Ophthalmol. 2002;86(4):418–23.
6. Arita R, Itoh K, Maeda S, Maeda K, Furuta A, Tomidokoro A, Aihara M, Amano S. Effects of long-term topical antiglaucoma medications on meibomian glands. Graefes Arch Clin Exp Ophthalmol. 2012;250(8):1181–5.
7. Lee SY, Wong TT, Chua J, Boo C, Soh YF, Tong L. Effect of chronic anti-glaucoma medications and trabeculectomy on tear osmolarity. Eye. 2013;27(10):1142–50.
8. Mastropasqua R, Agnifili L, Fasanella V, Curcio C, Brescia L, Lanzini M, Fresina M, Mastropasqua L, Marchini G. Corneoscleral limbus in glaucoma patients: in vivo confocal microscopy and immunocytological study. Invest Ophthalmol Vis Sci. 2015;56(3):2050–8.
9. Baudouin C. Allergic reaction to topical eye drops. Curr Opin Allergy Clin Immunol. 2005;5(5):459–63.
10. Pellinen P, Huhtala A, Tolonen A, Lokkila J, Mäenpää J, Uusitalo H. The cytotoxic effects of preserved and preservative-free prostaglandin analogs on human corneal and conjunctival

epithelium in vitro and the distribution of benzalkonium chloride homologs in ocular surface tissues in vivo. Curr Eye Res. 2012;37(2):145–54.
11. Gandolfi S, Paredes T, Goldberg I, Coote M, Wells A, Volksone L, Pillai MR, Stalmans I, Denis P. Travoprost Bak-Free Clinical Study Group. Comparison of a travoprost BAK-free formulation preserved with polyquaternium-1 with BAK-preserved travoprost in ocular hypertension or open-angle glaucoma. Eur J Ophthalmol. 2012;22(1):34–44.
12. Januleviciene I, Derkač I, Grybauskiene L, Paulauskaitė R, Gromnickaite R, Kuzmienė L. Effects of preservative-free tafluprost on tear film osmolarity, tolerability, and intraocular pressure in previously treated patients with open-angle glaucoma. Clin Ophthalmol. 2012;6:103–9.
13. Garcia-Feijoo J, Sampaolesi JR. A multicenter evaluation of ocular surface disease prevalence in patients with glaucoma. Clin Ophthalmol. 2012;6:441–6.
14. Baudouin C. Glaucoma and ocular surface disease: who, why and how to treat? View Glaucoma. 2013;8(1):4–10.
15. Cho HK, Park MH, Moon JI. The effect of additional topical cyclosporin or vitamin A on the ocular surface during antiglaucoma medication administration. Ophthalmic Res. 2012;48(3):139–45.
16. Saini M, Dhiman R, Dada T, Tandon R, Vanathi M. Topical cyclosporine to control ocular surface disease in patients with chronic glaucoma after long-term usage of topical ocular hypotensive medications. Eye. 2015;29(6):808–14.
17. Thorne JE, Anhalt GJ, Jabs DA. Mucous membrane pemphigoid and pseudopemphigoid. Ophthalmology. 2004;111(1):45–52.
18. Ahmed M, Zein G, Khawaja F, Foster CS. Ocular cicatricial pemphigoid: pathogenesis, diagnosis and treatment. Prog Retin Eye Res. 2004;23(6):579–92.
19. Tsai JH, Derby E, Holland EJ, Khatana AK. Incidence and prevalence of glaucoma in severe ocular surface disease. Cornea. 2006;25(5):530–2.
20. Holland EJ, Schwartz GS. The Paton lecture: ocular surface transplantation: 10 years' experience. Cornea. 2004;23(5):425–31.
21. Schwartz GS, Holland EJ. Iatrogenic limbal stem cell deficiency: when glaucoma management contributes to corneal disease. J Glaucoma. 2001;10(6):443–5.
22. Alvarenga LS, Mannis MJ, Brandt JD, Lee WB, Schwab IR, Lim MC. The long-term results of keratoplasty in eyes with a glaucoma drainage device. Am J Ophthalmol. 2004;138(2):200–5.
23. Lim KS. Corneal endothelial cell damage from glaucoma drainage device materials. Cornea. 2003;22(4):352–4.

Chapter 10
Comorbid Psychiatric and Inflammatory Conditions in Dry Eye Disease

Nisreen Ezuddin, Sarah Avila, and Anat Galor

Case #1: Ocular Surface Disease and Comorbid Psychiatric Conditions

VG is a 45-year-old white female evaluated in the clinic with complaints of increasing dryness and irritation in both eyes for the past several months. Symptoms are constant but vary in intensity over at time. On review of systems, the patient endorses fibromyalgia, depression, and anxiety, but she is not currently on any treatment. Her past medical history is otherwise unremarkable and she does not take any medications. The patient also denies tobacco, alcohol, or recreational drug use. Upon further questioning, she reports increased fatigue, weight gain, concentration problems, and significant sleep disruption over the past 3 weeks. She feels sad but denies suicidal or homicidal ideations.

On examination, her best-corrected visual acuity is 20/20 OU with normal intraocular pressures. Osmolarity testing (TearLab, San Diego) reveals a value of 293 mOsm/L OD and 295 mOsm/L OS. InflammaDry (RPS, Tampa) is negative with a blue band in the control center in both eyes. Evaluation of the external periocular skin is unremarkable. On slit lamp examination, the eyelid margins are clean, the sclera and conjunctiva are white and quiet, and the corneas are clear OU. On fluorescein examination, tear film breakup time (TFBUT) is 14 s and 15 s in the right and left eye, respectively. Tear lake is of normal volume. Schirmer's testing with anesthesia reveals 10 mm of wetting OD and 12 mm of wetting OS after 5 min. The remaining ocular examination is otherwise unremarkable.

N. Ezuddin, BS • S. Avila, BS • A. Galor, MD, MSPH (✉)
Miami Veterans Administration Medical Center, 1201 NW 16th St, Miami, FL 33125, USA

Bascom Palmer Eye Institute, University of Miami,
900 NW 17th Street, Miami, FL 33136, USA
e-mail: agalor@med.miami.edu

A.R. Djalilian (ed.), *Ocular Surface Disease*,
https://doi.org/10.1007/978-3-319-15823-5_10

A depression screening questionnaire (patient health questionnaire (PHQ-9)) was administered with a resulting score of 20 (range 0–27). This score corresponds to severe depression.

What Do These Findings Mean?

This patient has dry eye symptoms but a normal slit lamp exam. She also has concomitant symptoms of depression. The case of Mrs. G is not an uncommon one. Mental illness affects millions in the USA with anxiety disorders being the most common, affecting 40 million American adults over the age of 18, or 18% of the population. Anxiety and depression often coexist, and nearly half of patients with depression are also diagnosed with an anxiety disorder.

Symptoms of major depression include (1) sad, depressed, or irritable mood, (2) loss of interest or pleasure, (3) significant sleep loss/gain; (4) sleep disruption, (5) loss of energy/fatigue nearly every single day, (6) significant appetite changes, (7) thoughts of death or dying, (8) concentration/decision-making difficulties, and (9) worthlessness or excessive guilt. A major depressive episode is characterized as lasting at least 2 weeks with clear changes from a previous state that interferes with life [1].

Patients with depression often present to other physicians with concomitant physical symptoms. In a study of 1146 primary care patients with major depression, 69% reported an unexplained physical symptom as their chief complaint (defined as symptoms outside of the classification for DSM-IV and ICD-10) [2]. Dry eye symptoms may be one of several physical complaints reported by patients with depression. The direction of the relationship, however, has not been established as it is known that chronic pain can lead to depression. As such, depression may occur in patients with chronic ocular symptoms, or, conversely, as above, dry eye symptoms may be one of many physical manifestations of depression.

Irrespective, if a patient presents with unexplained dry eye symptoms, a clinical screening for depression is reasonable. There are many different ways to screen for depression, and multiple factors need to be considered in choosing the appropriate screen. Firstly, the screening modality should have diagnostic accuracy in the population being screened, and, secondly, the screening measure should be feasible, which includes the number of questions, response format, literacy level, and time it takes to administer [39]. An important screening instrument used by psychiatrists is the Beck Depression Inventory (BDI-II), which is a 21-item questionnaire that monitors for treatment response. The Beck Depression Inventory for Primary Care (BDI-PC) is an adaptation from the BDI-II, which includes a seven-item questionnaire with a cutoff of four points and has a sensitivity of 97% and specificity of 99% in identifying major depression in a primary care setting, as compared to the gold standard of the diagnostic interview [3, 4]. Table 10.1 shows a comparison of six different screening instruments used by physicians when screening for depression with the gold standard for comparison being a structured clinical interview.

Table 10.1 Comparison of depression screening instruments

Instrument	Sensitivity (%)	Specificity (%)	Items	Response format	Literacy level	Time to administer (min)
BDI	90	79	21	Four statements of symptom severity per item	Easy	2–5
EDPS	82	86	10	Four frequency ratings	Easy	<2
GDS	81	78	15	Yes or no	Easy	2–5
PHQ-2	83	90	2	Four frequency ratings	Average	<1
PHQ-9	88	88	9	Five frequency ratings	Average	<2
WHO-5	93	64	5	Five frequency ratings	Easy	<2

BDI beck depression inventory, *EPDS* Edinburgh postnatal depression scale, *GDS* geriatric depression scale, *PHQ-2* patient health questionnaire-2, *PHQ-9* patient health questionnaire-9, *WHO-5* World Health Organization well-being index

Mrs. G also carried a diagnosis of fibromyalgia. Fibromyalgia is a disease characterized by centralized pain manifesting as multifocal pain in different body regions at different times, not fully explained by injury or inflammation. Interestingly, some patients with fibromyalgia have also been found to have small fiber neuropathy on biopsy [5]. While widespread musculoskeletal pain is a hallmark of fibromyalgia, insomnia, cognitive disturbances (e.g., forgetfulness, decreased concentration), headache, irritable bowel syndrome, depression [6], and dry eye symptoms have also been found to be more common in patients with fibromyalgia [7, 8].

How Often Does Depression Coexist with Dry Eye?

Depression has been found to coexist with dry eye in a number of different population-based studies from Beijing [9], Korea [10], and the Netherlands [11]. In two population-based cross-sectional studies involving 2113 patients from Beijing and Korea, the results showed that depression correlated with dry eye symptoms (gritty, sandy, burning, dry), but did not correspond with dry eye signs of tear breakup time (TBUT) or Schirmer's test score [9, 10]. In a study utilizing the US Veterans Affairs (VA) national database, both post-traumatic stress disorder (odds ratio (OR) 1.92, 95% confidence interval (CI) 1.91–1.94) and depression (OR 1.92, 95% CI 1.91–1.94) were found to increase the risk of a dry eye diagnosis. These findings were robust when considering the effect of age, gender, and concomitant use of antidepressants and anxiolytics [12]. Regarding pain, in a cross-sectional study of 425 patients, the frequency of dry eye symptoms was higher in the subset of study participants with a chronic pain syndrome (irritable bowel syndrome (IBS), chronic pelvic pain, or fibromyalgia) than without it, but ocular signs were no worse [11].

What Are the Treatment Options in Comorbid Psychiatric and Pain Disorders?

Treatments for psychiatric conditions, like depression and anxiety, in patients with dry eyes are best approached by integrating pharmacological and nonpharmacological therapies (patient education, exercise therapy, cognitive behavioral therapy) while keeping the patient active in the process. These are based on the experiences in treating patients with fibromyalgia.

Pharmacologic Treatment

Pharmacologic treatments generally work by reducing the activity of excitatory neurotransmitters (such as glutamate) (e.g., pregabalin, gabapentin) or by increasing the activity of inhibitory neurotransmitters, such as norepinephrine, serotonin, and γ-aminobutyric acid or GABA (e.g., serotonin-norepinephrine reuptake inhibitors, which include duloxetine, milnacipran). After a diagnosis of depression or anxiety has been established, the next steps should be to determine whether treatment is needed or not, based on the clinical extent of severity, distress or impairment, and the patient's preference. If pharmacologic therapy is initiated, SSRIs or SNRIs are usually the first-line therapies given their reasonable side effect profile [13]. Table 10.2 gives a comparison of the SSRIs and SNRIs available in the treatment of depression and anxiety. After initiation of medication, changes in mood can be seen within 1–2 weeks [14–16].

Drugs listed in Table 10.2 have also been found effective in the treatment of fibromyalgia-associated pain and may be considered in patients with ocular surface pain. Currently, the best-studied medications include certain SNRIs (e.g., duloxetine and milnacipran), tricyclic antidepressants (e.g., amitriptyline), and anticonvulsants (e.g., gabapentin and pregabalin) [17–19]. Interestingly, other drugs frequently used to treat pain such as nonsteroidal anti-inflammatory drugs, opioids, and corticosteroids have not been shown effective in treating fibromyalgia pain. In fact, opioids have been shown to worsen fibromyalgia-related hyperalgesia and pain in other centralized pain states [20]. It is thought that the opioid system is hyperactive in fibromyalgia patients, possibly explaining why opioids are ineffective at treating pain symptoms. As such, another promising treatment in fibromyalgia is low-dose naltrexone [21]. Naltrexone is thought to suppress microglial activity and, thereby, decrease the production of proinflammatory factors, such as cytokines, excitatory amino acids, and nitric oxide, which can cause hyperalgesia, fatigue, and other symptoms of fibromyalgia [22, 23]. In addition, trigger point injections may be beneficial in the treatment of fibromyalgia [24, 25].

Table 10.2 Pharmacologic treatment for fibromyalgia-associated pain/anxiety which may be considered for ocular surface patients

Drug	Initial daily dose (oral, mg)	Daily dose range (oral)	Side effect profile/characteristics
Sertraline	25–50	50–150	Insomnia, agitation, GI upset, diarrhea
Fluoxetine	20	20–60	Insomnia, agitation, weight changes, takes weeks for effect
Paroxetine	20	20–50	Mild sedative, weakly anticholinergic
Citalopram	10	10–40	Can prolong QT interval, lower risk of insomnia and agitation
Duloxetine	30	60–120	Useful for treatment of comorbid pain conditions
Venlafaxine	75	75–225	Increased blood pressure (diastolic) and heart rate with increasing doses, greater risk of insomnia/agitation, useful for treatment of comorbid pain conditions
Buspirone	10 (divided doses)	10–60 (divided doses)	A nonbenzodiazepine anxiolytic, ineffective for comorbid major depression
Mirtazapine	15	15–60	Appetite stimulant, useful for anxiety with insomnia, sedating, atypical antidepressant
Quetiapine	25–50	50–300	Extrapyramidal symptoms, weight gain, metabolic side effects
Imipramine	75 (divided doses)	75–200 (divided doses)	Anticholinergic side effects, potential cardiotoxicity, TCA
Hydroxyzine	50 (bedtime)	25–50 TID	Anticholinergic side effects
Nortriptyline	10 (bedtime)	10–75	Anticholinergic side effects, dry mouth, dry eyes, somnolence, rarely tachycardia
Amitriptyline	5 (bedtime)	10–75	Anticholinergic side effects, dry mouth, dry eyes, somnolence, rarely tachycardia

Nonpharmacological Therapies

The best-studied nonpharmacological therapies are education, cognitive behavioral therapy, and exercise. For the initial treatment of unipolar major depression, numerous studies have shown that the efficacy of psychotherapy and pharmacologic treatment exceeds pharmacologic treatment alone. In fibromyalgia, other treatments include chiropractic manipulation, tai chi, yoga, acupuncture, and myofascial release therapy [26, 27]. Both transcutaneous and central neurostimulatory therapies have also been used to treat pain with some success in fibromyalgia [28, 29].

What Is an Appropriate Management of This Patient?

In this patient, a multi-specialist approach is required. The ophthalmologist should work with the patient's primary care physician and encourage a referral to a mental health professional. Despite good cross-sectional data associating mental illness and dry eye, no longitudinal data exist to guide therapy in this case. For example, it is not known what effect treating chronic non-ocular pain and depression/anxiety will have on dry eye symptoms. As such, it is advisable for the ophthalmologist to provide local therapy to improve ocular surface health, as needed, and to work in conjunction with other specialties that can address the non-ocular conditions associated with dry eye.

Case #2: Aqueous Deficient Dry Eye in the Setting of Systemic Immune Disease

A 49-year-old female with history of inflammatory arthritis on hydroxychloroquine therapy presented to the eye clinic with complaints of decreased vision, burning, and redness in both eyes. She uses preservative-free artificial tears up to 6–8 times a day without relief. She states her symptoms are worse upon awakening and while working on the computer for her secretarial job. Past medical history is significant for back and joint pain, which have been well controlled with hydroxychloroquine and ibuprofen as needed. She is otherwise healthy and takes no other medications.

On examination, her best-corrected visual acuity is 20/25 OU with normal intraocular pressures. Osmolarity testing reveals a value of 308 mOsm/L OD and 315 mOsm/L OS. Evaluation of the external periocular skin shows no rashes or skin findings. On slit lamp examination, moderate telangiectasias are observed on her lower eyelid margins, and the bulbar conjunctivas have mild hyperemia. On fluorescein examination, tear film breakup time (TFBUT) is 7 s and 9 s in the right and left eye, respectively. The patient has a decreased tear lake OU with 3+ punctate epithelial erosions in the inferior cornea. Schirmer's testing with anesthesia reveals 4 mm of wetting OD and 3 mm of wetting OS after 5 min. InflammaDry (RPS Technologies, Tampa) is positive with a moderate-strength band in both eyes. The remaining ocular examination is otherwise unremarkable.

What Do These Findings Mean?

These examination findings suggest that the patient has aqueous deficient dry eye (DE). The definition of dry eye provided by the 2007 international dry eye workshop (DEWS) report is "a multifactorial disease of the tears and ocular surface that results in symptoms of discomfort, visual disturbance, and tear firm instability with potential damage to the ocular surface. It is accompanied by increased osmolarity of the tear film and inflammation of the ocular surface" [30].

Given its multifactorial nature, no single test can identify all dry eye patients. A number of different diagnostic tests are used to evaluate different components of the ocular surface.

Tear Volume

Tear film volume can be examined using the slit lamp to observe the tear meniscus. An inferior tear meniscus height of less than 1 mm (in the absence of significant conjunctivochalasis obliterating the meniscus) suggests aqueous deficiency [30]. High-resolution anterior segment optical coherence tomography (OCT) has been more recently used to assess the inferior tear meniscus. The meniscus is first imaged with the machine, and the image is then used to calculate inferior tear meniscus volume [31].

A Schirmer strip can be used, either with an anesthetic (a measure of basal secretion) or without an anesthetic (a measure of basal secretion and reflex tearing) [30, 32] to measure tear production. The Schirmer's test is performed by placing a small strip of filter paper on the margin of the lower eyelid, leaving it in place for 5 min and measuring the length of the strip that is wet with tears. A value greater than 10 mm of wetting is considered adequate, and several cutoff values for dry eye have been recommended including less than 5 or 8 mm of wetting [30]. This is variable however, and other clinicians use a value of 7 mm for the Schirmer's test without anesthetic and 3 mm for the Schirmer's test with anesthetic [29].

Tear Film Stability

Fluorescein TFBUT measures tear film stability after a fluorescein dye drop is instilled in the tear film. Observation through the slit lamp can show the early breakup of the fluorescein across the cornea, seen as a dark spot forming through the tear film [30, 31]. A TFBUT less than the normal 10 s is a sign of rapid tear film breakup, an indicator of tear instability. Any perturbation in the tear film, including aqueous tear deficiency or lipid deficiency (meibomian gland dysfunction), can lead to an abnormal tear breakup time.

Epithelial Disruption

Aqueous deficiency can also lead to disruption of the corneal and conjunctival epithelial cells. Evaluation of epithelial cell health is performed with the instillation of topical dyes, such as fluorescein and lissamine green [30, 32].

Osmolarity

Elevated tear film osmolarity is another finding that may be present in DE. Tear hyperosmolarity results from aqueous evaporation from the ocular surface, which can occur due to low tear volume, fast evaporation, or a combination of both. In general, a value of 305 mOsm/L or greater is considered mildly elevated and of 318 mOsm/L or greater as severely elevated as shown in a study by Versura et al., with high positive predictive values and likelihood ratios [33]. A difference of 10 mOsm/L between the eyes or after repeated measurements in the same eye also suggests a dysfunctional tear film as a stable osmolarity measurement over time is one metric of a healthy tear film.

Inflammation

Levels of inflammatory mediators, such as interferon gamma, interleukin 1, interleukin 17, and others, have been shown to correlate with the severity of ocular surface disease [34]. Up until recently, however, measurement of inflammatory mediators on the ocular surface has not been routinely available. InflammaDry is a new diagnostic test that can detect matrix metalloproteinase-9 (MMP-9) on the ocular surface. The InflammaDry test of MMP9 should be performed prior to administering ocular anesthetic, topical dyes, or the Schirmer's test. Tear samples are collected from the palpebral conjunctiva with the sample collector fleece until it glistens, indicating that the sampling fleece is saturated. The sampling fleece is then placed within the test cassette with the addition of buffer solution. Within 10 min, if there is an MMP-9 antibody-antigen interaction on the immunoassay test strip, the result window will read positive with two lines (one blue and the other one red). The test provides a qualitative (yes/no) response. According to the manufacturer, the intensity of the red line is directly related to the amount of MMP-9 present. The lower detection limit of the test is 40 ng/mL [35]. The intensity of the band probably does provide some quantitative information, but this has not been validated.

Our impression is that this patient has moderate to severe dry eyes in the setting of a rheumatologic disease (rheumatoid arthritis). This raises the suspicion for Sjögren's syndrome.

What Further Evaluation Would You Consider for the Patient?

Thus, the presence of Sjögren's syndrome should be evaluated for by eliciting a thorough clinical history, examining the ocular surface and oral mucosa, and obtaining a serology panel, including rheumatoid factor (RF) and antinuclear antibodies (ANAs) which are sensitive for autoimmune diseases but not specific for Sjögren's. Within the ANA, a subset panel, the extractable nuclear antigens (ENAs), should be ordered to look for ANAs that bind to the ENAs, called anti-ENAs which include anti-RO (SS-A) and anti-La (SS-B) antibodies. Anti-RO (SS-A) and anti-La (SS-B) have a higher specificity for Sjögren's (positive in 70–95% and 60–90% of patients, respectively) [36]. Newer studies have identified additional antibodies in patients with SS to salivary gland protein 1 (SP-1), carbonic anhydrase 6 (CA6), and parotid secretory protein (PSP). Thus, SP-1, CA6, and PSP may be helpful in diagnosing other subsets of SS patients and perhaps aid in earlier diagnosis as recently shown in animal studies [37]. Negative serology, however, does not rule out SSs, and some patients with clinical evidence of SS may not have positive titers for these antibodies. In these cases, further testing may be necessary, including a salivary gland biopsy, performed by an ENT or oral surgeon.

Early diagnosis of SS is important given the risk of extraglandular manifestations, including cryoglobulinemia, vasculitis, anemia, leukopenia, and thrombocytopenia [38]. Patients with more severe sicca symptoms and those who develop extraglandular disease may need to be treated more aggressively with systemic medications such as hydroxychloroquine rather than the local measures used in those with milder sicca symptoms alone [39]. Although oral hydroxychloroquine has not been shown to improve dry eye, early institution of treatment is believed to improve salivary gland function [40] and may prevent progression to neoplastic transformation by modulating lymphoproliferation [41]. Rituximab has also been shown to be therapeutic in the treatment of severe extraglandular manifestations but also has not been shown to improve ocular symptoms so it is not recommended purely for ocular disease.

How Does Positive MMP Testing Affect Your Management of Patients with Ocular Surface Disease?

A positive MMP test provides objective evidence of inflammation on the ocular surface. Therefore, the patient should be given a trial of anti-inflammatory therapy. We typically start with a mild steroid such as loteprednol 0.05% or fluorometholone 0.01% (whenever available we prefer preservative-free steroids such as methylprednisolone) starting 2–3 times a day then tapering down to once a day by 1 month. If the patient feels improved on the steroids, then an anti-inflammatory agent such as cyclosporine 0.05% or lifitegrast is added while the steroids are tapered off or tapered down to once or twice a week.

Upon further questioning, the patient does report symptoms of dry mouth and a history of frequent dental caries. Serology comes back with high titers of +anti-RO and +anti-LA, and an official diagnosis of Sjögren's syndrome is made. She continued to use preservative-free artificial tears 6–8 times a day and has made lifestyle modifications such as sleeping with the fan off and increasing essential fatty acids in her diet. Given the inflammatory nature of her disease and the positive MMP testing, the patient was started on cyclosporine emulsion 0.05% BID OU and fluorometholone 0.01% BID for 1 month and then daily. The patient comes back to clinic after 2 months and reports that

her symptoms are improved but not eliminated. Her steroids are tapered down to one or twice a week.

The patient is offered a choice of punctal occlusion or serum tears as the next step and prefers to go with serum tears first. Patient is started on autologous serum tears 20% four times a day, and 3 months later, she reported a significant improvement in her dry eye symptoms. In addition, corneal staining improved in both eyes. This patient continues to be monitored for ocular surface disease (while also being monitored for hydroxychloroquine toxicity on a yearly basis).

References

1. American Psychiatric Association. Diagnostic and statistical manual of mental disorders. 5th ed. Arlington, VA: American Psychiatric Publishing; 2013.
2. Simon GE, VonKorff M, Piccinelli M, Fullerton C, Ormel J. An international study of the relation between somatic symptoms and depression. N Engl J Med. 1999;341:1329–35. doi:10.1056/NEJM199910283411801.
3. Williams JW Jr, Pignone M, Ramirez G, Perez Stellato C. Identifying depression in primary care: a literature synthesis of case-finding instruments. Gen Hosp Psychiatry. 2002;24:225–37.
4. Subica AM, et al. Factor structure and diagnostic validity of the Beck Depression Inventory-II with adult clinical inpatients: comparison to a gold-standard diagnostic interview. Psychol Assess. 2014;26:1106–15. doi:10.1037/a0036998.
5. Caro XJ, Winter EF, Dumas AJ. A subset of fibromyalgia patients have findings suggestive of chronic inflammatory demyelinating polyneuropathy and appear to respond to IVIg. Rheumatology. 2008;47:208–11. doi:10.1093/rheumatology/kem345.
6. Arnold LM, Gebke KB, Choy EH. Fibromyalgia: management strategies for primary care providers. Int J Clin Pract. 2016;70:99–112. doi:10.1111/ijcp.12757.
7. Clauw DJ. Pain management: Fibromyalgia drugs are 'as good as it gets' in chronic pain. Nat Rev Rheumatol. 2010;6:439–40. doi:10.1038/nrrheum.2010.120.
8. Anxiety and Depression. http://www.adaa.org/about-adaa/press-room/facts-statistics.
9. Labbe A, et al. Dry eye disease, dry eye symptoms and depression: the Beijing Eye Study. Br J Ophthalmol. 2013;97:1399–403. doi:10.1136/bjophthalmol-2013-303838.
10. Kim KW, et al. Association between depression and dry eye disease in an elderly population. Invest Ophthalmol Vis Sci. 2011;52:7954–8. doi:10.1167/iovs.11-8050.
11. Vehof J, Sillevis Smitt-Kamminga N, Kozareva D, Nibourg SA, Hammond CJ. Clinical characteristics of dry eye patients with chronic pain syndromes. Am J Ophthalmol. 2016;162:59–65 e52. doi:10.1016/j.ajo.2015.11.017.
12. Galor A, et al. Depression, post-traumatic stress disorder, and dry eye syndrome: a study utilizing the national United States Veterans Affairs administrative database. Am J Ophthalmol. 2012;154:340–346 e342. doi:10.1016/j.ajo.2012.02.009.
13. Anderson IM, et al. Evidence-based guidelines for treating depressive disorders with antidepressants: a revision of the 2000 British Association for Psychopharmacology guidelines. J Psychopharmacol. 2008;22:343–96. doi:10.1177/0269881107088441.
14. Uher R, et al. Early and delayed onset of response to antidepressants in individual trajectories of change during treatment of major depression: a secondary analysis of data from the Genome-Based Therapeutic Drugs for Depression (GENDEP) study. J Clin Psychiatry. 2011;72:1478–84. doi:10.4088/JCP.10m06419.
15. Papakostas GI, Perlis RH, Scalia MJ, Petersen TJ, Fava M. A meta-analysis of early sustained response rates between antidepressants and placebo for the treatment of major depressive disorder. J Clin Psychopharmacol. 2006;26:56–60.

16. Posternak MA, Zimmerman M. Is there a delay in the antidepressant effect? A meta-analysis. J Clin Psychiatry. 2005;66:148–58.
17. Hauser W, Bernardy K, Uceyler N, Sommer C. Treatment of fibromyalgia syndrome with antidepressants: a meta-analysis. JAMA. 2009;301:198–209. doi:10.1001/jama.2008.944.
18. Hauser W, Petzke F, Sommer C. Comparative efficacy and harms of duloxetine, milnacipran, and pregabalin in fibromyalgia syndrome. J Pain. 2010;11:505–21. doi:10.1016/j.jpain.2010.01.002.
19. Hauser W, Petzke F, Uceyler N, Sommer C. Comparative efficacy and acceptability of amitriptyline, duloxetine and milnacipran in fibromyalgia syndrome: a systematic review with meta-analysis. Rheumatology (Oxford). 2011;50:532–43. doi:10.1093/rheumatology/keq354.
20. Brummett CM, et al. Survey criteria for fibromyalgia independently predict increased postoperative opioid consumption after lower-extremity joint arthroplasty: a prospective, observational cohort study. Anesthesiology. 2013;119:1434–43. doi:10.1097/ALN.0b013e3182a8eb1f.
21. Hutchinson MR, et al. Non-stereoselective reversal of neuropathic pain by naloxone and naltrexone: involvement of toll-like receptor 4 (TLR4). Eur J Neurosci. 2008;28:20–9. doi:10.1111/j.1460-9568.2008.06321.x.
22. Myers JS. Proinflammatory cytokines and sickness behavior: implications for depression and cancer-related symptoms. Oncol Nurs Forum. 2008;35:802–7. doi:10.1188/08.ONF.802-807.
23. Watkins LR, et al. Norman Cousins Lecture. Glia as the "bad guys": implications for improving clinical pain control and the clinical utility of opioids. Brain Behav Immun. 2007;21:131–46. doi:10.1016/j.bbi.2006.10.011.
24. Goldenberg DL, Burckhardt C, Crofford L. Management of fibromyalgia syndrome. JAMA. 2004;292:2388–95. doi:10.1001/jama.292.19.2388.
25. Carville SF, et al. EULAR evidence-based recommendations for the management of fibromyalgia syndrome. Ann Rheum Dis. 2008;67:536–41. doi:10.1136/ard.2007.071522.
26. Mist SD, Firestone KA, Jones KD. Complementary and alternative exercise for fibromyalgia: a meta-analysis. J Pain Res. 2013;6:247–60. doi:10.2147/JPR.S32297.
27. Li YH, Wang FY, Feng CQ, Yang XF, Sun YH. Massage therapy for fibromyalgia: a systematic review and meta-analysis of randomized controlled trials. PLoS One. 2014;9:e89304. doi:10.1371/journal.pone.0089304.
28. Williams JA, Imamura M, Fregni F. Updates on the use of non-invasive brain stimulation in physical and rehabilitation medicine. J Rehabil Med. 2009;41:305–11. doi:10.2340/16501977-0356.
29. Hargrove JB, et al. A randomized placebo-controlled study of noninvasive cortical electrostimulation in the treatment of fibromyalgia patients. Pain Med. 2012;13:115–24. doi:10.1111/j.1526-4637.2011.01292.x.
30. The definition and classification of dry eye disease: report of the Definition and Classification Subcommittee of the International Dry Eye WorkShop. Ocul Surf. 2007;5:75–92.
31. Wang J, Palakuru JR, Aquavella JV. Correlations among upper and lower tear menisci, noninvasive tear break-up time, and the Schirmer test. Am J Ophthalmol. 2008;145:795–800. doi:10.1016/j.ajo.2007.12.035.
32. Methodologies to diagnose and monitor dry eye disease: report of the Diagnostic Methodology Subcommittee of the International Dry Eye WorkShop. Ocul Surf. 2007;5:108–152.
33. Versura P, Profazio V, Campos EC. Performance of tear osmolarity compared to previous diagnostic tests for dry eye diseases. Curr Eye Res. 2010;35:553–64. doi:10.3109/02713683.2010.484557.
34. Acera A, Rocha G, Vecino E, Lema I, Duran JA. Inflammatory markers in the tears of patients with ocular surface disease. Ophthalmic Res. 2008;40:315–21. doi:10.1159/000150445. 000150445 [pii]
35. Sambursky R, et al. Sensitivity and specificity of a point-of-care matrix metalloproteinase 9 immunoassay for diagnosing inflammation related to dry eye. JAMA Ophthalmol. 2013;131:24–8. doi:10.1001/jamaophthalmol.2013.561.
36. Kumar V, Abbas AK, Fausto N, Robbins SL, Cotran RS. Robbins and Cotran pathologic basis of disease. 7th ed. Philadelphia: Elsevier Saunders; 2005.

37. Shen L, et al. Novel autoantibodies in Sjogren's syndrome. Clin Immunol. 2012;145:251–5. doi:10.1016/j.clim.2012.09.013.
38. Alexander EL, Arnett FC, Provost TT, Stevens MB. Sjogren's syndrome: association of anti-Ro(SS-A) antibodies with vasculitis, hematologic abnormalities, and serologic hyperreactivity. Ann Intern Med. 1983;98:155–9.
39. Venables PJ. Management of patients presenting with Sjogren's syndrome. Best Pract Res Clin Rheumatol. 2006;20:791–807. doi:10.1016/j.berh.2006.05.003.
40. Dawson LJ, et al. Hydroxychloroquine therapy in patients with primary Sjogren's syndrome may improve salivary gland hypofunction by inhibition of glandular cholinesterase. Rheumatology (Oxford). 2005;44:449–55. doi:10.1093/rheumatology/keh506.
41. Fox RI, et al. Treatment of primary Sjogren's syndrome with hydroxychloroquine. Am J Med. 1988;85:62–7.

Chapter 11
Recognition and Management of Obstructive Sleep Apnea (OSA)-Related Eye Disease

Charles S. Bouchard

Case 1: History

ER is a 48-year-old Hispanic male who is referred for evaluation of a chief complaint of irritation in the right eye greater than left eye for about a year. The patient has been told he has a growth on both eyes as well. He also complains of some blurred vision and redness in both eyes with mild itching and some tearing, right eye greater than left eye.

His past medical history is significant for diabetes and rosacea. His family history is positive for hypertension, glaucoma, and snoring in his father and brother.

His past ocular history is significant for mild myopia, mild bilateral pterygium, and contact lens wear which has become more intolerant. A social history query from the patient and his spouse elicits snoring at night. He did not have any sleep preference side.

For his history of his present illness, he comes with a diagnosis of dry eye, pterygium, and blepharitis. He has been seen by several eye care providers, and his ocular irritation has been managed with a variety of topical mediations including preservative-free artificial tears, loteprednol (which has been somewhat helpful), cyclosporine ophthalmic emulsion (Restasis®), azithromycin, and olopatadine (Patanol®). He was also tried oral doxycycline and warm compresses. He stopped the doxycycline secondary to gastrointestinal upset.

Electronic supplementary material The online version of this chapter (doi:10.1007/978-3-319-15823-5_11) contains supplementary material, which is available to authorized users.

C.S. Bouchard, MD, MA
Loyola University Medical Center, 2160 S First Ave, Maywood, IL 60153, USA
e-mail: cboucha@lumc.edu

A.R. Djalilian (ed.), *Ocular Surface Disease*,
https://doi.org/10.1007/978-3-319-15823-5_11

What Is Your Approach to Patients with Ocular Complaints of Irritation, Burning, Fluctuating Vision, and Some Itching?

In these patients it is most important to first obtain a careful **history** of each symptom and their prior response to treatment. The use of the OSDI questionnaire is a good start, and the score of 32 suggested mild to moderate ocular surface disease [1]. For the history, are the symptoms gradual or sudden in onset, are they constant or intermittent, and are there changes in vision with the symptoms and with the use of eye drops? What has been the response to environmental changes in humidity, wind, air conditioning, as well as response to topical and oral medications? Do the symptoms improve with eye closure? Are the symptoms worse at the end of the day? Is there prolonged time spent on a computer? Is the level of the computer low or horizontal (lid fissures and tear evaporation) and do the symptoms change significantly with an elevated viewing angle? These are all critical history questions in evaluating the ocular surface disease patient. A careful snoring history needs to be obtained from both the patient and partner as a key element for the diagnosis of sleep apnea and lax eyelid condition (LEC) [2–5] (Fig. 11.1).

In discussing the nature of the ocular surface disease and its management with the patient, an important step is to address the patient's expectations. The **chronic nature** of the disease must be made clear and that completely eliminating the symptoms may not be possible but that definite but small improvements in symptoms are what we look for. The **goals of therapy** are to improve not eliminate the symptoms, and the improvement might be definite but slight. No response must be carefully distinguished from small improvements since the incremental improvement is the very goal of the various approaches to therapy.

Using the treatments at the **appropriate frequency** and duration is also important. Questioning the patient if the treatment helps or does not help is important. If the treatment helps, then what is the least frequent dose/regimen to provide this help

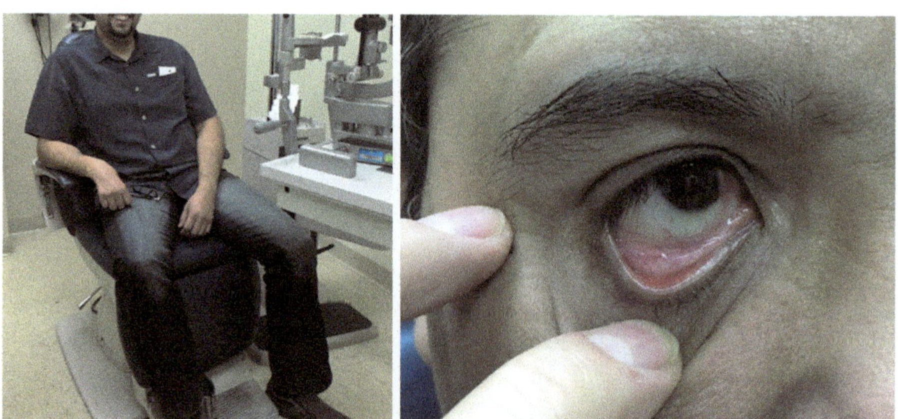

Fig. 11.1 Lax eyelid condition (LEC) in nonobese patient (Case 1) with sleep apnea (peak 70 s without breathing)

is key. The corollary of this approach is to stop treatments that do not help. The targeted **therapy schedule** should also be reviewed with the patient. For those treatments that the patient feels help, then the next step is to reduce the frequency of the treatment until they arrive at the least effective dose. Finally it is important to emphasize to patients that managing chronic ocular surface disease requires a **prophylactic approach**. They are used to prevent/reduce the symptoms. I use the sunscreen analogy. If you get sunburned and then run onto the house to put the sunscreen on and discover it not effective, that is not a problem with the sunscreen.

The ocular surface exam and diagnostic testing must also be equally sequence systematic and thorough [6]. This always includes an external exam, slit lamp exam, diagnostic testing, and immediate assessment of responses to drops (i.e., anesthetic). If patients deny improvement in symptoms following topical anesthetic, then other explanations for the symptoms need to be explored.

The **external exam** must include the skin type (Fitzpatrick scale), presence of rosacea, eyelid position (retraction, ptosis, lagophthalmos, entropion, ectropion), presence and degree of laxity (graded as % tarsal conjunctiva visible with moderate upper lid skin elevation [7]), direction of the eyelashes (eyelash ptosis, trichiasis), and resting blink frequency. Pen light exam of the eyelids, conjunctiva on manual lid retraction and elevation can also provide useful information (conjunctival subepithelial fibrosis, fornix shortening, symblepharon, pinguecula, and papillary reaction (from the light reflex off the bulbar conjunctiva)).

Slit lamp exam should focus on the *eyelid margins* including keratinization, meibomian glands (volume, plugging, thickening, vascularization, dropout), presence of demodex mites, and any subtle blond eyelashes. Next should be the *tear film* including meniscus, quality of the film (oily), and breakup time (BUT). The *conjunctival* exam should identify conjunctivochalasis, temporal lid parallel conjunctival folds (LIPCOFs) [8], lymphangiectasis, vascular dilation (focal and diffuse), and lissamine green staining presence and distribution (van Bijsterveld Index) [9]. The *corneal exam* should focus on the limbal neovascularization, presence and distribution of punctate staining, filaments, anterior basement membrane dystrophy, and focal keratitis. The anterior chamber and lens exams should also be documented.

Diagnostic testing should first include the findings from the ocular surface disease index (OSDI) [1], Schirmer (without anesthetic, 3 min), vital dye staining (fluorescein, Rose Bengal, lissamine green) of the cornea and bulbar and tarsal conjunctiva, tear breakup time (TBUT), and objective evaluation of the meibomian glands (plugging, volume, vascularization, thickening). Additional diagnostic testing options include the following: matrix metalloproteinase (MMP) testing (InflammaDry®), tear osmolarity (TearLab), Meibography (e.g., Lipiview®) impression cytology, and OCT quantitation of tear meniscus height [6].

On physical exam, the patient was a well-nourished man with normal habitus and BMI. His vision was 20/20 and 20/25 with spectacle correction. Pupil and confrontation visual field exams were normal.

On external exam your patient demonstrated eyelash ptosis, peau d'orange periocular skin changes, as well as rosacea, grade 2–3 eyelid laxity with medial canthal laxity [7]. The eyelid position demonstrated mild ptosis of the right eye with good levator function in both eyes. There was slight lower lid ectropion but

no entropion or misdirected lashes. The tarsal conjunctiva demonstrated 1−+ diffuse papillary conjunctivitis and the bulbar conjunctiva trace to 1+ injection.

Slit lamp exam demonstrated no keratinization of the lid margin or ocular surface, 2+ meibomian gland dysfunction with plugging, thickening, and mild gland dropout. No demodex mites were observed. There were no lid parallel conjunctival folds and no conjunctival lissamine staining, but a mild decreased BUT. The cornea demonstrated trace-1+ inferior fluorescein staining and minimal limbal vascularization. The rest of the slit lamp exam, anterior chamber, and lens were normal.

Fundus exam demonstrated a c/d ratio of .4 OU, with a normal posterior pole.

Diagnostic testing included a Schirmer 1 test result of 18 mm/20 mm without anesthetic at 3 min, a positive InflammaDry® testing for matrix metalloproteinase (MMP), and a tear osmolarity reading of 305 and 308.

At This Point, What Do You Conclude from the History and Exam?

In creating a differential diagnosis, it is also important to be systematic. We use the D4Vitamins mnemonic (Diet, Developmental, Drug, Degenerative, Vascular, Infectious, Traumatic/Toxic, Anoxic/Autoimmune, Metabolic, Endocrine, Neoplastic, Special) to run through the possibilities. This reduces the likelihood of overlooking a possible diagnosis by quickly jumping to conclusions from a few of the patient's complaints and some of the physical findings.

At this point, the patient has mild ocular surface disease with associated findings of rosacea and lax eyelids. There were no dietary restrictions in the history, and there were no findings to support vascular, infectious, metabolic, endocrine, neoplastic, and traumatic etiologies. He was not taking long-term preserved topical agents suggesting that a toxic etiology less likely. A Schirmer result of 18/20 rules out aqueous tear deficiency. A grade 2 mild laxity finding with a positive history of snoring suggests lax eyelid syndrome with possible sleep apnea even though the patient was not overweight. This is also supported by a positive family history of snoring. A sleep study was recommended.

Additional *review of systems* uncovers that the patient had a sleep study after his wife noticed that he would stop breathing at night and she would have to shake him to wake him up and get him to start breathing. Following the sleep study, he reported a peak apneic episode of 70 s (see video attached).

Floppy Eyelid Syndrome and Sleep Apnea

Floppy eyelid syndrome (FES) was first reported by Culbertson in 1981 and later by Parunovic and characterized by overweight young men with distensible eyelids and chronic conjunctivitis [3, 4]. Netland (1994) reported the histological findings of a reduction in elastin in the eyelid of FES patients [10]. Schlotzer (2005) further characterized the involvement of MMP in FES in addition to elastin reduction [11]. Series (2004) reported elastin disorganization in the soft palate of patients with snoring that underwent uvulopalatopharyngectomy [12]. Although it was unclear if the elastin changes were the cause or result of the snoring trauma, this finding suggests a possible systemic elastin dysfunction in these patients.

Woog first reported the association of sleep apnea and the lax eyelids in 1990 [13]. Multiple papers have reported this relationship, and Chambe in 2012 reported a 35% incidence of OSA in patients with FES [14]. Others have reported 90–100% of patients with FES have OSAS [15–19]. There might be a genetic association in OSA [20] (Fig. 11.2).

Van den Bosch (1994) introduced the condition of "lax eyelid syndrome" (LES) with similar findings in nonobese individuals of any sex [2]. Finally, Fowler and Dutton (2010) broadened the finding of eyelid laxity and associated findings and divided the laxity into three categories: lax eyelid condition (LEC), lax eyelids of any age without associated eye findings; lax eyelid syndrome (LES), adding ocular surface changes conjunctivitis to the LEC; and finally floppy eyelid syndrome, FES in overweight men [5]. The association of eyelid laxity with ocular surface disease is well documented [21–26] (Figs. 11.3, 11.4 and 11.5).

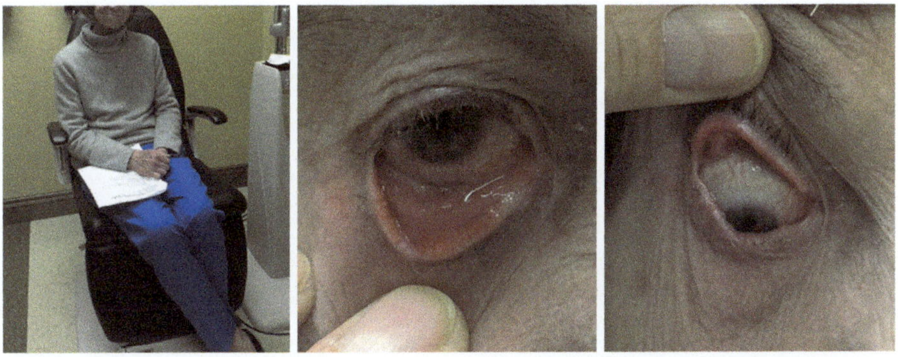

Fig. 11.2 Nonobese patient with glaucoma, lax eye syndrome (LES), and OSAS (Case 2)

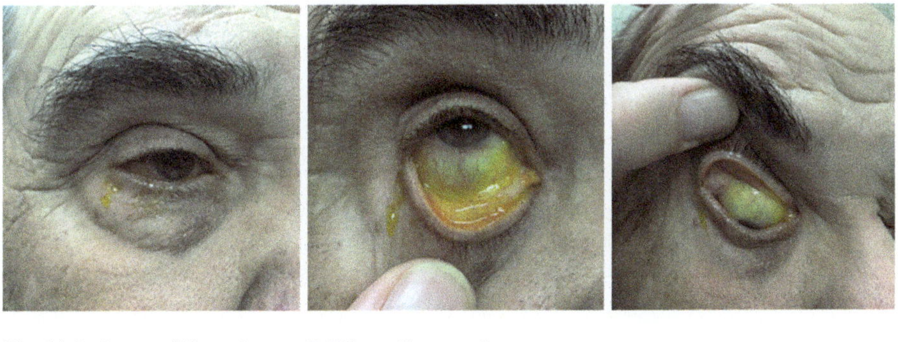

Fig. 11.3 Lax eyelid syndrome (LES), undiagnosed

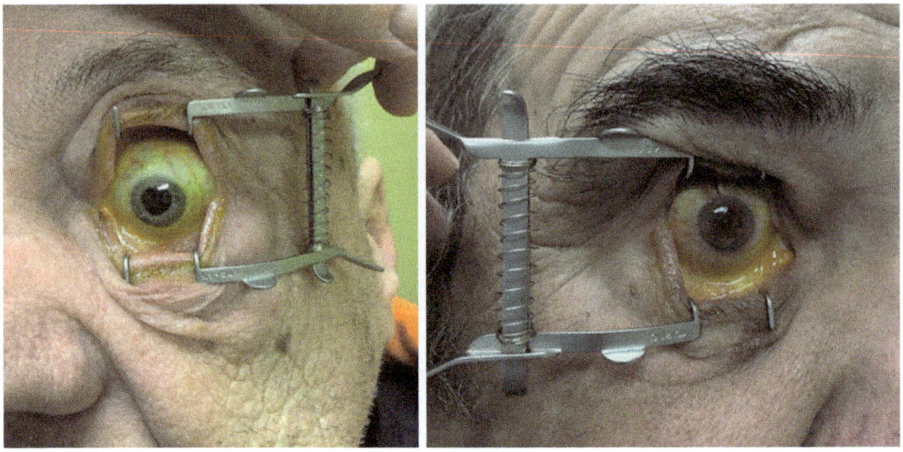

Fig. 11.4 Laxometer device for quantitating lid laxity

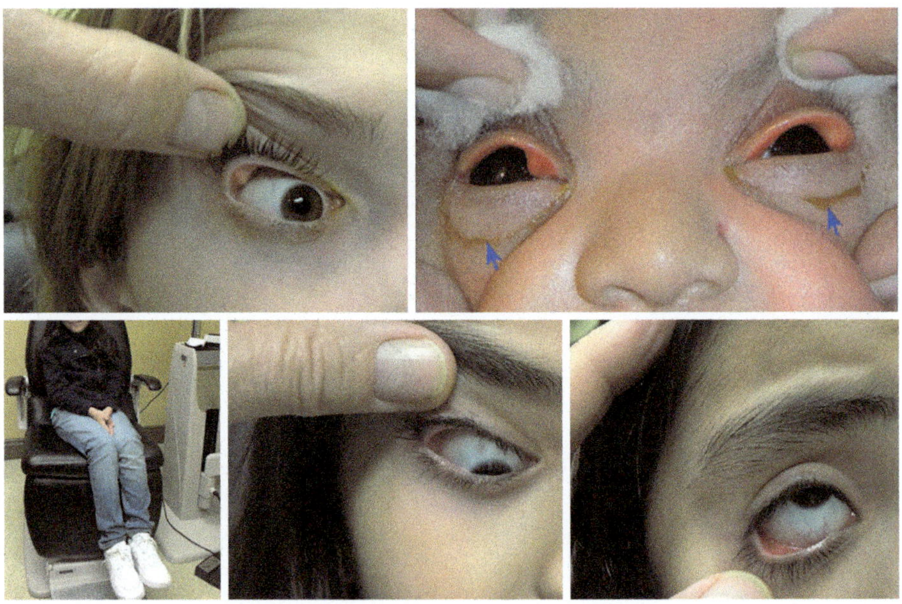

Fig. 11.5 Lax eyelid condition (LEC) (any age)

What Is the Association Between Ocular Surface Disease, Sleep Apnea And Floppy (Lax) Eyelid Syndrome?

The ocular surface changes are definitely associated with floppy eyelids. Acar et al. reported on 280 patients with OSAHS with OHS severity determined by AHI Index [27]. They all underwent a complete eye exam with Schirmer, TBUT, and ocular surface staining. Each patient also completed the OSDI questionnaire. FES was present in 23% of the non OHSH group, 41.7% in the mild OSHS group, 66.7% in the moderate, and 74.6% in the severe OSAS group. The OSDI questionnaire, Schirmer test, TBUT, and corneal staining all demonstrated a significant correlation with the severity of the OSAS.

What Are the Next Steps in the Management of This Patient?

The chronic low-grade inflammation associated with the chronic papillary conjunctivitis associated with lax eyelid syndrome may be due in part to elevation in MMP in the tear film. The inflammatory mediators associated with the rosacea blepharoconjunctivitis probably also contribute to the process. OSDI, TBUT, and ocular surface staining need to be carefully evaluated in patients with FES and OSAH [22]. Treatment needs to be directed toward reducing inflammation and repair the eyelid to globe apposition. This can be accomplished through lateral canthal ligament tightening and or full thickness wedge resection. Management of the meibomian gland dysfunction with topical azithromycin 1% (AzaSite®), compresses, and tetracyclines may also help [28, 29].

What Were the Outcomes of the Management?

The diagnosis of lax eyelid syndrome (LES) was made, and the patient had an upper lid wedge resection and lateral canthal tightening [30, 31]. There was better apposition of the lid against the globe. The signs and symptoms improved over 2–3-week period. The punctate keratitis and discharge resolved. The lateral lower lid ectropion improved as well. The lash ptosis also improved slightly. Histological specimens demonstrated moderate subconjunctival chronic inflammatory infiltrate especially around the accessory lacrimal tissue with bacterial colonies on the conjunctival surface [10, 11]. The tarsal plate demonstrated lipomatous atrophy, and the dermis showed severe elastic degeneration. Demodex brevis was present in the meibomian glands.

Summary and Conclusions

1. **Evaluation of all patients with complaints of chronic irritation should include a careful evaluation of the eyelid laxity including distraction test of both the upper and lower lids as well as tarsal conjunctival inflammation.**
2. **Patients with complaints of chronic irritation with a normal Schirmer and who are unresponsive to frequent topical preservative-free tear drops should**

suggest a diagnosis other than aqueous tear deficiency (lax eyelids, allergic conjunctivitis, conjunctival chalasis, etc.).

3. **Identification of lax eyelids should prompt an evaluation of sleep apnea and the many associated ocular (and systemic) neurovascular diseases associated with sleep apnea (glaucoma, ischemic optic neuropathy, papilledema, retinal vein occlusion).**

Case 2

A 66-year-old Caucasian woman was referred for a glaucoma management. Her past medical history is significant for diabetes, hypertension, hypercholesterolemia, and atrial fibrillation. She denies a family history of glaucoma. Her ocular medications included brimonidine/timolol drops (Combigan®), latanoprost (Xalatan®), and preservative-free artificial tears. Her systemic medications included amiodarone, atorvastatin, and enalapril (Vasotec).

On external exam she had mild rosacea and bilateral slight lash ptosis. She had moderate lid laxity (grade 2), with mild papillary conjunctivitis .

Slit lamp exam demonstrated mild papillary conjunctivitis, mild arcus, and mild nuclear sclerotic cataract. There was no punctate staining and the Schirmer was 18 both eyes.

Fundus exam demonstrated an optic nerve cup to disk ratio of 0.7 in both eyes. The remainder of her fundus exam demonstrated mild vascular attenuation and a normal macula. Her applanation pressures were 14 and 15. Humphrey visual field testing demonstrated bilateral superior arcuate scotomas. OCT testing demonstrated moderate NFL loss bilaterally.

Remembering the Mechanical and Ischemic Causes of Glaucoma, What Other Tests Might Be Helpful to Explain the Progressive Visual Loss with Pressures in the Mid to Low Teens?

Carotid ultrasounds, CT, and MRI imaging were normal. Diurnal and nocturnal IOP measurements were all less than 17. A 24-h electrocardiogram demonstrated intermittent atrial fibrillation. She was started on amiodarone with resolution of the atrial fibrillation. Over several years her HVF continued to worsen in spite of pressures less than 15 mmHg.

Upon further questioning, the patient reported a history of daytime fatigue, difficulty concentrating, and some morning headache. She admits to snoring occasionally, and her spouse confirms that the snoring occurs more regularly.

What Are the Next Steps in the Diagnosis and/or Management of This Patient?

The history of snoring and daytime fatigue as well as her lax eyelids should prompt a suspicion of sleep apnea [32–35]. The patient was sent for a polysomnography (PSG), and she was diagnosed with obstructive sleep apnea syndrome (OSAS). Upper airway obstruction can be classified into three categories: (1) OSAS, the most severe associated with complete cessation of airflow associated with daytime sleepiness, (2) sleep hypopnea, and (3) upper airway resistance syndrome which is snoring without a significant decrease in airflow. Not all patients with OSA have daytime sleepiness and are described as having OSA. Most patients do not remember waking at night during the apneic episode, which makes the diagnosis more difficult. OSAS is defined as > 5 apnea/hypopnea events (AHI)/hour, and severity is graded as mild, moderate, and severe. The respiratory disturbance index (RDI) measures the number of events/hour. Symptoms of OSAS include daytime sleepiness, daytime headaches, difficulty concentrating, and memory problems (Faridi et al.). In sleep apnea, the patient does not remember awakening. The Joint National Committee on the Prevention, Detection, Evaluation and Treatment of High Blood Pressure identify OSAS as a treatable secondary cause of hypertension [36]. OSAS is also associated with pulmonary hypertension, myocardial infarction, cardiac arrhythmia, congestive heart failure, stroke, cardiac related mortality, and all-cause mortality [37, 38]. The Sleep Heart Health Study (SHHS) concluded that there was a definite relationship between RDI in patients with OSAS and stroke, heart failure, and vascular disease [39].

Glaucoma is a progressive optic neuropathy, an ocular neurodegenerative disorder that is characterized by optic nerve changes and characteristic visual field changes. Vascular risk factors include a variety of diseases associated with reduced blood flow and ischemia. Several of these disease including migraine, Raynaud's phenomenon, atrial fibrillation, and reduced nocturnal blood pressure can lead to decreased ocular perfusion pressure. These are just risk factors and not necessarily causes of the optic neuropathy. Although lowering IOP is the only established modifiable risk factor, it is well known that deterioration in the visual field can occur despite good IOP control stimulation a search into other modifiable factors. Faridi et al. published an excellent review of the role of sleep apnea and glaucoma [40].

In 1982, Walsh and Montplaisir first reported the association between glaucoma and OSAS [41]. During sleep, local and systemic vascular alterations also occur in that are balanced by local autoregulation in order to maintain homeostasis. However, in OSA, the normal physiological balance is upset. OSA is a potentially modifiable risk factor, which has been increasingly associated with glaucoma independent of intraocular pressure. OSAS is a common but often unrecognized disorder [42]. Because of the chronic intermittent hypoxia, OSAS has been increasingly associated with increasing risk of neurovascular disease (diabetes) including pulmonary, cardiovascular (atherosclerosis, heart disease, peripheral neuropathy), and cerebrovascular disease (stroke, cognitive decline, depression, headache, and nonarteritic ischemic optic neuropathy NION) [43–46]. The relationship between OSAS and glaucoma risk is controversial. Many studies support that the OSAS has also been known to be associated with glaucomatous optic neuropathy with 5.7–27% of glaucoma patients having OSAS [47–57]. Several studies have failed to demonstrate a relationship between OSAS and glaucoma [58–62]. Associations between RDI and VF indices have been reported. Shi et al. performed a meta-analysis of papers reporting the association of OSAS and glaucoma [63]. They reviewed 16 cross-sectional (six case control and nine cohorts) clinical studies with 2,278,832 participants. Pooled odd ratios were calculated for the association of OSAS and glaucoma. They found an adjusted hazard ratio of glaucoma in this OSAS population of 1.67 (95% CI = 1.30–2.17). Muniesa et al. found that FES was a risk factor for glaucoma in the OSA population [64].

Role of Vascular System in Glaucoma in Patients with OSAS

Perfusion Pressure (Blood Pressure: IOP)

The role of blood flow and ischemia in the pathophysiology of glaucoma is not well known. Drance reported in 1972 a series of NTG patients with about a third with a history of hemodynamic shock [65]. Progressive VF loss in the setting of normal or low IOP also suggests other factors than IOP. Low nocturnal perfusion pressure as a risk factor for glaucoma has support from several large studies [66]. The EMGT reported a decrease in risk of glaucoma with an elevation in systolic blood pressure [66]. The role of perfusion pressure in OSAS is also unclear. With a decrease in sympathetic tone at night, the normal blood pressure decreases by 10–20% or 15 mm. This is balanced by increase in ocular blood pressure from the supine position. There are conflicting reports regarding the role of lower systemic blood pressure in the pathophysiology of NTG due to local autoregulatory mechanisms. OSAS can alter the blood flow to the optic nerve and thus affect perfusion pressure. Mojon reported that the severity of the OSAS correlated with the severity of the glaucomatous nerve damage. OSAS associated with increased sympathetic tone can lead to vascular endothelial dysregulation from hypoxia mediated changes and can also affect optic nerve head blood flow.

Patients with a greater decrease in nocturnal blood pressure can be associated with progressive field loss [67].

The mechanical and vascular theories supporting the pathophysiology of glaucoma have support from OSAS. From the vascular theory, upper airway collapse leads to the hypoxia that stimulates sympathetic activation resulting in many effects including renin-angiotensin system activation and elevation in blood pressure.

Factors which can effect ocular perfusion and possibly glaucoma progression include: low blood pressure, IOP fluctuation, low intracranial pressure, and OSAS. CPAP can actually normalize the IOP as well as restore normal blood pressure [68]. The apnea-hypopnea index (AHI) was 60 and her respiratory disturbance index (RDI) with a peak apnea of 70 s and an oxygen saturation of 64%.

Hypopnea leads to hypoxia, which in combination with hypertension can lead to endothelial damage, decreasing responsiveness to nitric oxide. This results in autonomic dysfunction/altered blood flow from a vasodilation and vasoconstriction imbalance.

Hypoxia and subsequent reperfusion lead to oxidative stress, an inflammation with increased inflammatory markers and reactive oxygen species.

Autonomic Dysfunction

The increase in sympathetic tone in OSAS associated with intermittent hypoxic episodes is thought to result in endothelial damage [69]. Elevated levels of plasma and urine levels of catecholamines are found in OSAS. OSAS affects the vascular endothelium through oxidative stress, inflammation, atherosclerosis, and a decrease in nitric oxide [70, 71]. The vasoconstrictor endothelin-1 has been shown to upregulate in OSAS and in NTG [72]. OSAS then has a role in vascular regulation.

Ischemia

Although atherosclerosis and carotid vessel disease are not associated with glaucoma, silent cerebrovascular infarcts are elevated in patients with NTG [73]. Intermittent hypoxia, associated with vasospastic-induced ischemia such as migraine, has also been associated with LTG as reported by the Collaborative Normal Tension Glaucoma (CNTG) study. Hypoxia-induced platelet activation present in OSAS patients can be reduced with CPAP therapy [74].

Inflammation and Oxidative Stress

Intermittent hypoxia and reperfusion injury found in OSAS patients both systemically and in the eyelids result in inflammatory changes predisposing to glaucomatous damage.

Hypercapnia

Apnea results in peripheral vasoconstriction and then regional vasodilation of the cerebral and myocardial circulation. The post-apneic hyperventilation leads to hypocapnia and peripheral vasodilation. The lack of subsequent vasodilation in the ophthalmic vessels in glaucomatous eyes could then lead to a cerebrovascular "steal" from the blood flow to the optic nerve head. The hypercapnia also increases intracranial pressure as well as cause metabolic stress and acidosis.

Role of IOP in OSAS and Glaucoma

The mechanism for a mechanical cause is predicated on the pressure and structure of the lamina. IOP in normal and glaucoma patients peaks during the nighttime with elevations being unknown or unmeasured. IOP is determined by the amount of aqueous humor formation, the resistance of the outflow tracks, and the episcleral venous pressure. Aqueous formation decreases at night with a lower metabolic rate, but the episcleral venous pressure increases in the supine position. The stages of sleep and the autonomic nervous regulation of the hemodynamics also play a role. Although increases in systolic blood pressure might increase IOP, the amount is negligible. Inspiratory effort with closed glottis might actually lower episcleral venous pressure and lower IOP. One study found no change in IOP after prolonged apnea with NTG patients and OSAS. So the contribution to glaucomatous changed from IOP is probably minimal.

In addition to glaucoma, OSAS has also been associated with a variety of ocular diseases including: anterior ischemic optic neuropathy (AION), bilateral disk edema secondary to increase in intracranial hypertension, lax eyelids and lax eyelid syndrome, ptosis, papillary conjunctivitis, filamentary keratopathy, retinal vascular tortuosity, and central serous chorioretinopathy [33, 75–77].

What Are the Next Approaches to Therapy?

The patient was started on continuous positive airway pressure (CPAP) therapy. Her visual fields were monitored every 6 months and demonstrated no progression over 3-year period. This finding has been previously reported by Kremmer et al. [78].

Summary and Conclusions

1. **Glaucoma, as a progressive optic neuropathy, has both ocular and systemic risk factors and vascular risk factors that lead to reduced perfusion pressure including: migraine, atrial fibrillation, and nocturnal blood pressure reduction.**
2. **OSAS characterized by intermittent hypoxia is a modifiable risk factor for glaucoma for its non-IOP associated mechanisms including a reduction in optic nerve head perfusion pressure, autonomic dysfunction, ischemia, vascular inflammation, and oxidative stress.**

3. **The diagnosis and severity of OSAS, often overlooked, should be suspected in association of low-tension glaucoma and progressive HVF loss in the setting of normal/low IOP (Kremmer et al.).**
4. **Symptoms of OSAS (snoring, daytime sleepiness, daytime headaches, difficulty concentrating, and memory problems) should be investigated in patients with glaucoma.**
5. **CPAP may slow the progression of visual field loss in patients with OSAS and well-controlled IOP.**
6. **Ophthalmologists, otolaryngologists, and sleep physicians need to better understand the relationships between eye disease and OSAS.**

Case 3

A 61-year-old black male with a 10-year history of diabetes, hypertension, and hyperlipidemia presents with a chief complaint of sudden onset of peripheral vision loss in the right eye, which he noticed upon awakening in the morning. The visual change had been stable for 1 week. He denied prior episodes of transient vision loss in that eye. He denied any other associated ocular complaints. He denied history of migraine, collagen vascular disease, carotid artery disease, or endocrine disorder. He denied use of erectile dysfunction drugs.

On exam his visual acuity was 20/60. Pupil exam was normal. Confrontations visual field exam demonstrated a right peripheral field loss. Applanation pressures were 18 mmHg in both eyes.

External exam demonstrated grade 2 lax eyelids and mild lash ptosis.

Slit lamp exam demonstrated mild tarsal papillary conjunctivitis, mild bilateral bulbar conjunctival injection, mild conjunctivochalasis, normal corneas, and mild cataract.

Fundus exam demonstrated a branch retinal vein occlusion in the left eye. This was confirmed by fluorescein angiography. High-speed and high-resolution spectral domain OCT demonstrated a decreased mean choroidal thickness of 201 μm (324 μm in controls).

What Are the Risk Factors for Branch Retinal Vein Occlusion?

There are many well-known risk factors for retinal vein occlusion including hypertension and diabetes. Stem in 2013 reported on 494,165 enrollees over 55 years of age in a managed care network from 2001 to 2009 [79]. Black patients, prior dx stroke, and hypercoagulable state all had elevated risk for CRVO. Patients with end organ damage from diabetes or hypertension also had elevated risk for CRVO.

The seminal work by Sohan Singh Hayreh (1974) suggested a potential mechanism for vein occlusion which includes a hypoxia-induced vasodilation of the central retinal artery which compresses the central retinal vein sheath [80]. Hypercapnia-induced cerebral vasodilation leads to increased intracranial pressure, papilledema, and elevated venous pressure at the optic nerve head. This results in a slowing of the venous circulation. Elevated venous pressure leads to plasma leaving the vascular compartment with an increase in local viscosity. Fluctuations in oxygen and carbon dioxide function as metabolic stresses and overwhelm the autoregulatory capacity of the optic nerve head and retina. In sleep apnea, arousal from sleep associated with sympathetic stimulation can result in severe hemodynamic disturbances. In addition, platelet aggregability, endothelial dysfunction, and inflammation also play a role. These same mechanisms are also in operation for ischemic optic neuropathy [43, 80–82].

What Is the Significance of Choroidal Thinning in This Patient?

Thinning of the choroid as measured by OCT has been demonstrated in pathological myopia, age-related macular degeneration, glaucoma and diabetic retinopathy, and increased in Vogt-Koyanagi-Harada disease and central serous chorioretinopathy [83–85]. Choroidal thinning has also been demonstrated in patients with OSAS [86, 87]. Presumably, hypoxia and reperfusion episodes are responsible for the changes in OSAS, where they result in oxidative stress, inflammation, damage to vascular endothelium, and decreased responsiveness to nitric oxide. Insufficient vasodilation of vessels may then lead to a decrease in choroidal blood flow. Unlike retinal and optic nerve head vasculature, the choroidal circulation is subject to autonomic regulation. The impaired sympathetic autoregulation of the choroid in severe OSAS may be responsible for the thinner choroidal thickness vs. control. Chronic hypoxia and abnormal blood flow can lead to retinal cell damage, edema, pigment epithelial damage, blood-retinal barrier breakdown, and increased choroidal exudation to the retina. Sildenafil citrate has been shown to increase choroidal thickness due too secondary vasodilatory effect on the choroidal circulation [88]. Our patient denies this however.

Xin proposed a sympathetic nervous regulatory disorder in OSAS from the chronic intermittent hypoxia [86]. Mason et al. found patients with clinically significant macular edema have high prevalence of OSAS [89].

What Are the Known Systemic and Ocular Diseases Associated with OSAS?

The known systemic diseases associated with OSAS include hypertension, myocardial infarction, stroke, cardiac arrhythmia, and abnormal glucose metabolism. Ocular neurovascular diseases include glaucoma, nonarteritic anterior ischemic optic neuropathy (NAION), visual field defects, papilledema, and floppy eyelid syndrome.

Retinal vein occlusion has been reported in a large Taiwanese study of 35,634 patients (5965 patients with OSA and 29,669 controls). Patients with OSA had a 1.94-fold increase in incidence of RVO independent of age, gender, and comorbidities [90]. The pathogenesis is thought to result from a slowdown of retinal circulation. Glacet-Bernard et al. reported on 63 consecutive patients with RVO, with 30 patients having 2 of 3 risk factors: cardiovascular disease, snoring, and daytime sleepiness [91]. Seventy-seven percent of those (23 of 30) had OSAS by PSG. Mean age was 56.3 and mean follow-up 15 months (range 6–24 months). Of the 30 patients, 23 had CRVO, 5 had BRVO, and 2 had hemi central vein occlusion.

Summary and Conclusions

1. **Obstructive sleep apnea should be suspected in all vasculopathic patients with neurovascular ocular disease and especially in those who develop retinal vascular occlusion.**
2. **A careful personal history of snoring and daytime sleepiness should alert the clinician of the possibility of sleep apnea. A family history of snoring should also be elicited.**
3. **Careful examination of the laxity of the eyelids will increase the clinical support for the diagnosis of OSA.**

Acknowledgements *Financial Disclosures*: Charles Bouchard does not have any financial disclosures regarding the contents discussed in this chapter. *Conflict of Interest*: Charles Bouchard does not have any conflicts of interest regarding the contents discussed in this chapter.

References

1. Schiffman RM, Christianson MD, Jacobsen G, Hirsch JD, Reis BL. Reliability and validity of the ocular surface disease index. Arch Ophthalmol. 2000;118:615–21.
2. van den Bosch WA, Lemij HG. The lax eyelid syndrome. Br J Ophthalmol. 1994;78:666–70.
3. Culbertson WW, Ostler HB. The floppy eyelid syndrome. Am J Ophthalmol. 1981;92:568–75.
4. Parunovic A. Floppy eyelid syndrome. Br J Ophthalmol. 1983;67:264–6.
5. Fowler AM, Jonathan JD. Floppy eyelid syndrome as a subset of lax eyelid conditions: relationships and clinical relevance (an ASOPRS thesis). Ophthal Plast Reconstr Surg. 2010;26:195–204.
6. Messmer EM. The pathophysiology, diagnosis and treatment of dry eye disease. Dtsch Arztebl Int. 2015;112:71–82.
7. Liu DT, Di Pascuale MA, Sawai J, Gao YY, Tseng SC. Tear film dynamics in floppy eyelid syndrome. Invest Ophthalmol Vis Sci. 2005;46:1188–94.
8. Hoh H, Schirra F, Kienecker C, Ruprecht KW. Lid-parallel conjunctival folds are a sure diagnostic sign of dry eye. Ophthalmologe. 1995;92:802–8.
9. Lemp MA, Baudouin C, Baum J, Dogru M, Foulks GN, Kinoshita S et al. The definition and classification of dry eye disease: report of the Definition and Classification Subcommittee of the International Dry Eye Workshop. Ocul Surf. 2007;5(2):75–92.

10. Netland PA, Sugrue SP, Albert DM, Shore JW. Histopathologic features of the floppy eyelid syndrome. Involvement of tarsal elastin. Ophthalmology. 1994;101:174–81.
11. Schlotzer-Schrehardt U, Stojkovic M, Hofmann-Rummelt C, Cursiefen C, Kruse FE, et al. The Pathogenesis of floppy eyelid syndrome: involvement of matrix metalloproteinases in elastic fiber degradation. Ophthalmology. 2005;112:694–704.
12. Series F, Chakir J, Boivin D. Influence of weight and sleep apnea on the immunological and structural features of the uvula. Am J Respir Crit Care Med. 2004;170:1114–9.
13. Woog JJ. Obstructive sleep apnea and the floppy eyelid syndrome. Am J Ophthalmol. 1990;110:314–5.
14. Chambe J, Laib S, Hubbard J, Erhardt C, Ruppert E, et al. Floppy eyelid syndrome is associated with obstructive sleep apnoea: a prospective study on 127 patients. J Sleep Res. 2012;21:308–15.
15. Muniesa MJ, Huerva V, Sanchez-de-la-Torre M, Martinez M, Jurjo C, et al. The relationship between floppy eyelid syndrome and obstructive sleep apnoea. Br J Ophthalmol. 2013;97:1387–90.
16. Robert PY, Adenis JP, Tapie P, Melloni B. Eyelid hyperlaxity and obstructive sleep apnea (O.S.A.) syndrome. Eur J Ophthalmol. 1997;7:211–5.
17. Karger RA, White WA, Park W, Rosales AG, McLaren JW, et al. Prevalence of floppy eyelid syndrome in obstructive sleep apnea–hypopnea syndrome. Ophthalmology. 2006;113:1669–974.
18. Bouchard C, Maki S, Undevia N, Gaynes B, Price R, et al. The association of systemic and ocular disease and the under diagnosis of floppy eyelid syndrome in patients with obstructive sleep apnea. Invest Ophthalmol Vis Sci. 2014;55:1465.
19. Beis PG, Brozou CG, Gourgoulianis KI, Pastaka C, Chatzoulis DZ, et al. The floppy eyelid syndrome: evaluating lid laxity and its correlation to sleep apnea syndrome and body mass index. ISRN Ophthalmol. 2012;20:1–4.
20. Yin T, Li NF, Heizhati M, Zhang J, Zhang J, et al. Association of glucose transporter 4 genetic polymorphisms with obstructive sleep apnea syndrome in Han Chinese general population: a cross-sectional study. Lipids Health Dis. 2014;13:12–21.
21. Leibovitch I, Selva D. Floppy eyelid syndrome: clinical features and the association with obstructive sleep apnea. Sleep Med. 2006;7:117–22.
22. Culbertson WW, Tseng SC. Corneal disorders in floppy eyelid syndrome. Cornea. 1994;139:33–42.
23. Pihlblad MS, Schaefer DP. Eyelid laxity, obesity, and obstructive sleep apnea in keratoconus. Cornea. 2013;32:1232–6.
24. Mastrota KM. Impact of floppy eyelid syndrome in ocular surface and dry eye disease. Optom Vis Sci. 2008;85:814–6.
25. Ezra DG, Beaconsfield M, Sira M, Bunce C, Wormald R, et al. The associations of floppy eyelid syndrome: a case control study. Ophthalmology. 2010;117:831–8.
26. Acar M, Firat H, Yuceege M, Ardic S. Long-term effects of PAP on ocular surface in obstructive sleep apnea syndrome. Can J Ophthalmol. 2014;49:217–21.
27. Acar M, Firat H, Acar U, Ardic S. Ocular surface assessment in patients with obstructive sleep apnea–hypopnea syndrome. Sleep Breath. 2013;17:583–8.
28. Veldman P, Colby K. Current evidence for topical azithromycin 1% ophthalmic solution in the treatment of blepharitis-associated ocular dryness. Int Ophthalmol Clin. 2011;51:43–52.
29. Chan HH, Lee SSY, Tong LT. Use of tetracyclines and macrolides in dry eyes and blepharitis: a systematic review. J Symptoms Signs. 2014;3:204–13.
30. Ezra DG, Beaconsfield M, Collin R. Floppy eyelid syndrome: stretching the limits. Surv Ophthalmol. 2010;55:35–46.
31. Ezra DG, Beaconsfield M, Sira M, Bunce C, Shah-Desai S, et al. Long-term outcomes of surgical approaches to the treatment of floppy eyelid syndrome. Ophthalmology. 2010;117:839–46.
32. Madani M, Madani F. Epidemiology, pathophysiology, and clinical features of obstructive sleep apnea. Oral Maxillofacial Surg Clin N Am. 2009;21:369–75.
33. Waller EA, Bendel RE, Kaplan J. Sleep disorders and the eye. Mayo Clin Proc. 2008;83:1251–61.

34. Abdal H, Pizzimenti JJ, Purvis CC. The eye in sleep apnea syndrome. Sleep Med. 2006;7:107–15.
35. Cheung N, Wong TY. Obesity and eye diseases. Surv Ophthalmol. 2007;52:180–95.
36. Chobanian AV, Bakris GL, Black HR, Cushman WC, Green LA, et al. The Seventh report of the Joint National Committee on prevention, detection, evaluation, and treatment of high blood pressure: the JNC 7 report. JAMA. 2003;289:2560–72.
37. De Torres-Alba F, Gemma D, Armada-Romero E, Rey-Blas JR, López-de-Sá E, et al. Obstructive sleep apnea and coronary artery disease: from pathophysiology to clinical implications. Pulm Med. 2013;2013:1–9.
38. Yaggi HK, Concato J, Kernan WN, Lichtman JH, Brass LM, et al. Obstructive sleep apnea as a risk factor for stroke and death. N Engl J Med. 2005;353:2034–41.
39. Gottlieb DJ, Yenokyan G, Newman AB, O'Connor GT, Punjabi NM. Prospective study of obstructive sleep apnea and incident coronary heart disease and heart failure: the sleep heart health study. Circulation. 2010;122:352–60.
40. Faridi O, Park SC, Liebmann JM, Ritch R. Glaucoma and obstructive sleep apnoea syndrome. Clin Experiment Ophthalmol. 2012;40:408–19.
41. Walsh JT, Montplaisir J. Familial glaucoma with sleep apnoea: a new syndrome? Thorax. 1982;37:845–9.
42. Mannarino MR, Di Filippo F, Pirro M. Obstructive sleep apnea syndrome. Eur J Int Med. 2012;23:586–93.
43. Bilgin G, Koban Y, Arnold AC. Nonarteritic anterior ischemic optic neuropathy and obstructive sleep apnea. J Neuroophthalmol. 2013;33:232–4.
44. Koehler U, Cassel W, Hildebrandt O, Kesper K, Kianinejad P, et al. Obstructive sleep apnea in neurological diseases: specially as a risk factor for stroke. Nervenarzt. 2014;85:35–42.
45. Li M, Hou WS, Zhang XW, Tang ZY. Obstructive sleep apnea and risk of stroke: a meta-analysis of prospective studies. Int J Cardiol. 2014;172:466–9.
46. Banerjee D, Leong WB, Arora T, Nolen M, Punamiya V, et al. The potential association between obstructive sleep apnea and diabetic retinopathy in severe obesity-the role of hypoxemia. PLoS One. 2013;8:e79521.
47. Sergi M, Salerno DE, Rizzi M, Blini M, Andreoli A, et al. Prevalence of normal tension glaucoma in obstructive sleep apnea syndrome patients. J Glaucoma. 2007;16:42–6.
48. Mojon DS, Hess CQ, Goldblum D, Fleischhauer J, Koerner F, et al. High prevalence of glaucoma in patients with sleep apnea syndrome. Ophthalmology. 1999;106:1009–12.
49. Mojon DS, Hess CW, Goldblum D, Bohnke M, Korner F, et al. Primary open-angle glaucoma is associated with sleep apnea syndrome. Ophthalmologica. 2000;214:115–8.
50. Lin PW, Friedman MW, Lin HC, Chang HW, Wilson M, et al. Normal tension glaucoma in patients with obstructive sleep apnea/hypopnea syndrome. J Glaucoma. 2011;20:553–8.
51. Bendel RE, Kaplan J, Heckman M, Fredrickson PA, Lin SC. Prevalence of glaucoma in patients with obstructive sleep apnea—a cross-sectional case series. Eye. 2008;22(9):1105.
52. Karakucuk S, Goktas S, Aksu M, Erdogan N, Demirci S, et al. Ocular blood flow in patients with obstructive sleep apnea syndrome (OSAS). Graefes Arch Clin Exp Ophthalmol. 2008;246:129–34.
53. Boyle-Walker M, Semes LP, Clay OJ, Liu L, Furh P. Sleep apnea syndrome represents a risk for glaucoma in a veterans' affairs population. ISRN Ophthalmol. 2011;2011:920767.
54. Blumen Ohana E, Blumen MB, Bluwol E, Derri M, Chabolle F, et al. Primary open angle glaucoma and snoring: prevalence of OSAS. Eur Ann Otorhinolaryngol Head Neck Dis. 2010;127:159–64.
55. Onen SH, Mouriaux F, Berramdane L, Dascotte JC, Kulik JF, et al. High prevalence of sleep-disordered breathing in patients with primary open-angle glaucoma. Acta Ophthalmol Scand. 2000;78:638–41.
56. Tsang CSL, Chong SL, Ho CK, Li MF. Moderate to severe obstructive sleep apnoea patients is associated with higher incidence of visual field defects. Eye. 2006;20:38–42.

57. Kargi SH, Altin R, Koksal KL, Cinar F, et al. Retinal nerve fibre layer measurements are reduced in patients with obstructive sleep apnea syndrome. Eye. 2005;19:575–9.
58. Girkin CA, McGwin G Jr, McNeal SF, Owsley C. Is there an association between pre-existing sleep apnoea and the development of glaucoma? Br J Ophthalmol. 2006;90:679–81.
59. Roberts TV, Hodge C, Graham SL, Burlutsky G, Mitchell P. Prevalence of nocturnal oxygen desaturation and self-reported sleep-disordered breathing in glaucoma. J Glaucoma. 2009;18:114–8.
60. Khandgave TP, Puthran N, Ingole AB, Nicholson AD. The assessment of sleep apnea as a risk factor in glaucoma. J Clin Diagn Res. 2013;7:1391–3.
61. Kadyan A, Asghar J, Dowson L. Ocular findings in sleep apnoea patients using continuous positive airway pressure. Eye. 2009;24:843–50.
62. Geyer O, Cohen N, Segev E, Rath EZ, Melamud L, et al. The prevalence of glaucoma in patients with sleep apnea syndrome: same as in the general population. Am J Ophthalmol. 2003;136(6):1093.
63. Shi Y, Liu P, Guan J, Su K. Association between glaucoma and obstructive sleep apnea syndrome: a meta-analysis and systemic review. PLoS One. 2015;10:e0115625.
64. Muniesa M, Sanchez-de-la-Torre M, Huerva V, Lumbierres M, Barbé F. Floppy eyelid syndrome as an indicator of the presence of glaucoma in patients with obstructive sleep apnea. J Glaucoma. 2014;23:81–5.
65. Drance SM. Some factors in the production of low tension glaucoma. Br J Ophthalmol. 1972;56:229–42.
66. Leske MC. Ocular perfusion pressure and glaucoma: clinical trial and epidemiologic findings. Curr Opin Ophthalmol. 2009;20:73–8.
67. Graham SL, Drance SM. Nocturnal hypotension role in glaucoma progression. Surv Ophthalmol. 1999;43:S10–6.
68. Pepin JL, Chiquet C, Tamisier R, Levy P, Almanjoumi A, et al. Frequent loss of nyctohemeral rhythm of intraocular pressure restored by nCPAP treatment in patients with severe apnea. Arch Ophthalmol. 2010;128:1257–63.
69. Fletcher EC. Sympathetic overactivity in the etiology of hypertension of obstructive sleep apnea. Sleep. 2003;26:15–9.
70. Jelic S, Padeletti M, Kawut SM, Higgins C, Canfield SM, et al. Inflammation, oxidative stress, and repair capacity of the vascular endothelium in obstructive sleep apnea. Circulation. 2008;117:2270–8.
71. Kato M, Roberts-Thomson P, Phillips BG, Haynes WG, Winnicki M, et al. Impairment of endothelium-dependent vasodilation of resistance vessels in patients with obstructive sleep apnea. Circulation 2000;102:2607–2610.
72. Priou P, Gagnadoux F, Tesse A, Mastronardi ML, Agouni A, et al. Endothelial dysfunction and circulating microparticles from patients with obstructive sleep apnea. Am J Pathol. 2010;177:974–83.
73. Suzuki J, Tomidokoro A, Araie M, Tomita G, Yamagami J, et al. Visual field damage in normal-tension glaucoma patients with or without ischemic changes in cerebral magnetic resonance imaging. Jpn J Ophthalmol. 2004;48(4):340.
74. Hui DS, Ko FW, Fok JP, Chan MC, Li TS, et al. The effects of nasal continuous positive airway pressure on platelet activation in obstructive sleep apnea syndrome. Chest. 2004;125:1768–75.
75. Stein JD, Kim DS, Mundy KM, Talwar N, Nan B, et al. The association between glaucomatous and other causes of optic neuropathy and sleep apnea. Am J Ophthalmol. 2011;152:989–98.
76. Mojon DS, Hedges TR III, Ehrenberg B, Karam EZ, Goldblum D, et al. Association between sleep apnea syndrome and nonarteritic anterior ischemic optic neuropathy. Arch Ophthalmol. 2002;120(5):601.
77. Palombi K, Renard E, Levy P, Chiquet C, Deschaux C, et al. Non-arteritic anterior ischaemic optic neuropathy is nearly systematically associated with obstructive sleep apnoea. Br J Ophthalmol. 2006;90:879–82.

78. Kremmer S, Niederdraing N, Ayertey HD, Steuhl KP, Selbach JM. Obstructive sleep apnea syndrome, normal tension glaucoma, and nCPAP therapy – a short note. Sleep. 2003;26(2):161.
79. Stem MS, Talwar N, Comer G, Stein JD. A longitudinal analysis of risk factors associated with central retinal vein occlusion. Ophthalmology. 2013;120:362–70.
80. Hayreh SS. Anatomy and physiology of the optic nerve head. Trans Am Acad Ophthalmol Otolaryngol. 1974;78:240–54.
81. Hayreh SS. Acute ischemic disorders of the optic nerve. Pathogenesis, clinical manifestations and management. Ophthalmol Clin North Am. 1996;9:407–42.
82. Archer EL, Pepin S. Obstructive sleep apnea and nonarteritic anterior ischemic optic neuropathy: evidence for an association. J Clin Sleep Med. 2013;9:613–8.
83. Chung SE, Kang SW, Lee JH, Kim YT. Choroidal thickness in polypoidal choroidal vasculopathy and exudative age-related macular degeneration. Ophthalmology. 2011;118(5):840.
84. Esmaeelpour M, Povazay B, Hermann B, Hofer B, Kajic V, et al. Mapping choroidal and retinal thickness variation in type 2 diabetes using three-dimensional 1060-nm optical coherence tomography. Invest Ophthalmol Vis Sci. 2011;52:5311–6.
85. Immura Y, Fujiwara T, Margolis R, Spaide RF. Enhanced depth imaging optical coherence tomography of the choroid in central serous chorioretinopathy. Retina. 2009;29:1469–73.
86. Xin C, Wang J, Zhang W, Wang L, Peng X. Retinal and choroidal thickness evaluation by SD-OCT in adults with obstructive sleep apnea-hypopnea syndrome (OSAS). Eye. 2014;28:415–21.
87. Karalezlli A, Eroglu FC, Kivanc T, Dogan R. Evaluation of choroidal thickness using spectral-domain optical coherence tomography in patients with severe obstructive sleep apnea syndrome: a comparative study. Int J Ophthalmol. 2014;7:1030–4.
88. Kim DY, Silverman RH, Chan RV, Khanifar AA, Rondeau M, et al. Measurement of choroidal perfusion and thickness following systemic sildenafil (Viagra®). Acta Ophthalmol. 2013;91:183–8.
89. Mason RH, West SD, Kiire CA, Groves DC, Lipinski HJ, et al. High prevalence of sleep disordered breathing in patients with diabetic macular edema. Retina. 2012;32:1791–8.
90. Chou KT, Huang CC, Tsai DC, Chen YM, Perng DW, et al. Sleep apnea and risk of retinal vein occlusion: a nationwide population-based study of Taiwanese. Am J Ophthalmol. 2012;154:200–5.
91. Glace-Bernard A, Lereaux les Jardins G, Lasry S, Coscas G, et al. Obstructive sleep apnea among patients with retinal vein occlusion. Arch Ophthalmol. 2010;128:1533–8.

Chapter 12
Diagnosis and Management of Cicatricial Conjunctivitis

Robert T. Swan, Jennifer Cao, and C. Stephen Foster

Case 1

GG is a 59-year-old female referred to you for chronic conjunctivitis. She is employed as a manager at a telecommunications company. Her past medical history is significant for thalassemia with mild, stable anemia and gastric reflux treated with esomeprazole. Otherwise she is healthy and takes no other systemic medications. She does not have a history of seasonal allergies. She has no family history of eye disease.

Her past ocular history is significant for contact lens wear of which she is now intolerant. Approximately 8 months ago, she was seen by her orthopedist who noted that both of her eyes were injected. Soon after, she developed symptoms of burning and tearing but not itching. Her primary doctor diagnosed viral conjunctivitis and recommended erythromycin ointment. When that proved ineffective, she was referred to an ophthalmologist. There she was diagnosed with allergic conjunctivitis, dry eyes, blepharitis, and meibomian gland dysfunction (MGD).

Over the next 7 months, her symptoms have been refractory to topical treatment with preserved and non-preserved artificial tears, olopatadine, cyclosporine ophthalmic emulsion (Restasis), azithromycin, loteprednol, and prednisolone

R.T. Swan, MD • J. Cao, MD
Massachusetts Eye Research and Surgery Institution (MERSI),
1440 Main Street, Suite 201, Waltham, MA 02451, USA

Ocular Immunology and Uveitis Foundation, Waltham, MA, USA

C.S. Foster, MD, FACS (✉)
Massachusetts Eye Research and Surgery Institution (MERSI),
1440 Main Street, Suite 201, Waltham, MA 02451, USA

Ocular Immunology and Uveitis Foundation, Waltham, MA, USA

Harvard Medical School, Boston, MA, USA
e-mail: sfoster@mersi.com

A.R. Djalilian (ed.), *Ocular Surface Disease*,
https://doi.org/10.1007/978-3-319-15823-5_12

eye drops. Autologous serum tears provided some temporary relief but have been cost prohibitive. Brief courses of oral prednisone (60 mg) and oral doxycycline have been ineffective. Difluprednate has partially improved her symptoms. Its chronic use has led to steroid-induced ocular hypertension requiring brimonidine. She is currently using difluprednate (Durezol) 1 time a day, brimonidine 2 times a day, and Restasis 2 times a day, all in both eyes. On this regimen her eyes are still symptomatic and uncomfortable. In addition, the glare while driving at night is becoming intolerable. You are the third eye doctor she has seen, and she traveled a long way to come to your office.

What Is Your Examination Approach to Chronic, Intractable Ocular Surface Symptoms?

It is important to examine the entire anterior segment. While emphasis tends to be placed on bulbar conjunctiva and cornea, one must also pay close attention to the eyelid margin, eyelid position, and laxity, the direction of eyelashes, and the palpebral conjunctiva (via eyelid eversion). The inability to tolerate contact lenses is most commonly attributed to "dry eye," but other causes of ocular inflammation can be present. Schirmer testing and lissamine green staining patterns can be very helpful.

On examination her vision is 20/25 in each eye without correction. Her pupils are equally reactive without an afferent pupillary defect. Her intraocular pressure is 22 in each eye. Evaluation of the periocular skin shows no evidence of rash or other lesions. There is no trichiasis. There is no significant lid laxity or lagophthalmos. The meibomian glands and the eyelid margin appear normal. Her conjunctiva is diffusely injected bilaterally. On upper eyelid eversion, there is a mild papillary reaction with subepithelial fibrosis seen bilaterally. Examination of the inferior palpebral conjunctiva reveals bilateral subepithelial fibrosis. Lower eyelid retraction with the eye in upgaze reveals a mild (~25 %) forniceal foreshortening bilaterally. No conjunctival granulomas are seen. Sclera appears normal. Her corneas have numerous punctate epithelial erosions. Her anterior chamber is quiet and iris normal in each eye. She has a 2+ posterior subcapsular cataract bilaterally. Her optic nerve cup-to-disc ratio is 0.2 bilaterally. The remainder of her dilated fundus exam is normal.

What Diagnosis Do These Findings Suggest? What Additional History Would This Exam Prompt You to Obtain?

This patient has chronic cicatrizing conjunctivitis. If not looked for, the telltale signs of subepithelial fibrosis and forniceal foreshortening often go unrecognized, and this condition smolders along for months to years with symptomatic inflammation despite multiple treatments. Often it is symblepharon formation that prompts recognition and referral, though this is a later, more advanced finding.

Subepithelial fibrosis forms under the palpebral conjunctiva one to two millimeters inside of the lid margin. It appears as fine interweaving strands with a white glistening appearance running parallel to the lid margin (Fig. 12.1). Generally, the fornix is not fully visualized even with downward traction on the lower lid while the patient is in far upgaze. If one can easily flatten the fornix in such a manner, it is likely that it is foreshortened (Fig. 12.2).

When these findings of cicatrizing conjunctivitis are discovered, the first diagnostic consideration is whether it is the result of a historical event or is reflective of an active process. Patients should be questioned about previous episodes of severe conjunctivitis, chemical injuries, a history of Stevens-Johnson syndrome (SJS), or prior chronic use of topical glaucoma medications, particularly pilocarpine [1].

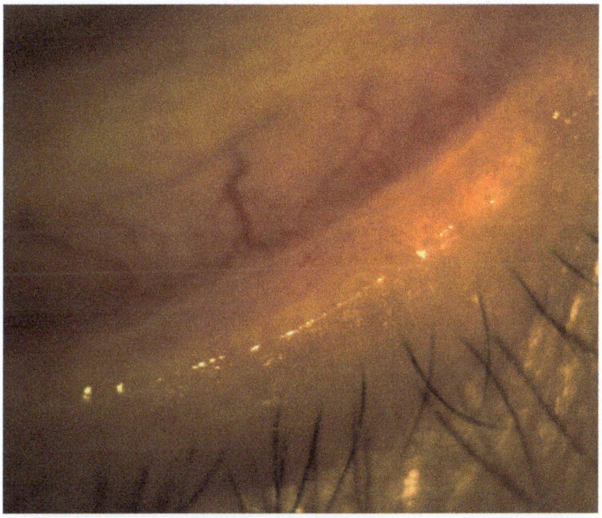

Fig. 12.1 This is a representative photograph of subepithelial fibrosis

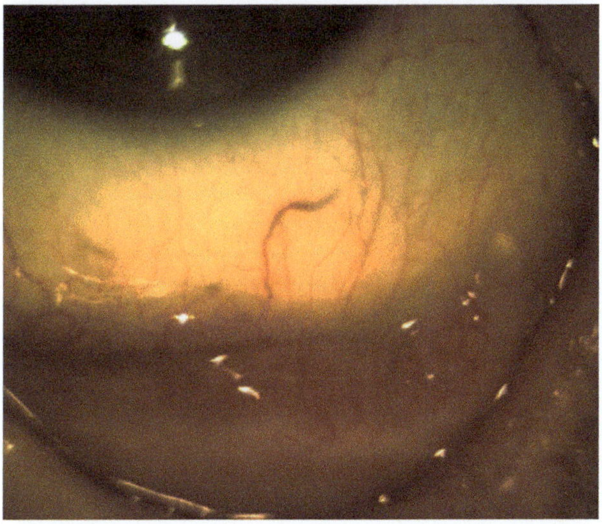

Fig. 12.2 This is a representative photograph of forniceal foreshortening. Note that traction on the eyelid puts tension on the bulbar conjunctiva

These episodes can result in conjunctival scarring that, in general, is not progressive. A rare but important exception here is an autoimmune-mediated progressive scarring found in some patients with SJS long after resolution of the acute episode [2].

Active, progressive cicatrizing conjunctivitis has many reported etiologies. Of those with autoimmune etiologies, ocular cicatricial pemphigoid (OCP) is likely the most common with an estimated incidence of 1:12,000 to 1:60,000 [3]. Rosacea with MGD and atopic disease are both common entities in general ophthalmic practice, but, in especially severe forms, each can be the primary cause of conjunctival cicatrization [4, 5]. Importantly, even mild to moderate MGD or atopy can combine with OCP to form a more refractory disease.

Several systemic inflammatory syndromes have also been described as rare causes of cicatrizing conjunctivitis. These include (but are not limited to) Sjögren's syndrome, granulomatosis with polyangiitis (GPA) (formerly Wegener's granulomatosis), and sarcoidosis [1, 6–8]. Paraneoplastic cases have also been reported [9]. Trachoma causes chronic conjunctival scarring resulting in a cicatricial entropion that then causes mechanical damage to the ocular surface. Worldwide, it is the most common infectious cause of blindness [10]. While extremely rare in the USA, trachoma should be considered in recent immigrants from endemic areas.

OCP is defined as a slow but relentless progression of conjunctival scarring eventually leading to corneal involvement and blindness [11, 12]. It is a bilateral disease but in some cases can be markedly asymmetric. The four stages of the disease have been described (Table 12.1). It falls under the spectrum of diseases classified as mucous membrane pemphigoid (MMP) [13]. In these disorders antibodies are

Table 12.1 Evaluation and treatment of ocular cicatricial pemphigoid

Foster staging system for OCP	Stage 1—Chronic conjunctivitis accompanied by subconjunctival fibrosis
	Stage 2—Conjunctival fornix foreshortening due to cicatrization
	Stage 3—Presence of symblephara, entropion, trichiasis, keratopathy
	Stage 4—Corneal keratinization, ankyloblepharon, severe dry eye
Cicatrizing conjunctivitis workup	1. Serologic evaluation for underlying disorder (GPA, Sjögren's syndrome, sarcoidosis, atopy)
	2. Conjunctival biopsy for histopathology and immunofluorescence
	3. Collaborative investigation of other potentially involved mucous membranes
OCP treatment	Early—antimetabolites (AZA, MTX, MMF)
	Advanced or progressive—combination IVIg and rituximab (preferred) or CYC
Confounding and aggravating factors	Atopy
	Meibomian gland dysfunction
	Trichiasis
	Topical medications, particularly preservatives

OCP ocular cicatricial pemphigoid, *GPA* granulomatosis with polyangiitis, *AZA* azathioprine, *MTX* methotrexate, *MMF* mycophenolate mofetil, *IVIg* intravenous immunoglobulin, *CYC* cyclophosphamide formed to various glycoproteins in mucous membrane basement membrane zones (BMZ) resulting in chronic inflammation and scarring of mucous membranes. OCP can occur as an isolated condition or in combination with other mucous membrane involvement. The gold standard for diagnosis of OCP remains a conjunctival biopsy demonstrating immunoglobulin or complement deposition at the epithelial BMZ. False negatives are common and do not rule out the condition [14].

Though this patient's current condition started with a presumed viral conjunctivitis, the conjunctivitis itself was never noted to be especially severe; rather it has simply lingered. Now identified as cicatrizing, a thorough history and review of systems should be performed to look for an occult underlying systemic inflammatory process with focus on involvement of other mucous membranes. Patients will often not mention oral or vaginal lesions without prompting. Special emphasis should be placed on dysphagia and breathing abnormalities as these may signal occult involvement in the esophagus or larynx. Involvement of these areas has been estimated to be 5–15% [15]. Laryngeal strictures are of particular importance as they can be life-threatening if not diagnosed. Though uncommon, OCP has been reported as a manifestation of a para-neoplastic process; however, routine workup for occult malignancy is not indicated (beyond age-appropriate routine screening tests).

The patient denies a history of trauma, chemical injury, SJS, or previous severe conjunctivitis. Additional review of systems for this patient reveals mild dysphagia for which she underwent an endoscopy that showed mild idiopathic scarring of the esophagus. This was attributed to reflux and prompted treatment with esomeprazole. With this medication and some dietary modifications, no other treatment has been necessary. She has no other mucous membrane lesions. There are no signs or symptoms suggest an underlying connective tissue or vasculitic disorder. Baseline anterior segment photographs are taken.

What Are Your Next Diagnostic Steps?

Patients with cicatrizing conjunctivitis should have a serologic workup for baseline studies and mimicking etiologies (ESR, CBC, comprehensive metabolic panel, serum IgE, ANA, SS-A, SS-B, ANCA, ACE/lysozyme). A conjunctival biopsy can be performed on any part of the bulbar conjunctiva. Several specific reports of technique have been described [1, 14, 16]. Briefly, this can be done by using a bleb of subconjunctival lidocaine for both anesthesia and demarcation of the tissue from underlying Tenon's capsule. The biopsy is taken using forceps and scissors after which antibiotic ointment and a pressure patch are applied. The biopsy needs to be large enough to allow proper pathologic interpretation.

Blood work is drawn, and the bulbar conjunctival biopsy is taken from the inferior nasal quadrant. It is completed on the same day given the patient's travel distance. It is approximately 3 × 4 mm in size. Forceps are used to place the tissue on gauze soaked in normal saline.

In What Solution(S) Will You Deliver the Biopsy to Pathology? What Type of Pathologist Would Be Best Equipped to Read It? What Pathologic Studies Will You Request?

As with most biopsies done on ocular tissue, it is best to communicate with the pathologist in advance to make sure he/she is comfortable and experienced in conjunctival tissue processing and interpretation. In addition to ocular pathologists who have significant experience processing and interpreting conjunctival tissue, immunofluorescence is commonly performed by dermatopathologists.

As biopsy specimens are often reflexively placed in formalin, it is emphasized that immunofluorescence often cannot be performed well on specimens delivered in this solution. Michel's solution or normal saline can be used. It is important to communicate with the pathologist regarding his/her individual preferences.

The histologic pattern of inflammation should be evaluated, specifically whether there are granulomatous features to suggest conditions such as sarcoidosis or GPA. The presence of goblet cells should be noted. The number/location of mast cells is also of importance, specifically if there are excessive numbers or excessive degranulation that might suggest an atopic component. Immunofluorescence should be used to evaluate for linear staining of immunoglobulins or complement at the epithelial basement membrane zone (BMZ).

The conjunctival tissue was large enough to be cut in half. Half was placed in formalin for histopathology and the other half in Michel's solution for immunofluorescence. The specimen was brought to pathology promptly. As the appointment ends, the patient is perturbed that you have not made any modifications to her therapy nor have you extensively discussed the individual items on your differential diagnosis.

We inform our patients that there are many causes of cicatricial conjunctivitis and that we prefer to not go into extensive discussions on diagnosis or therapeutic decisions until the return of the serologies and biopsy. This sometimes frustrates patients, as they want immediate answers. As many patients have failed multiple therapies before being referred, we discuss the importance of having as much information as possible before deciding on the next step.

In 2 weeks, she returns. The serologic workup is negative for systemic disorders. Histopathologic evaluation of the conjunctiva reveals a mononuclear lymphocytic infiltrate in the stroma, decreased goblet cells, and a normal mast cell population without significant degranulation. There is no evidence of granulomatous inflammation. Immunofluorescence shows positive linear staining of IgG, IgA, and complement (C3) at the epithelial BMZ.

What Is the Most Likely Diagnosis?

The clinical exam and biopsy are consistent with ocular cicatricial pemphigoid (OCP). Given her history of esophageal scarring, you contact the GI specialist to make sure he is aware of the possibility of mucous membrane pemphigoid.

What If the Immunofluorescence Results Had Been Equivocal?

Avidin-biotin complex (ABC) staining has been shown to increase the sensitivity of biopsy results that are negative or equivocal on immunofluorescence [1]. This is routinely done in our lab in instances where there is a high clinical suspicion.

If ABC staining is not available, a second biopsy could be considered. Yet, some patients are not excited about a second biopsy, and at times it can still be negative. For those biopsy-negative patients in whom the clinical condition looks and progresses in a manner typical for OCP, we offer systemic therapy. A common misconception is that negative results rule out OCP. Chronic cicatricial conjunctivitis, regardless of biopsy results, needs to be treated systemically to control the inflammation. Patients whose biopsy does not show classic pemphigoid are still at great risk of vision loss from chronic cicatrization.

1. *Assuming no known drug allergies, what therapeutic options would you present to the patient? Is there an option that is contraindicated?*
2. *What can one do if one is not comfortable prescribing and monitoring immunomodulatory therapy (IMT)? Is there a topical alternative?*
3. *How long will it take to know the full clinical effect of the medication? How will you know if the patient is in remission?*

Systemic treatment is required for OCP. For non-vision threatening cases, we prefer the use of an antimetabolite with a proven track record in this disease: methotrexate (MTX), mycophenolate mofetil (MMF), or azathioprine (AZA) [17, 18]. In the past, we have used dapsone for mild cases, but this has fallen out of favor in our practice given the high incidence of hemolytic anemia while on this medication and the safety of alternatives [19]. This patient's thalassemia would be a relative contraindication to dapsone.

Many ophthalmologists are not experienced, comfortable, or motivated to prescribe and monitor IMT. Yet it is increasingly recognized how important these steroid-sparing therapies are for ocular inflammatory disease. In such cases, we recommend a close collaboration with a rheumatology or hematology colleague who can prescribe and monitor the medication. The ophthalmologist must take the leading role in communicating the status of the ocular inflammation and, if necessary, the need to increase or change therapy.

We monitor treatment efficacy by improvement in both subjective symptoms and objective conjunctival injection. We consider remission to be a white and quiet eye. This underscores the need for periodic anterior segment photography. We allow 6 weeks for an antimetabolite to reach full effect. After 3 weeks of therapy, we will attempt to taper any corticosteroids (oral or topical) that have been used as a bridge in therapy. In patients who only partially respond to the starting dose, the dose can be increased. Here we wait an additional 6 weeks to know the full effect of the increased dose. If a patient is not tolerating a medication, we will discontinue it and move along to another.

As she does not drink alcohol, she was started on 15 mg of methotrexate weekly with daily folic acid supplementation. After 1 month she reported clinical improvement, and Durezol was finally tapered. Off Durezol her IOP improved and so brimonidine was discontinued as well. At this time she tells

you that her eyes feel "wonderful." She reports she has not been using artificial tears and, if possible, would like to discontinue Restasis. She would also like to resume contact lens wear.

What Is the Relationship Between Dry Eye Syndrome and OCP? Can She Stop Restasis? What About Resuming Her Contact Lenses?

Often, tearing in patients with OCP is felt secondary to "dry eye" and is often treated reflexively as an aqueous deficiency. However, OCP itself does not cause a true aqueous deficiency until late stages [1]. As she is doing so well, it is reasonable to trial off Restasis with restarting for worsening symptoms. There is no contraindication to contact lenses so long as they are well tolerated.

Now 3 months into remission, she returns for follow-up. Her glare symptoms have progressed, and she is extremely anxious for cataract surgery.

When Will You Perform This Surgery? What Perioperative Changes to Systemic Therapy Will You Make? How Will the OCP Affect Your Surgical Approach to the Cataract Surgery?

Ocular surgery should not be performed on patients with OCP until remission is achieved. For traditional extracapsular cataract surgery, we recommend waiting for 6 months at the very least [1]. There are no data on optimal length of remission for patients undergoing phacoemulsification. Here we prefer a minimum of 3 months of remission. In all patients, no matter how long the remission, perioperative high-dose prednisone should be used. We typically start with 60 mg of prednisone for 3 days before surgery with a taper of 10 mg every 4 days after surgery. The patient should continue all current IMT as well.

Regarding surgical technique, exposure can be difficult in these patients, as a normal speculum may not fit. In such cases we use a 6-0 silk suture through the lid margins for retraction. If possible a clear corneal incision should be made to avoid manipulation of the conjunctiva [20].

Postoperatively these patients can develop abrupt but persistent corneal epithelial defects that, when finally resolved, leave the patient with poor vision secondary to corneal scarring and thinning [21, 22]. For this reason, we recommend reexamining these patients every 1–2 weeks postoperatively. If conjunctival scarring progresses, high-dose prednisone should be reinitiated and systemic therapy increased. If a corneal epithelial defect develops, amniotic membrane grafting or tarsorrhaphy should be considered early if there are no signs of improvement with aggressive lubrication [21]. We do not recommend operating on the second eye until it is clear that the first eye is completely healed. Ultimately, despite best efforts, outcomes after cataract surgery in patients with OCP are not as favorable as in normal patients

[20, 23]. Thus, the threshold to proceed with surgery should be higher and the patient well informed about a potentially difficult postoperative period.

She waits for an additional 3 months before having uneventful cataract surgery in both eyes (2 months apart). She has now achieved 1 year of remission. She is not having any side effects from the methotrexate but does not like the idea of being "on medication."

These situations are common. We make sure patients know upfront that we intend to continue therapy for a minimum of 2 years following full steroid-free remission before attempting to taper. Attempting to taper medication earlier is a mistake and will almost inevitably result in a relapse. To address her concern of taking methotrexate, we discuss the long history of experience and safety (with proper monitoring) that the medical community has with this medication.

Once 2 years of steroid-free remission is achieved, medication is slowly tapered. Her methotrexate dose is reduced by 5 mg every 6–12 weeks. Once off medication, we monitor patients at 3-month intervals with slow extension over time. If there is a relapse, she will return to her previous dose for another 2 years before trying to taper again.

Case 2

CC is a 65-year-old female with bilateral chronic cicatrizing conjunctivitis that has been refractory to treatment. She is referred to you for assistance with a nonhealing corneal epithelial defect of the right eye. In addition to her work as an attorney, she has previously been employed as a model. She has not been able to work recently due to her chronic ocular injection. Her medical history is significant for hypertension controlled with lisinopril. Review of systems is negative for dyspnea, dysphagia, or lesions of other mucous membranes. She has occasional diarrhea and an occasional rash from rosacea. She does not recall ever having a herpes simplex (HSV) lesion.

About 15 years ago, she had an uneventful cosmetic blepharoplasty of all four lids. Three years ago she had cataract surgery of both eyes. About 18 months ago, she developed chronic tearing of the right eye with a sensation of dryness, irritation, and visible injection of both eyes. She was initially diagnosed with dry eye syndrome and MGD. Restasis and oral doxycycline (100 mg by mouth twice daily) were started, and punctual plugs were placed. She could not tolerate doxycycline due to nausea.

Despite these treatments, the conjunctival inflammation persisted, and she was referred to a cornea specialist whom she first saw 12 months ago. The specialist noted numerous inferior symblephara creating a significantly blunted fornix. A conjunctival biopsy was not performed given the high clinical suspicion of OCP. At that visit, the patient was started on mycophenolate mofetil (MMF) 1 gram twice daily that improved but did not resolve her symptoms. The irritation, dryness, and injection persisted bilaterally, albeit to a lesser extent.

Her corneas had no documented pathology until 6 months ago when epitheliopathy was seen on the right cornea. 3 months ago she developed a central

epithelial defect of the right eye. This defect has persisted despite amniotic membrane grafts, a brief trial of oral prednisone, and valacyclovir. She recalls the oral prednisone helped her symptoms, but her epithelial defect continued. A bandage contact lens has been helpful to decrease her irritation. She is currently instilling prednisolone four times a day to the right eye.

On examination her vision is 20/400 OD, 20/30 OS. Her pupils are equal. Her IOP is 12 OU. The slit lamp examination reveals numerous symblephara in the inferior fornices (Fig. 12.3), now only 25% of normal depth. There is 2+ conjunctival injection bilaterally. The right corneal epithelium has been replaced with hazy, irregular conjunctival epithelium. There is superficial neovascularization and a 2.5 mm epithelial defect centrally (Fig. 12.4). There is no associated infiltrate or stromal thinning seen. The left cornea appears normal.

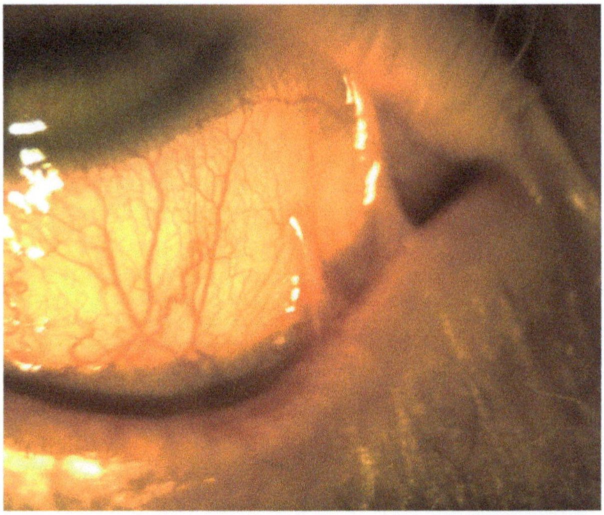

Fig. 12.3 Inflamed conjunctiva with inferior symblephara

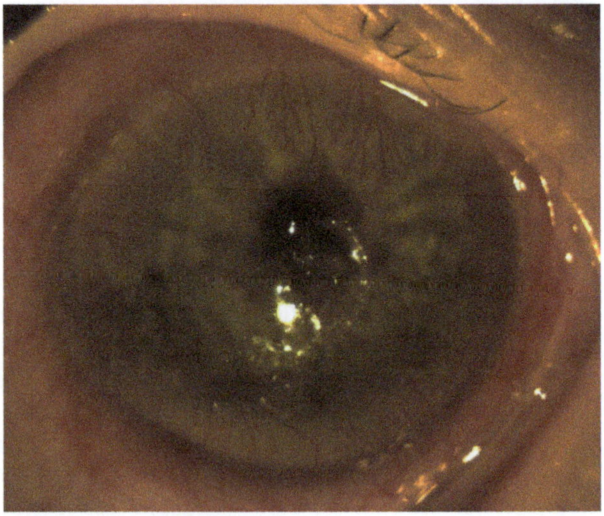

Fig. 12.4 Neovascularization of cornea (limbal stem cell failure) due to chronic inflammation and a central epithelial defect in the same patient

The anterior chambers appear quiet and irides appear normal. She is pseudophakic bilaterally. The details of the right fundus are obscured by the corneal haze. The left fundus appears normal. B-scan ultrasonography of the right eye is normal.

What Additional Workup Would You Recommend? What Temporizing Measures Can You Offer While the Workup Is Pending?

Though the patient and referring doctor place understandable emphasis on the right corneal epithelial defect, closure will require control of the underlying systemic disease. Her clinical appearance is consistent with OCP though other mimicking systemic inflammatory conditions need to be ruled out. This starts with a thorough review of systems and a serologic workup. If a provider prefers, this can be done in collaboration with a rheumatologist. HSV titers in adults are frequently positive, but can be helpful to exclude herpetic infection if negative. From her history and exam, it appears that the epithelial defect is resulting from the conjunctivalization of the cornea secondary to limbal stem cell deficiency, not HSV.

Her right eye has been blinded and her left eye is at risk. The underlying process is both active and idiopathic. For this reason, a conjunctival biopsy should be performed to better characterize the underlying inflammation and attempt to definitively diagnose OCP. As she is functionally monocular at this time, biopsy should be performed on the right eye. Given the significant inferior scarring, an alternate part of the bulbar conjunctiva can be chosen as a biopsy site. If in addition to an epithelial defect, there is concern for corneal ulceration, a conjunctival resection of the adjacent limbus could be both therapeutic and diagnostic.

Pending the results of the workup, temporizing measures should be instituted. The topical corticosteroid drops have been ineffective and increase risk of infection or thinning in an eye with a chronic epithelial defect. She should be transitioned to high-dose oral prednisone. MMF, though clearly not completely effective, should be continued for now. Antibiotic ophthalmic ointment given 4 times a day will keep the surface lubricated and act as prophylaxis from infection.

Anterior segment photographs are obtained. Combination bacitracin/polymyxin B ophthalmic ointment to the right eye four times a day was initiated. Oral prednisone at 60 mg daily is started and steroid drops are discontinued. Rheumatology consultation reports presence of Raynaud's phenomenon, but otherwise there is no evidence of an underlying connective tissue or vasculitic disease. Serologic workup (including Sjögren's antibodies, sarcoidosis, GPA and HSV titers) is negative. A conjunctival biopsy is performed in the superior bulbar conjunctiva of the right eye. Histopathology shows no granulomatous or atopic features. Immunofluorescence demonstrates IgA staining at the BMZ confirming the diagnosis of OCP. Valacyclovir is discontinued given lack of efficacy and negative serologies.

What Are Your Systemic Treatment Recommendations? What Are Your Ocular Treatment Recommendations?

Systemic:

This patient's condition has remained active bilaterally despite IMT. In patients who fail antimetabolite therapies or who present with severe, imminently vision-threatening disease, aggressive immunosuppression is required.

In our experience with advanced and/or rapidly progressive OCP, the best method to quickly halt disease activity is our protocol of rituximab and intravenous immunoglobulin (IVIg) [24]. We give rituximab (375 mg/m^2) weekly for eight consecutive weeks followed by at least four monthly injections. After this, we consider extension based on clinical response. This rituximab protocol is in contrast to rheumatoid arthritis protocols involving two infusions every 6 months. For ocular inflammation, IVIg requires dosing of 2 mg/kg [25]. IVIg at this dose results in a larger protein load which can cause patients to develop severe post-infusion headaches. To avoid this, we recommend dividing the dose over 3 days and giving each infusion slowly over 6 h. Systemic IgA deficiency needs to be ruled out before giving IVIg and can be added to the initial serologic workup. Rheumatologists and oncologists are experienced with these medications and can assist with the infusions if preferred.

Ocular:

The epithelial defect will not heal until the systemic disease is under control. She should continue antibiotic ointment four times a day. If there is concern for a corneal melt, amniotic membrane grafting may temporarily halt the process. Treatment of the underlying MGD is important. She should perform warm compresses and eyelid massage twice daily. Lower doses of doxycycline have shown efficacy in MGD and may be more tolerable then her previous regimen [26]. As she is functionally monocular, polycarbonate safety glasses should be recommended.

Her private insurance company has approved IVIg but denied the request for rituximab as well as a subsequent appeal.

What Other Treatment Options Can You Offer Her? What Guidance Can You Give Her on Insurance Appeals?

Until the recognition of the superiority of combination IVIg and rituximab, cyclophosphamide (CYC) was our mainstay of therapy for severe or recalcitrant cases [19, 24, 27]. Indeed, efficacy with CYC continues to be reported, with lower-dose protocols for elderly patients described [28]. However, CYC carries additional risks of malignancy and hemorrhagic cystitis which limits long-term use. Monotherapy with IVIg has been beneficial in certain CYC failures [25]. Of those with disease activity despite IVIg alone, remission has occurred with addition of rituximab [24].

Regardless of proven efficacy, expensive off-label treatments for rare orphan diseases are a recipe for insurance company denials. To be the best advocate for your patient, you should document (both in the chart and with anterior segment photography) that this condition is vision threatening. Appeals to the insurance company should include copies of appropriate supporting medical literature. Finally, for those patients who have failed multiple tiers of appeals, a healthcare attorney may be helpful.

IVIg was started when approval was obtained. This patient hired a healthcare attorney who sent reports to the State Attorney General and the Insurance Commission of the State. Following this, approval was gained for rituximab. She is started on 8 weekly rituximab infusions along with monthly IVIg. There is a clear response seen after the third week of rituximab, and at that time the prednisone was tapered to 10 mg/week. Concurrently, MMF was gradually tapered over the next 2 months. After 2 months of IVIg/rituximab therapy, her conjunctiva is white and quiet. She is declared to be in remission. New baseline anterior segment photographs are taken. Her rituximab is extended to monthly. She continues monthly IVIg.

With systemic therapy and aggressive ocular lubrication, her right corneal defect has been resolved. Her vision in that eye remains poor (count fingers at 4 ft) due to the conjunctivalization of the cornea. She is anxious for the vision in the right eye to be "back to normal" through any means possible.

What Are Potential Options for Visual Rehabilitation of the Right Cornea? What Are the Main Barriers to a Successful Outcome? What Would You Ultimately Recommend?

Although surgical options for visual rehabilitation exist, the overall prognosis for eyes with advanced OCP is very poor. This is due to a combination of colluding elements. First, the symblepharon create a difficult anterior segment access surgically. Additionally there is difficulty retaining a contact lens postoperatively. Often in these patients, there can be an incomplete blink leading to exposure. In late stages of OCP, there is also a superimposed aqueous tear deficiency. Finally, limbal stem cell deficiency can develop, as it has in this patient.

Experience with penetrating keratoplasty (PK) in OCP patients has revealed that, although sometimes necessary for tectonic purposes, visual restoration is limited even under optimal circumstances [29].

Keratoprosthesis (Kpro) can conceivably provide a clear visual axis despite these factors. However, the typical Type 1 Boston Kpro is at high risk of melting or infection due to a compromised fornix that is unable to retain a contact lens [30]. The literature suggests that the Type 2 Boston Kpro affords slightly better outcomes in OCP patients compared to the Type 1, though the overall survival is low in both groups [31]. Our experience with the Type 2 Kpro has not been as positive, and as such we continue to favor the Type 1 Kpro in carefully selected patients. There is also a high risk of glaucoma in all Kpro patients [32]. With the conjunctival scarring, glaucoma surgery can become complicated.

For all of these reasons, Kpro should be considered a last resort, and patients must be ready to commit to very frequent, life-long monitoring. In addition, a detailed informed consent needs to be clear about the high probability of potential complications and that, as these complications mount, there is a real risk of losing all vision or even the eye itself.

We thus reserve such heroic efforts to extremely motivated patients who are otherwise bilaterally blind. We would not consider or recommend surgery given the excellent vision in the left eye. In the future, there may be developments that change this view. One option being investigated for complete limbal stem cell deficiency is cultivation and ocular transplantation of autologous oral epithelial mucosa [33]. Although promising for patients with SJS, to date there has not been lasting improvement in visual acuity in study patients with OCP [33].

You decline to operate on the right eye, explaining that the significant risks outweigh the possibility of limited improvement in vision. Assuming she stays in remission, how should her therapy be adjusted in the future?

The primary goal in these vision-threatening situations is stability. Often, there is little room for progression without blindness. If a patient remains stable on a regimen, the intervals of medications can be cautiously extended. We have reported the efficacy of an IVIg protocol adapted from a consensus statement on MMP treatment [25, 34]. At this time, we wait for at least 6 months (and often 12 months) of stable remission on monthly IVIg before slowly extending the interval. We extend intervals in 2-week increments. We confirm stability at the new interval for a minimum of two infusions before extending again. Ultimately, if a patient has been stable for two 16-week intervals, IVIg can be discontinued with close observation every 3 months [25].

One year later, she continues to be in remission on monthly rituximab and IVIg. The rituximab is discontinued. After another 3 months of remission, the IVIg is extended to 6 weeks. As time goes on, her interval will be slowly extended providing she remains in stable remission. If she relapses, we will reinitiate rituximab and return to monthly IVIg.

In our experience one must remain ever watchful for signs of relapse and maintain a low threshold to restart therapy. A study of long-term outcomes of patients with severe OCP treated with conventional immunosuppression (usually CYC) showed 46% of these patients could not be tapered completely off medication without relapse [19]. There are no long-term data on relapse rates with combination rituximab/IVIg treatment.

Case 3

NH is a 48-year-old male referred for chronic progressive cicatrization of both eyes. He reports significant ocular itching, irritation, and tearing symptoms of gradual onset over the last 2 years. After developing symblephara, he had a conjunctival biopsy elsewhere which he recalls was negative for pemphigoid. Three months ago, mycophenolate (MMF) 1 g twice daily was started as a therapeutic trial after documentation of progressive disease activity and concern that the biopsy represented a false negative. Despite treatment his condition has worsened and now he has an entropion with symptomatic trichiasis. He is anxious to have this surgically repaired, but the oculoplastic surgeon has requested that you assist in optimizing his ocular surface first. He tells you he

is healthy except for environmental allergies to "everything." He takes an over-the-counter oral antihistamine everyday but has not tried eye drops. He is trying to quit smoking. He is employed as a computer programmer.

On examination vision is 20/50 OU with equal pupils and IOP of 15 OU. Examination of the eyelids reveals a bilateral mild inward rotation of the lower lid margin with a few misdirected lashes in contact with the cornea (Fig. 12.5). The periocular skin is eczematous. The lid margin itself has numerous telangiectasias and severe meibomian gland dysfunction. The conjunctiva is 2+ injected, and there is subepithelial fibrosis, a blunted fornix, and symblephara bilaterally (Fig. 12.6). Eversion of the upper eyelids reveals a papillary conjunctivitis. The cornea has peripheral neovascularization bilaterally, but his visual axis is clear. The anterior chamber is quiet. There is a trace PSC bilaterally. Dilated fundus exam is normal.

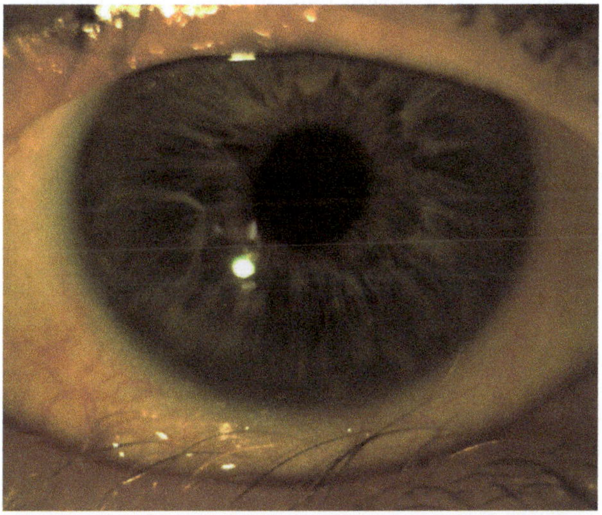

Fig. 12.5 Conjunctival injection and entropion of the lower lid

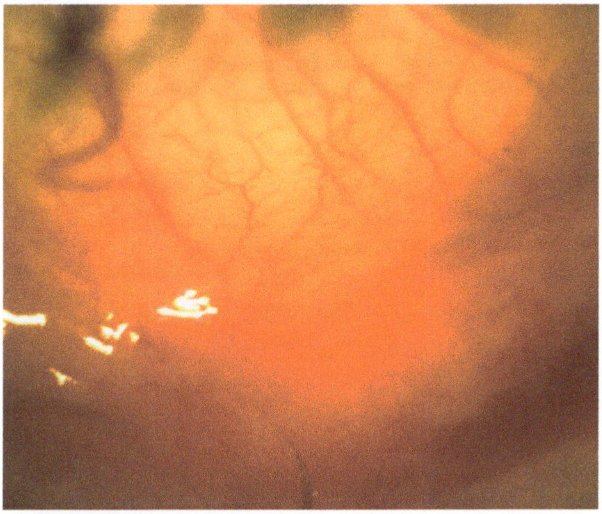

Fig. 12.6 Inflammation and scarring of the inferior conjunctival fornix in the same patient

What Further History Is Required? What Serologic Studies (In Addition to the Standard Workup) Should Be Performed? Should the Biopsy Be Repeated?

While it is possible that MMF simply was not effective, this patient has numerous potential saboteurs. These include ocular surface irritation from smoking and computer over use, allergic conjunctivitis, mechanical irritation from trichiasis, and significant meibomian gland dysfunction. Also there is the lack of a clear diagnosis for the cicatrizing conjunctivitis. Atopic disease and rosacea can each be a primary cause of cicatrizing conjunctivitis as well as act in combination with OCP to make a particularly recalcitrant clinical scenario [5, 35]. Once present, trichiasis itself can be a source of additional inflammation.

Allergic conjunctivitis and dry periocular skin described here can each be a manifestation of an underlying atopic disposition. If asked, atopic patients will often relate a history of childhood eczema, asthma, and/or allergic rhinitis (hay fever), all components of the atopic triad. If atopy is of concern, a serologic workup should include quantitative IgE and an absolute eosinophil count [36].

Prior to repeating a conjunctival biopsy, one should make effort to find the pathology report from the original biopsy. There is more to a report than "positive" and "negative."

The patient does reveal a history of eczema as a child but does not recall asthma. He used to get allergy injections but stopped several years ago when his job became more demanding. His serologies show elevation of IgE and absolute eosinophil count but are otherwise negative. The patient signs a release of information so you can obtain the conjunctival biopsy report.

What Information Will You Look for in the Body of the Report? Does It Matter Who Read the Biopsy?

As with any clinical test, the first question is that of reliability. You will need to decide whether to base your treatment on this report. Was the sample processed properly? Is the pathologist experienced in reading conjunctival biopsies of patients with cicatrizing conjunctivitis?

In this case, the report comes from a reliable, experienced pathologist. The histopathology report mentions mast cell degranulation in the stroma and that an eosinophil is seen in the epithelium. No granulomatous features are noted. Immunofluorescence is negative for epithelial BMZ staining but positive for IgE stromal staining. Follow-up ABC staining was performed and is also negative.

How Does This "Negative" Report Change Your Management? Is It Possible the Report Represented a False Negative for OCP?

Excessive degranulation populations of mast cells (especially if degranulating) and epithelial eosinophils are both abnormal and strongly support the clinical suspicion of an atopic process.

The possibility of a false negative for pemphigoid should always be kept in mind. Conjunctival biopsies require expert handling and interpretation. Even under optimal conditions, false negatives can and do occur. In a patient with a high pretest probability of cicatricial pemphigoid, a therapeutic trial of IMT is reasonable and appropriate even if the biopsy is negative. At this point, with the information available, the atopic component should be the primary focus of future therapies.

How Will You Treat the Atopic Disease?

Treatment of allergic conjunctivitis can be challenging and is discussed more thoroughly elsewhere in this text. We will comment briefly on two important principles in this regard. First, that with vision-threatening atopic disease, close collaboration with an allergist is essential. Second, that identification, removal, and avoidance of aggravating environmental factors is the foundation of all other therapies [5].

This patient is urgently referred back to his former allergist. He will continue the oral antihistamine. He will start therapy with a topical combination antihistamine/mast cell stabilizer. A brief course of topical corticosteroids is given as well to decrease the amount of inflammation.

How Will You Address the Other Contributors to Inflammation Control (Meibomian Gland Dysfunction, Trichiasis, Dry Eye, Smoking)?

Meibomian gland disease (MGD) treatment is essential to control the underlying condition. A correlation between worsening MGD and increased tear production, possibly as a compensatory mechanism, has been described [37]. Warm compresses and eyelid massage are mainstays of initial treatment. The method of massage is important. Many patients simply rub their eyes. They should be instructed in the anatomic orientation of the meibomian glands and the need to massage vertically to maximize the effort. The use of doxycycline should also be considered.

With his occupation, computer overuse syndrome with both accommodative and evaporative components is to be expected. Smoking has also been described as an ocular irritant [38]. The patient can be educated on periodic breaks and smoking cessation.

Trichiasis does not automatically require epilation. If the lashes are long and not symptomatic, they can be monitored. In patients with active OCP, we prefer frequent epilation to avoid any trauma to the eyelid or conjunctiva. A bandage or scleral contact lens can be helpful if there is enough fornix and the patient tolerates it [39, 40]. Soft contact lenses (bandage) are particularly useful in patients with cicatricial entropion/trichiasis, and whenever possible patients are encouraged to use them on a daily basis to protect the cornea from epithelial defects and to minimize inflammation induced by the lashes. Once disease remission is achieved, hyfrecation or other surgical procedures can be considered.

If there is persistent inflammation despite therapy, the effect of trichiasis can be evaluated by epilating the lashes, filling eye with ointment, patching, and reevaluating the patient in several hours. With this treatment, trichiasis-induced injection will decrease.

Though he has partial improvement with oral and topical antihistamines, his symptoms recur (though less then at presentation) whenever steroid drops are tapered. The patient is actively working with his allergist.

Are There Are Other Ophthalmic Treatment Options? If These Fail And/Or Vision Is at Risk, Is There a Systemic IMT Modality That Could Offer a Favorable Response?

Calcineurin inhibitors are the next step. Topical options with demonstrated efficacy in atopic disease include Restasis and tacrolimus ophthalmic ointment [41, 42]. If Restasis is ineffective, compounded cyclosporine 1% ophthalmic solution can be trialed [43]. Finally, oral cyclosporine has been used to achieve remission in patients with otherwise intractable, vision-threatening atopic disease [5, 35].

What Is the Utility of Cyclosporine for OCP?

Neither cyclosporine nor tacrolimus has efficacy in OCP [1]. We have used it rarely as supplemental treatment in patients with an otherwise refractory atopic component to the conjunctivitis.

What About the Entropion? When Would You Recommend Treating This? What If the Patient Had OCP?

There is no literature specifically examining the repair of entropion secondary to atopic disease. Our preference is to await the results of the biopsy to both support the suspicion of an atopic etiology and exclude OCP. Given that he is symptomatic, that this appears to be an atopic process, and that there is very low likelihood of concomitant OCP, we would recommend early entropion repair while other therapies are being implemented.

Entropion repair on patients with uncontrolled, active OCP can lead to significant progression of the disease [44]. Outcomes are best when the disease is firmly in remission for at least a year [40]. Even with remission, we still recommend high-dose perioperative prednisone use in these patients. This delay can be very frustrating to patients, and it is important to communicate the risk reduction that it is achieving.

Through the combined efforts of you and the allergist, his underlying conjunctival inflammation is now under better control. He now chronically uses Restasis and topical and oral antihistamines. He uses tacrolimus ophthalmic ointment during spring and fall when he is most symptomatic. His now occasional flares are treated with steroid drops. He is more comfortable following entropion repair. In his gratitude, he does you the courtesy of referring his two brothers with similar symptoms to your practice.

Summary

Chronic cicatrizing conjunctivitis can have many etiologies. Evaluation of active disease requires a complete review of systems, serologic testing, and a conjunctival biopsy. Important causes of active, progressive disease include OCP, atopic disease, and rosacea. In some cases these etiologies can combine to make the disease stubborn. Additionally, systemic disorders such as Sjögren's syndrome, sarcoidosis, and GPA can uncommonly manifest this way. Trachoma, though commonly worldwide, is extremely rare in the USA.

OCP is a systemic disease requiring systemic treatment. It may occur in isolation or with involvement (sometimes occult) of other mucous membranes. We use the Foster staging system for OCP [1]. Diagnosis prior to symblepharon formation requires a high clinical suspicion and recognition of subepithelial fibrosis and forniceal foreshortening (both of which can be subtle). We routinely look for these features in patients with chronic, intractable conjunctival inflammation.

Following serologic testing and confirmatory biopsy, we advocate a stepladder approach to therapy. We typically begin with antimetabolite therapy. In progressive, advanced, or imminently vision-threatening disease, we favor combination of IVIg and rituximab. Following induction of steroid-free remission, treatment should continue at least 2 more years before tapering is attempted. We periodically obtain anterior segment photographs to evaluate the effect of treatment.

In addition to treatment of the underlying systemic process, focus on aggravating factors such as atopy, meibomian gland dysfunction, and trichiasis should be addressed. The level of conjunctival injection is the most important measure of disease activity. It is best to assess this before any drops are placed by the technician. The goal of treatment is have the conjunctival injection to be less than 0.5+. Topical steroids are not typically used as a long-term treatment and is not able to alter the course of the disease. However, it may be used adjunctively as pulse therapy. Non-preserved (e.g., dexamathasone or methylprednisolone) or non-BAK-preserved drops (e.g., difluprednate) may be preferable. Oral doxycycline or minocycline may have a small additive effect in patient receiving oral immunosuppressive agents and may be used adjunctively.

No intraocular or periocular surgery should be performed until remission is achieved. Though challenging, gaining comfort treating this potentially blinding disease is a worthwhile endeavor and can be as rewarding to the provider as it is beneficial to the patient.

Acknowledgments *Financial Disclosures*: None of the authors have any financial disclosures regarding the contents discussed in this manuscript. *Conflict of Interest*: None of the authors have any conflicts of interest with the contents discussed in this manuscript.

References

1. Foster CS. Cicatricial pemphigoid. Trans Am Ophthalmol Soc. 1986;84:527–663.
2. Foster CS, Fong LP, Azar D, Kenyon KR. Episodic conjunctival inflammation after Stevens-Johnson syndrome. Ophthalmology. 1988;95(4):453–62.
3. Kirzhner M, Jakobiec FA. Ocular cicatricial pemphigoid: a review of clinical features, immunopathology, differential diagnosis, and current management. Semin Ophthalmol. 2011;26(4-5):270–7.
4. Ravage ZB, Beck AP, Macsai MS, Ching SS. Ocular rosacea can mimic trachoma: a case of cicatrizing conjunctivitis. Cornea. 2004;23(6):630–1.
5. Foster CS, Calonge M. Atopic keratoconjunctivitis. Ophthalmology. 1990;97(8):992–1000.
6. Geggel HS, Mensher JH. Cicatricial conjunctivitis in sarcoidosis: recognition and treatment. Ann Ophthalmol. 1989;21(3):92–4.
7. Nguyen DQ, Harper J, Hiscott P, Quah SA, Jacob A, Kaye SB. The significance of cicatricial conjunctivitis in Wegener's granulomatosis. Nephrol Dial Transplant. 2006;21(11):3342–3.
8. Miserocchi E, Waheed NK, Baltatzis S, Foster CS. Chronic cicatrizing conjunctivitis in a patient with ocular cicatricial pemphigoid and fatal Wegener granulomatosis. Am J Ophthalmol. 2001;132(6):923–4.
9. Ahuero AE, Jakobiec FA, Bhat P, Ciralsky JB, Papaliodis GN. Paraneoplastic conjunctival cicatrization: two different pathogenic types. Ophthalmology. 2010;117(4):659–64.
10. Taylor HR, Burton MJ, Haddad D, West S, Wright H. Trachoma. Lancet. 2014;384(9960):2142–52.

11. Foster CS, Sainz De La Maza M. Ocular cicatricial pemphigoid review. Curr Opin Allergy Clin Immunol. 2004;4(5):435–9.
12. Faraj HG, Hoang-Xuan T. Chronic cicatrizing conjunctivitis. Curr Opin Ophthalmol. 2001;12(4):250–7.
13. Eschle-Meniconi ME, Ahmad SR, Foster CS. Mucous membrane pemphigoid: an update. Curr Opin Ophthalmol. 2005;16(5):303–7.
14. Bernauer W, Elder MJ, Leonard JN, Wright P, Dart JK. The value of biopsies in the evaluation of chronic progressive conjunctival cicatrisation. Graefes Arch Clin Exp Ophthalmol. 1994;232(9):533–7.
15. Schempf U, Plentz R, Stueker D, et al. Scarring mucous membrane pemphigoid presenting as double stenosis of the larynx and esophagus: precautions during therapy can avoid complications. Endoscopy. 2014;46(Suppl 1):E617–8.
16. Grau AE, Setterfield J, Saw VP. How to do conjunctival and buccal biopsies to investigate cicatrising conjunctivitis: improving the diagnosis of ocular mucous membrane pemphigoid. Br J Ophthalmol. 2013;97(4):530–1.
17. Saw VP, Dart JK, Rauz S, et al. Immunosuppressive therapy for ocular mucous membrane pemphigoid strategies and outcomes. Ophthalmology. 2008;115(2):253–61, e251.
18. McCluskey P, Chang JH, Singh R, Wakefield D. Methotrexate therapy for ocular cicatricial pemphigoid. Ophthalmology. 2004;111(4):796–801.
19. Miserocchi E, Baltatzis S, Roque MR, Ahmed AR, Foster CS. The effect of treatment and its related side effects in patients with severe ocular cicatricial pemphigoid. Ophthalmology. 2002;109(1):111–8.
20. Geerling G, Dart JK. Management and outcome of cataract surgery in ocular cicatricial pemphigoid. Graefes Arch Clin Exp Ophthalmol. 2000;238(2):112–8.
21. Puranik CJ, Murthy SI, Taneja M, Sangwan VS. Outcomes of cataract surgery in ocular cicatricial pemphigoid. Ocul Immunol Inflamm. 2013;21(6):449–54.
22. Bissen-Miyajima H, Monden Y, Shimazaki J, Tsubota K. Cataract surgery combined with ocular surface reconstruction in patients with severe cicatricial keratoconjunctivitis. J Cataract Refract Surg. 2002;28(8):1379–85.
23. Sainz de la Maza M, Tauber J, Foster CS. Cataract surgery in ocular cicatricial pemphigoid. Ophthalmology. 1988;95(4):481–6.
24. Foster CS, Chang PY, Ahmed AR. Combination of rituximab and intravenous immunoglobulin for recalcitrant ocular cicatricial pemphigoid: a preliminary report. Ophthalmology. 2010;117(5):861–9.
25. Sami N, Letko E, Androudi S, Daoud Y, Foster CS, Ahmed AR. Intravenous immunoglobulin therapy in patients with ocular-cicatricial pemphigoid: a long-term follow-up. Ophthalmology. 2004;111(7):1380–2.
26. Sobolewska B, Doycheva D, Deuter C, Pfeffer I, Schaller M, Zierhut M. Treatment of ocular rosacea with once-daily low-dose doxycycline. Cornea. 2014;33(3):257–60.
27. Suelves AM, Arcinue CA, Gonzalez-Martin JM, Kruh JN, Foster CS. Analysis of a novel protocol of pulsed intravenous cyclophosphamide for recalcitrant or severe ocular inflammatory disease. Ophthalmology. 2013;120(6):1201–9.
28. Friedman J, Marcovich AL, Kleinmann G, Schattner A. Low-dose pulsed intravenous cyclophosphamide for severe ocular cicatricial pemphigoid in elderly patients. Cornea. 2014;33(10):1066–70.
29. Tugal-Tutkun I, Akova YA, Foster CS. Penetrating keratoplasty in cicatrizing conjunctival diseases. Ophthalmology. 1995;102(4):576–85.
30. Palioura S, Kim B, Dohlman CH, Chodosh J. The Boston keratoprosthesis type I in mucous membrane pemphigoid. Cornea. 2013;32(7):956–61.
31. Pujari S, Siddique SS, Dohlman CH, Chodosh J. The Boston keratoprosthesis type II: the Massachusetts eye and ear infirmary experience. Cornea. 2011;30(12):1298–303.
32. Ahmad S, Akpek EK, Gehlbach PL, Dunlap K, Ramulu PY. Predictors of visual outcomes following Boston type 1 keratoprosthesis implantation. Am J Ophthalmol. 2015;159(4):739–47.

33. Sotozono C, Inatomi T, Nakamura T, et al. Visual improvement after cultivated oral mucosal epithelial transplantation. Ophthalmology. 2013;120(1):193–200.
34. Ahmed AR, Dahl MV. Consensus statement on the use of intravenous immunoglobulin therapy in the treatment of autoimmune mucocutaneous blistering diseases. Arch Dermatol. 2003;139(8):1051–9.
35. Power WJ, Tugal-Tutkun I, Foster CS. Long-term follow-up of patients with atopic keratoconjunctivitis. Ophthalmology. 1998;105(4):637–42.
36. Wakamatsu TH, Satake Y, Igarashi A, et al. IgE and eosinophil cationic protein (ECP) as markers of severity in the diagnosis of atopic keratoconjunctivitis. Br J Ophthalmol. 2012;96(4):581–6.
37. Arita R, Morishige N, Koh S, et al. Increased tear fluid production as a compensatory response to meibomian gland loss: a multicenter cross-sectional study. Ophthalmology. 2015;122(5):925–33.
38. Matsumoto Y, Dogru M, Goto E, et al. Alterations of the tear film and ocular surface health in chronic smokers. Eye. 2008;22(7):961–8.
39. Schornack MM, Baratz KH. Ocular cicatricial pemphigoid: the role of scleral lenses in disease management. Cornea. 2009;28(10):1170–2.
40. Gibbons A, Johnson TE, Wester ST, et al. Management of patients with confirmed and presumed mucous membrane pemphigoid undergoing entropion repair. Am J Ophthalmol. 2015;159(5):846–52, e842.
41. Nivenius E, van der Ploeg I, Jung K, Chryssanthou E, van Hage M, Montan PG. Tacrolimus ointment vs steroid ointment for eyelid dermatitis in patients with atopic keratoconjunctivitis. Eye. 2007;21(7):968–75.
42. Gonzalez-Lopez JJ, Lopez-Alcalde J, Morcillo Laiz R, Fernandez Buenaga R, Rebolleda Fernandez G. Topical cyclosporine for atopic keratoconjunctivitis. Cochrane Database Syst Rev. 2012;9:CD009078.
43. Tesse R, Spadavecchia L, Fanelli P, et al. Treatment of severe vernal keratoconjunctivitis with 1% topical cyclosporine in an Italian cohort of 197 children. Pediatr Allergy Immunol. 2010;21(2 Pt 1):330–5.
44. Hatton MP, Raizman M, Foster CS. Exacerbation of undiagnosed ocular cicatricial pemphigoid after repair of involutional entropion. Ophthal Plast Reconstr Surg. 2008;24(2):165–6.

Chapter 13
Scleral Lenses in the Management of Ocular Surface Disease

Ellen Shorter and Victoria Butcko

Case 1

A 64-year-old male patient was referred for evaluation. He had a history of chronic lymphocytic leukemia with previous allogenic stem cell transplantation. His chief complaint was eye irritation with foreign body sensation in the left eye greater than right.

Previous ocular history included severe dry eye syndrome secondary to chronic ocular graft-versus-host disease (GVHD), filamentary keratitis, superior limbic keratoconjunctivitis, and resolved corneal epithelial defect in the left eye. Current ocular medications included preservative-free artificial tears tid OU, oral doxycycline 20 mg bid, and 50% autologous serum tears qid OU. Previous ocular treatment included topical cyclosporine 0.05%, punctal occlusion, topical steroids, and soft bandage contact lenses.

He had trace scurf, lid margin telangiectasia, 1+ meibomian gland inspissation, and silicone punctal plugs present in all four puncta. On lid eversion, there was 1+ hyperemia and mild fibrosis of the upper tarsal plates. There was 1+ diffuse conjunctival injection and conjunctival chalasis with fluorescein staining along the superior bulbar conjunctiva and limbus in both eyes. The right cornea had 1+ inferior punctate corneal staining with inferior filaments and 2+ superior limbal punctate staining. The left eye had 3+ diffuse punctate staining with filaments and 3+ superior limbal punctate staining.

E. Shorter, OD (✉)
University of Illinois at Chicago, 1855 W. Taylor Street, Chicago, IL 60612, USA
e-mail: eshorter@uic.edu

V. Butcko, OD
The Jesse Brown VA Medical Center, Chicago, IL 60612, USA

A.R. Djalilian (ed.), *Ocular Surface Disease*,
https://doi.org/10.1007/978-3-319-15823-5_13

What Additional Therapeutic Measures Would You Consider for This Patient?

This patient has severe dry eye secondary to chronic ocular GVHD. He has been on maximal therapy but still continues to be debilitated by his symptoms. He could benefit from a large-diameter gas-permeable scleral lens or prosthetic replacement of the ocular surface ecosystem (PROSE) device. The goals of fitting a therapeutic scleral lens or PROSE device is to improve ocular comfort and support the ocular surface that has been unresponsive to traditional ocular surface disease treatment (Fig. 13.1).

When initial topical therapy and lid hygiene management cannot adequately relieve a patient's symptoms, gas-permeable scleral lenses are an option to improve the ocular surface, provide symptomatic relief of dry eye symptoms, and improve visual acuity [1]. The large diameter of the device covers the ocular surface and bathes the cornea and conjunctival tissue in a fluid reservoir. This environment promotes healing of the surface epitheliopathy while improving pain and photophobia associated with chronic ocular GVHD [2].

Graft-versus-host disease (GVHD) describes inflammatory manifestations that occur after transplant when there is activation of donor T cells causing an extensive inflammatory reaction often affecting multiple organ systems. GVHD can be described as acute, occurring within the first 100 days of transplant, or chronic. Acute GVHD most often involves the mucous membranes of the mouth and intestinal tract, liver, and skin. Chronic GVHD occurs in 60–70% of patients [3].

Ocular manifestations of GVHD are commonly relapsing and remitting and affect an estimated 25% [4] to 50% [5] of individuals with systemic GVHD. One of the most common ocular sequelae, as seen in our patient, is keratoconjunctivitis sicca. This complication has been reported to occur in 53% of individuals with

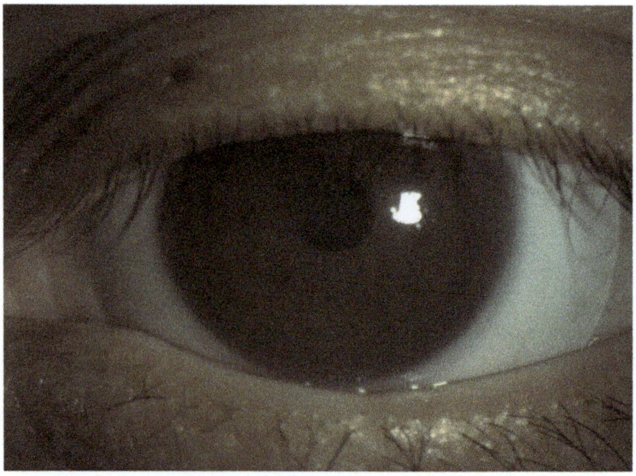

Fig. 13.1 Image of a patient's well-fit scleral lens

chronic GVHD [6]. Lacrimal gland dysfunction causes severe aqueous deficiency and is usually complicated by meibomian gland dysfunction. Additional findings can include scleroderma-like eyelid changes, filamentary keratitis, and corneal ulcers [7].**The patient was evaluated and fit with 18.2 mm diagnostic scleral lenses in office. His comfort and lens fit were evaluated after a settling period of 30 min. The first set of lenses were ordered.**

What Are the Key Components for Evaluating the Fit of a Scleral Lens or PROSE Device?

First, it is essential to determine if the lens completely clears and vaults over the cornea. If there is complete corneal clearance, next evaluate the limbal area to ensure limbal clearance. If central or limbal touch is suspected, fluorescein dye can be applied to the bowl of the lens, and a thin, white light optic section can help identify areas of touch. Lastly, evaluate the haptic portion of the lens that rests on the sclera. The haptic should not compress the blood vessels and should align with the sclera avoiding both edge impingement and excessive edge lift. Once appropriate corneal vault is achieved, a spherical over-refraction should be performed to obtain best corrected visual acuity.

The patient returned 2 weeks later and was trained on safe lens handling and instructed to use preservative-free saline to fill the bowl of the lens. Visual acuity was 20/20 OD/OS, and he reported immediate relief in his dry eye symptoms.

Therapeutic scleral contact lens fits have proved efficacious at improving dry eye symptoms with a high rate of continuation of scleral lens wear in patients with GVHD (90%) over an average of 32 months [8].

What Are Some Special Considerations with Scleral Lenses in Patients with Severe Ocular Surface Disease?

Patients with OSD should be monitored closely. We typically schedule follow-up visits 1 week after the initial lenses are dispensed and then every few weeks as needed. Patients may need to be seen more frequently if they experience issues with lens application and removal or require many lens modifications to improve fit. At each visit, we measure visual acuity, evaluate the fit, and ensure there is adequate corneal and limbal clearance. We also monitor the conjunctiva for areas of compression, stain, or signs of haptic tightness. These issues could cause inadequate tear film exchange and lead to corneal edema or neovascularization from hypoxia. Topical therapies, including immunosuppressive therapies or serum tears, may also be tapered or eliminated in some patients.

It should be emphasized that only non-preserved solutions should be used to fill the bowl of the lens. We recommend prescribing 0.9% inhalation sodium chloride solution available in 3 mL or 5 mL sterile unit vials. Another option is preservative-free buffered ophthalmic saline that is available in a larger 4 ounce bottle. In general, topical medications should be used without the scleral lens in place. If you prescribe medications to be placed directly in the bowl of the device, care should be taken to use preservative-free formulations. If the patient is using autologous serum tears, we generally encourage them to continue their use before and after lens wear or overtop of the lens. In some circumstances, you may recommend they place a drop of serum tears directly into the bowl of the lens before application; however, you should monitor for complications or infection.

Despite having a good scleral lens fit, patients with severe ocular surface disease often experience issues with lens fogging. The fogging can be due to poor surface wetting or buildup of debris in the fluid under the lens. This can contribute to progressive blurring of the vision after a few hours of lens wear. If the fogging is related to the lens surface, the patient can increase the frequency of artificial tears or remove and reapply the lens. A trial of off-label Mucomyst (10% *N*-acetylcysteine) eye drops may be tried to inhibit mucus buildup on the surface. Clouding of the tear film reservoir can be seen in patients with scleral lenses that have areas of corneal touch, excessive edge lift, or, alternatively, tight edges with poor fluid exchange. If fluorescein dye placed on the surface immediately seeps beneath the edge, the haptic can be tightened in that area. Some of these cases may represent inflammatory cells or epithelial cells. We have anecdotally noticed that loose conjunctiva (chalasis) may contribute to the collection of cells and debris in the reservoir.

Discussion

Bandage soft contact lenses can also be considered in the management of chronic ocular GVHD. Russo et al. found that extended wear silicone hydrogel lenses provided symptomatic relief but did not improve the condition of the ocular surface [9]. Another study of extended wear bandage soft contact lenses found improvement in manifestations of ocular GVHD with less punctate epithelial erosions in 58% of patients after 2 weeks [10]. While neither study reported any complications, consideration must be given to the use of prophylactic antibiotics given the risk of microbial keratitis with extended wear soft lens use on an already compromised epithelium (e.g., ofloxacin or polymyxin-trimethoprim 1–2 times a day). We have used daily wear soft lenses successfully in ocular GVHD patients, particularly if they have a history of contact lens wear in the past. Overall, soft lenses improve patient symptoms however seem less effective for improving signs compared to scleral lenses. In our experience, most patients with severe disease are ultimately transitioned to scleral devices.

Consistent with current literature, this patient reported immediate improvement of ocular surface disease symptoms. He felt a relief from burning, less grittiness, decreased eye pain, and decreased foreign body sensation with the gas-permeable scleral lenses. In this particular case, when conventional therapy had failed to alleviate symptoms, the gas-permeable scleral lenses provided much needed relief to the patient while also protecting the cornea and conjunctiva from desiccation and blink-related trauma [2].

Case 2

A 78-year-old male patient was referred due to complaints of contact lens intolerance and decreased lens wear time. He had a history of keratoconus with previous penetrating keratoplasty surgery in both eyes 35 years ago, pseudophakia, ocular hypertension, and dry eye syndrome. He complained of constant, severe, burning eye pain. His ocular medications included fluorometholone 0.1 % qd OU, bimatoprost 0.01 % qhs OU, timolol qam OS, cyclosporine 0.05 % bid OU, and preserved artificial tears q2h.

Best corrected visual acuity with 9.5 mm corneal gas-permeable lenses was 20/20 in both eyes. Vision was correctable to 20/30 in both eyes with a manifest refraction of – 5.25 + 6.00 × 173 OD and – 6.00 + 5.25 × 120 OS.

On slit lamp examination, there was severe lid telangiectasia and gland inspissation with thick, turbid meibum that could not be expressed. There was 1+ diffuse bulbar conjunctiva injection and corneal grafts with inferior ectasia and 1+ punctate staining. The gas-permeable lenses were flat-fitting with central corneal touch and excessive edge lift.

Intraocular pressures were 16 mmHg OD and 15 mmHg and pachymetry was 584 OD and 534 OS. The dilated fundus exam was normal with healthy optic nerves and cup-to-disc ratios of 0.25 in the right eye and 0.3 in the left eye.

Given the Patient's History of Corneal Ectasia, What Type of Optical Correction Would You Consider?

Spectacles and soft contact lenses are considered; however, they are not ideal for this patient due to high amounts of refractive astigmatism and irregular corneal astigmatism. Gas-permeable lenses are a better option as they mask corneal irregularity and generally provide superior visual clarity.

The decision was made to refit his corneal gas permeable lenses and reduce corneal bearing. We discussed a range of corrective options available including small-diameter gas-permeable, piggyback lens systems, hybrid and large-diameter gas-permeable lenses including scleral lenses, or PROSE devices.

What Recommendations Would You Make for This Patient Based on His Dry Eye Symptoms and Clinical Findings of Meibomian Gland Dysfunction?

The patient was instructed to discontinue all benzalkonium chloride (BAK) preserved artificial tears and instructed to use preservative-free artificial tears. Education on meibomian gland dysfunction and lid hygiene was provided, and warm compresses with lid cleaning were initiated.

At the follow-up visit, he reported clear vision with his new corneal gas-permeable lenses but continued to experience eye and eyelid pain. He described the soreness as severe and constant, occurring with or without lenses on.

In consultation with his cornea and glaucoma specialists, a plan was made to reduce all preserved ophthalmic medications. Humphrey 24–2 visual field exams were full, but given his history of intraocular pressures in the mid-30s, prophylactic therapy was continued. Timolol was changed to a preservative-free formulation and bimatoprost was discontinued. Fluorometholone 0.1% was replaced with preservative-free loteprednol 0.5% (ointment), and preservative-free erythromycin ointment was added for use at bedtime.

If Further Intraocular Pressure Lowering Is Necessary, What Other Alternative Treatments Would You Consider?

A number of topical glaucoma medications are available in preservative-free formulations including timolol, dorzolamide/timolol combination, and prostaglandin analog tafluprost. Additional options such as Alphagan®P with Purite (Allergan, Dublin, Ireland) and Travatan Z® with SofZia (Alcon, Fort Worth, Texas) have a less irritating, vanishing preservative. If additional intraocular pressure lowering is deemed necessary, oral agents, argon laser trabeculoplasty, selective laser trabeculoplasty, or glaucoma surgeries could also be considered.

Despite aggressive therapy, the patient had ongoing eyelid inflammation and eye pain.

What Other Therapies Are Available for the Management of Meibomian Gland Dysfunction?

Systemic tetracycline or topical azithromycin treatment can also be used. Low-dose doxycycline has been shown to be as effective as high-dose doxycycline at decreasing subjective symptoms for patients with chronic meibomian gland dysfunction with fewer reported side effects [11]. Topical azithromycin 1% (Akorn, Lake Forest, Illinois) can also be prescribed for patients who remain symptomatic as it has been shown to increase tear film stability [12]. A 2-week treatment of topical treatment has been shown to significantly reduce the signs and symptoms of posterior blepharitis compared to warm compresses alone [13]. Meibomian gland intraductal probing (Maskin Meibomian Gland Intraductal Probe, Rhein Medical, St Petersburg, Florida) and LipiFlow® thermal pulsation system (TearScience, Morrisville, NC) are additional therapies available for meibomian gland dysfunction refractory to traditional therapies. These treatments can be costly as they are not widely covered by insurance plans.

Our patient underwent Maskin meibomian gland intraductal probing. His eyelids showed rapid improvement of the lid margin inflammation and improved meibum flow. Maintenance with frequent warm compresses and lid cleaning was recommended.

The patient was evaluated for PROSE treatment in both eyes. The goals of treatment were to support the ocular surface while maintaining clear visual acuity. Using PROSE devices, he achieved clear, comfortable vision with all-day wear.

Large-diameter gas-permeable lenses are an excellent option for patients with corneal irregularity and ocular surface disease. They play an important role in improving visual acuity in patients with ectasia when traditional modalities have failed. Scleral lenses have been shown to improve best corrected visual acuity from 20/40 to 20/20 in patients with keratoconus after an average of only 2.8 fitting visits [14]. PROSE treatment can improve visual acuity and visual function in patients with irregular corneas. PROSE treatment has been shown to improve Ocular Surface Disease Index scores by 79% in patients with irregular astigmatism after penetrating keratoplasty and improve logarithm of minimal angle of resolution vision 88% in patients with keratoconus [15].

We strongly encourage patients with advanced corneal ectasia be evaluated for a large-diameter gas-permeable lens prior to proceeding with penetrating keratoplasty. A comparative study of patients with ectasia who underwent either keratoplasty or PROSE treatment found that eyes with advanced corneal ectasia can be fit successfully with PROSE devices with better and more rapid visual acuity outcomes compared to keratoplasty [16].

Scleral devices can provide long-term visual rehabilitation while maintaining ocular comfort. A review of 63 patients' (107) eyes fit with scleral lenses for keratoconus, post-keratoplasty astigmatism, and corneal scarring found that 78% of patients reported good comfort and 75% continued scleral lens use after 3 months [17]. An additional series of patients with corneal ectasia from the Boston Foundation for Sight reported 88% of eyes had continued daily device use after 6 months and 26.6 point improvement in NEI VFQ-25 scores [18].

Case 3

A 55-year-old female was referred for evaluation of a non-healing epithelial defect. She had a history of aneurysm with CN VI and CN VII palsy resulting in severe exposure keratopathy. Treatment required a 6 mm permanent lateral tarsorrhaphy and gold weight eyelid implant. The ocular surface remained

stable for many years with 20/200 visual acuity. After complications arose from migration of the gold weight requiring removal, she presented with a non-healing 1.5 × 3 mm persistent epithelial defect in the left eye.

What Initial Treatment Do You Consider for a Patient with a Non-healing Epithelial Defect?

The initial therapy for an epithelial defect typically includes frequent lubrication and soft bandage contact lens application with prophylactic antibiotics. If the defect remains despite treatment, it is important to eliminate potential medicamentosa from topical ophthalmic medications. If this is ruled out, punctal occlusion may be helpful in addition to pressure patching or even tarsorrhaphy as was done previously with this patient.

There are also a number of newer therapies that can be considered for a persistent epithelial defect that has been refractory to traditional therapies. Surface healing may be achieved with the addition of autologous serum drops, amniotic membrane grafts, and scleral lenses or PROSE treatment. Autologous serum tears have been shown effective in 47–83% of cases where persistent epithelial defects did not resolve with standard therapy [19]. Amniotic membrane grafting can be used to reduce inflammation, vascularization, and scarring of the cornea while promoting reepithelialization. Prokera (Bio-Tissue, Miami, FL), a self-retaining amniotic membrane device, is readily available and can easily be placed in office [19].

What Is the Role of PROSE Treatment in Patients with Persistent Epithelial Defects?

PROSE treatment has been shown to be very effective for patients with non-healing epithelial defects. The device completely bathes the ocular surface in sterile saline providing a healthy environment for the cornea to promote rapid healing. Within the fluid-filled chamber of the PROSE device, there is a continuous fluid-tear interchange under that haptic to provide oxygen to the compromised corneal surface [19].

A retrospective review showed eight eyes with non-healing defects refractory to traditional therapy were treated with a fluid-ventilated, gas-permeable PROSE devices. A standardized protocol was used with continuous PROSE wear and was followed until re-epithelialization was achieved. The devices were removed briefly daily for cleaning, disinfection, and replacement of the fluid reservoir with preservative-free saline and one drop of preservative-free fourth-generation fluoroquinolone antibiotic for prophylaxis. Once cornea re-epithelialization was achieved, the patient was transitioned to daily device wear. All eyes achieved resolution of the persistent epithelial defects without any cases of microbial keratitis [20]. Another series of patients with persistent epithelial defects from BostonSight using PROSE treatment with overnight wear and prophylactic moxifloxacin reported complete re-epithelialization in 17/20 eyes after a median duration of 8.5 days without any complications of microbial keratitis [21]. Continuous wear of a scleral or PROSE device can promote healing of epithelial defects that have been unresponsive to traditional therapies; however, patients require close clinical monitoring and fourth-generation topical fluoroquinolone use.

Over the course of 2 months, the epithelial defect failed to heal despite frequent lubrication, overnight patching, bandage contact lens, debridement, and autologous serum tears. PROSE treatment was discussed and an in-office consultation was scheduled. The goal of treatment was to heal the epithelial defect and to support the ocular surface. A PROSE device was applied in office with some difficulty due to partial lateral tarsorrhaphy. Visual acuity was 20/40 with an 18 mm trial device. A smaller device was considered; however, a partial reversal of the tarsorrhaphy was performed.

The patient was able to safely apply and remove the PROSE device with the assistance of a lighted stand and plunger. She was unable to return for daily monitoring so the decision was made to limit the device use to daytime with prophylactic moxifloxacin 0.5% and erythromycin 0.5% ointment at bedtime.

What Type of Follow Up Schedule Would You Recommend for This Patient?

Patients with slowly healing or non-healing epithelial defects require very close monitoring due to risk of infectious keratitis and corneal melt. As seen with this patient, concurrent prophylactic antibiotic therapy was warranted. She was educated on the signs and symptoms of infection and scheduled for follow-up twice weekly.

After 4 weeks of daily wear with the PROSE device, the persistent epithelial defect resolved and her vision was correctable to 20/25 in the left eye.

Acknowledgments *Financial Disclosures*: None of the authors have any financial disclosures regarding the contents discussed in this manuscript. *Conflict of Interest*: None of the authors have any conflicts of interest with the contents discussed in this manuscript.

References

1. Jacobs DS, Rosenthal P. Boston scleral lens prosthetic device for treatment of severe dry eye in chronic graft-versus-host disease. Cornea. 2007;26(10):1195–9. doi:10.1097/ICO.0b013e318155743d.
2. Schornack MM, Baratz KH, Patel SV, Maguire LJ. Jupiter scleral lenses in the management of chronic graft versus host disease. Eye Contact Lens. 2008;34(6):302–5. doi:10.1097/ICL.0b013e318188e205.

3. Lee SJ, Vogelsang G, Flowers MED. Chronic graft-versus-host disease. Biol Blood Marrow Transplant. 2003;9(4):215–33. doi:10.1053/bbmt.2003.50026.
4. Lin X, Cavanagh H. Ocular manifestations of graft-versus-host disease: 10 years' experience. Clin Ophthalmol. 2015;9:1209–13.
5. Westeneng AC, Hettinga Y, Lokhorst H, Verdonck L, van Dorp S, Rothova A. Ocular graft-versus-host disease after allogeneic stem cell transplantation. Cornea. 2010;29(7):758–63. doi:10.1097/ICO.0b013e3181ca321c.
6. Allan EJ, Flowers MED, Lin MP, Bensinger RE, Martin PJ, Wu MC. Visual acuity and anterior segment findings in chronic graft-versus-host disease. Cornea. 2011;30:1392–7. doi:10.1097/ICO.0b013e31820ce6d0.
7. Nassar A, Tabbara KF, Aljurf M. Ocular manifestations of graft-versus-host disease. Saudi J Ophthalmol. 2013;27(3):215–22. doi:10.1016/j.sjopt.2013.06.007.
8. Schornack MM, Pyle J, Patel SV. Scleral lenses in the management of ocular surface disease. Ophthalmology. 2014;121(7):1398–405. doi:10.1016/j.ophtha.2014.01.028.
9. Russo PA, Bouchard CS, Galasso JM. Extended-wear silicone hydrogel soft contact lenses in the management of moderate to severe dry eye signs and symptoms secondary to graft-versus-host disease. Eye Contact Lens. 2007;33(3):144–7. doi:10.1097/01.icl.0000244154.76214.2d.
10. Inamoto Y, Sun Y-C, Flowers MED, et al. Bandage soft contact lenses for ocular graft-versus-host disease. Biol Blood Marrow Transplant. 2015;21(11):2002–7.
11. Yoo S-E, Lee D-C, Chang M-H. The effect of low-dose doxycycline therapy in chronic meibomian gland dysfunction. Korean J Ophthalmol. 2005;19:258–63. doi:10.3341/kjo.2005.19.4.258.
12. Foulks GN, Borchman D, Yappert MC, Kakar S. Topical azithromycin and oral doxycycline therapy of meibomian gland dysfunction: a comparative clinical and spectroscopic pilot study. Cornea. 2013;32(1):44–53. doi:10.1097/ICO.0b013e318254205f.
13. Luchs J. Efficacy of topical azithromycin ophthalmic solution 1% in the treatment of posterior blepharitis. Adv Ther. 2008;25(9):858–70. doi:10.1007/s12325-008-0096-9.
14. Schornack MM, Patel SV. Scleral lenses in the management of keratoconus. Eye Contact Lens. 2010;36(1):39–44. doi:10.1097/ICL.0b013e3181c786a6.
15. Lee JC, Chiu GB, Bach D, Bababeygy SR, Irvine J, Heur M. Functional and visual improvement with prosthetic replacement of the ocular surface ecosystem scleral lenses for irregular corneas. Cornea. 2013;32:1540–3. doi:10.1097/ICO.0b013e3182a73802.
16. DeLoss KS, Fatteh NH, Hood CT. Prosthetic replacement of the ocular surface ecosystem (PROSE) scleral device compared to keratoplasty for the treatment of corneal ectasia. Am J Ophthalmol. 2014;158(5):974–982.e2. doi:10.1016/j.ajo.2014.07.016.
17. Pecego M, Barnett M, Mannis MJ, Durbin-Johnson B. Jupiter scleral lenses: the UC Davis eye center experience. Eye Contact Lens. 2012;38(3):179–82. doi:10.1097/ICL.0b013e31824daa5e.
18. Baran I, Bradley JA, Alipour F, Rosenthal P, Le HG, Jacobs DS. PROSE treatment of corneal ectasia. Cont Lens Anterior Eye. 2012;35(5):222–7. doi:10.1016/j.clae.2012.04.003.
19. Katzman LR, Jeng BH. Management strategies for persistent epithelial defects of the cornea. Saudi J Ophthalmol. 2014;28(3):168–72. doi:10.1016/j.sjopt.2014.06.011.
20. Ciralsky JB, Chapman KO, Rosenblatt MI, et al. Treatment of refractory persistent corneal epithelial defects: a standardized approach using continuous wear PROSE therapy. Ocul Immunol Inflamm. 2014;23(3):219–24. doi:10.3109/09273948.2014.894084.
21. Lim P, Ridges R, Jacobs DS, Rosenthal P. Treatment of persistent corneal epithelial defect with overnight wear of a prosthetic device for the ocular surface. Am J Ophthalmol. 2013;156(6):1095–101. doi:10.1016/j.ajo.2013.06.006.

Chapter 14
Recent Advances in Conjunctivochalasis

Anny M.S. Cheng and Scheffer C.G. Tseng

Ocular surface health is maintained by a stable tear film, which requires both compositional and hydrodynamic factors [1]. The former comprises adequate production of mucins and aqueous tears. The latter includes the eyelids, with blinking to allow tear spread and clearance, whereas the eyelids close to avoid exposure. The stability and spread of the tear film requires coordinating effects between both compositional and hydrodynamic elements in the ocular defense system [1]. The compositional elements are comprised of the lacrimal glands, the meibomian glands, and the ocular surface epithelium to provide aqueous, lipid, and mucins in the tear fluid, respectively, while the hydrodynamic elements include tear spread, drainage, and evaporation, which are controlled by eyelid blinking and closure [1]. With each blink, tears spread from the conjunctival cul-de-sac in the fornix (third compartment) to the tear meniscus (second compartment) and finally to the preocular tear film (first compartment) [2, 3]. Also through blinking, the tear fluid is cleared into the nasal lacrimal drainage system.

Conjunctivochalasis (CCh) is defined as a disease process leading to the formation of a loose and redundant conjunctival fold interspersed between the globe and eyelids [4]. Advances have been made in the pathogenesis of CCh as a disease that is characterized by overexpression of matrix metalloproteinase (MMP) by CCh fibroblasts [5, 6]. The redundant conjunctival folds of CCh Conjunctivochalasis (CCh) redundant conjunctival fold interfere the tear flow by blocking the tear drainage puncta [7], disrupting continuity of the tear meniscus [4, 7, 8], and extending

A.M.S. Cheng, MD
Ocular Surface Center and Ocular Surface Research and Education Foundation,
7000 SW 97th Avenue, Suite 213, Miami, FL 33173, USA

Florida International University, Herbert Wertheim College of Medicine,
Miami, FL 33173, USA

S.C.G. Tseng, MD, PhD (✉)
Ocular Surface Center and Ocular Surface Research and Education Foundation,
7000 SW 97th Avenue, Suite 213, Miami, FL 33173, USA
e-mail: stseng@ocularsurface.com

A.R. Djalilian (ed.), *Ocular Surface Disease*,
https://doi.org/10.1007/978-3-319-15823-5_14

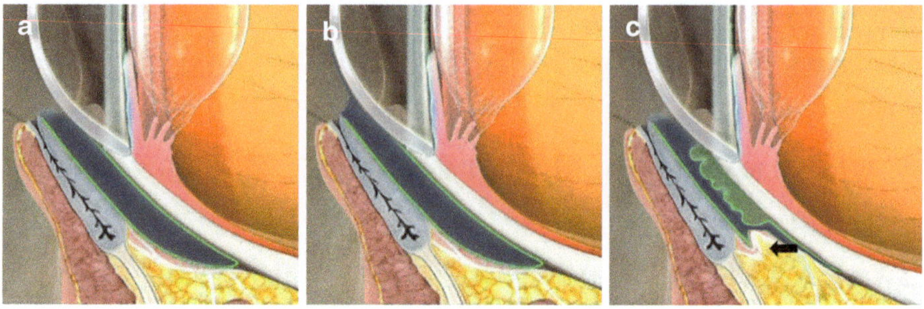

Fig. 14.1 Schematic demonstration of tear flow obliterated by CCh. Under the normal circumstance, the fornix tear reservoir depicted in *dark blue* is responsible for delivering tear fluids to the tear meniscus (**a**) and preocular surface (**b**) by blinking. In CCh, tear spread and fornix tear reservoir are obliterated by loose and wrinkled conjunctiva (**c**, *green*) and prolapse fat (**c**, *arrow*) due to degenerated Tenon's capsule (Taken with permission from Cheng et al. [9])

from the lid margin/meniscus locale to the fornix [9] to obliterate the tear flow from the fornix reservoir to the tear meniscus [10] (Fig. 14.1). Because CCh is highly prevalent [11] and age-dependent [11, 12], it can be a common but overlooked cause of ocular discomfort and may associate with tear instability that clinically mimics dry eye [reviewed in [4]]. Because both CCh and aqueous tear-deficient (ATD) dry eye are common in older populations, their coexistence makes it difficult to discern genuine dry eye from dry eye secondary to CCh. Furthermore, the aforementioned pathogenesis of CCh in perturbing the tear spread strongly suggests that the severity of dry eye can be aggravated by CCh. Herein, we illustrate three cases to highlight our proposed rationale in laying down a practical and logical algorithm for managing ocular surface diseases that manifest CCh.

Case #1

A 49-year-old female presented with ocular irritation, blurry vision, dryness, and tearing in both eyes for 6 years. She had been unsuccessfully treated with various topical concomitant medications including artificial tears, lubricants, conventional steroid, and cyclosporine. Her nasolacrimal drainage system was patent as confirmed by multiple times of probing and irrigation. Upon first office visit, slit lamp examination showed redundant conjunctival tissue interposed between the lid margin and the eye globe and an uneven but high tear meniscus (Fig. 14.2a). Her eyelids showed intact closure and blinking. All four puncta were swollen by inflammation and collapsed into a slit-like open appearance (Fig. 14.2b). Her tarsal and conjunctiva were diffusely injected (Fig. 14.2c, d).

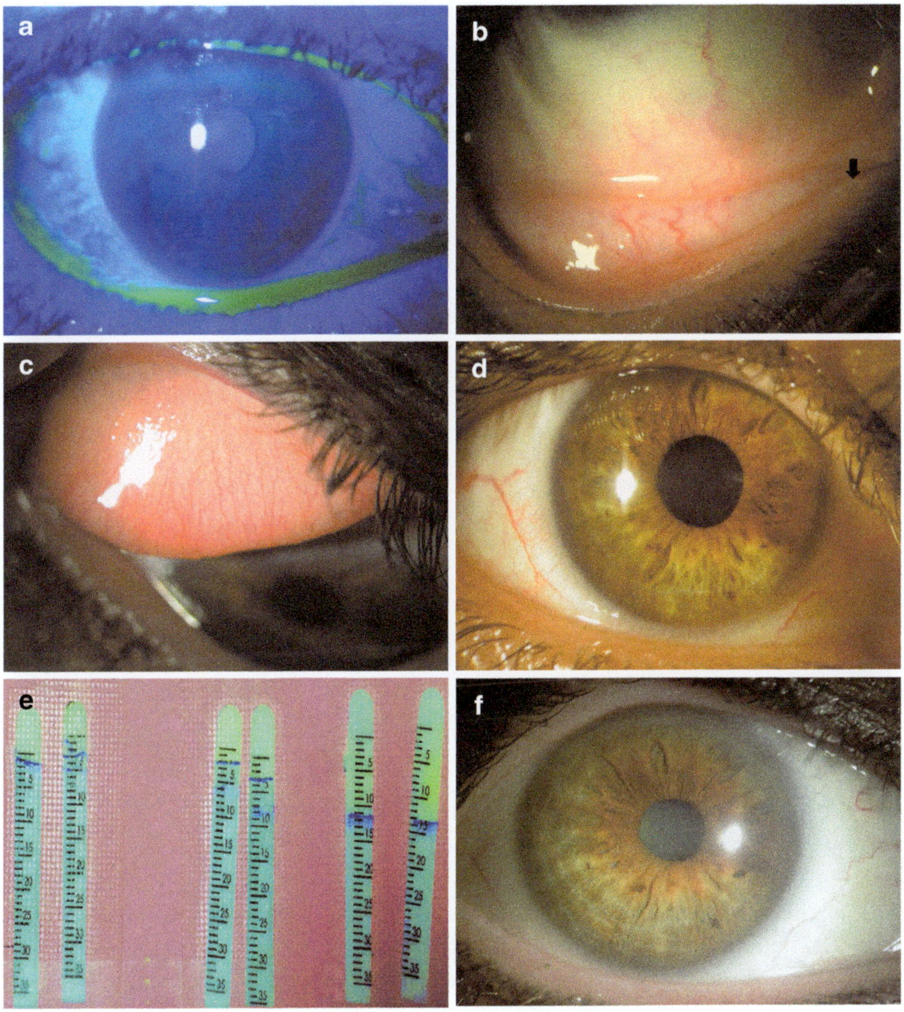

Fig. 14.2 Case #1. Although CCh is highlighted by conjunctival folds clinically resulting in a discontinuous tear meniscus (**a**), it can also be accompanied by swollen puncta (**b**, *arrow*), tarsal papillary reaction (**c**), and conjunctival injection most notable at above the lid margin (**d**), suggesting chronic ocular surface inflammation. FCT showed delayed tear clearance (**e**). After surgery, this eye recovered smooth, non-inflamed conjunctival surface (**f**), continuous tear meniscus (**g**), and non-swollen puncta (**h**, *arrow*). Repeat FCT revealed improved tear clearance but same low basal wetting length, i.e., 2 and 3 mm for OD and OS, respectively, for the first two pairs of strips (**i**). To resolve the remaining symptoms which were due to ATD dry eye, punctal occlusion by plug was performed (**j**)

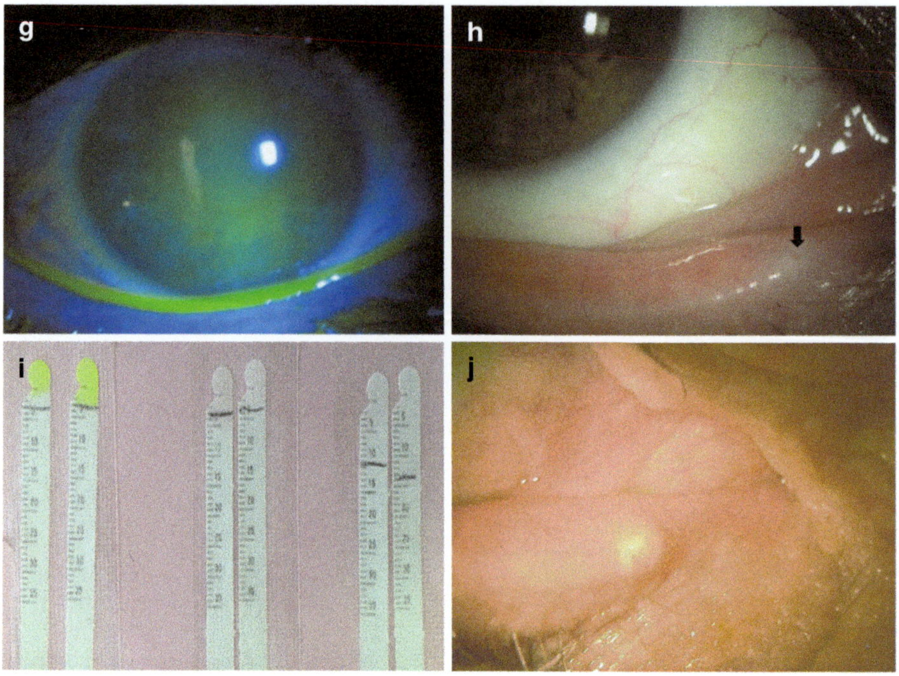

Fig. 14.2 (continued)

Why Did This CCh Patient Complain of Tearing While There was Patent Nasolacrimal Drainage?

The complaint of tearing is most likely resulted from delay tear clearance (DTC). Given that the aqueous tear fluid is cleared through punctum by the eyelid blinking pumping force and stable tear flow, DTC can arise from punctal occlusion, interference with the tear flow, or deficiency of any element in the hydrodynamic reflex. Nevertheless, DTC can also develop in cases of severe ATD to allow the tear meniscus to drop below the level discontiguous to the punctum [13]. Taken together, tear clearance is the convergent point of both hydrodynamic and compositional factors [1]. DTC also occurs when mucosal inflammation and swelling of the ocular surface impose a functional block of tear clearance [14]. One common cause of such mucosal swelling is chronic ocular surface inflammation inflicted by CCh. Conjunctival folds in CCh potentially can also block the punctum [7] besides interrupting the continuity of the tear meniscus [4, 7, 8], interfering with the tear flow from the fornix to the tear meniscus [10] and depleting the fornix tear reservoir [9]. DTC also aggravates ocular surface inflammation, which can then aggravate CCh because DTC also increased inflammatory cytokines in tear levels to upregulate expression of MMPs by CCh fibroblasts [15, 16]. Because DTC is worse during sleep due to the lack of blinking, inflammatory symptoms caused by CCh tend to be worse in the morning upon awakening and are frequently associated with swollen puncta in CCh [8, 14].

How Can One Measure Tear Clearance?

Measurement of tear clearance is indeed a useful clinical test to assess the status of ocular surface defense. The ocular tear volume is traditionally assessed by the Schirmer test, which is known to have a wide range of false positive and negative rates as well as lack of standardization [17–19]. Following application of 5 μL of Fluroress® (Akorn Inc., Abita Springs, LA, USA), which contains anesthetics, fluorescein clearance test (FCT) was performed by applying the Schirmer paper strip for 1 min every 10 min for a total of 30 min, at which time nasal stimulation is performed. Hence, FCT at one setting can determine basal tearing, reflex tearing, and tear clearance [14]. Because the paper strip is bent over the tear meniscus to reach the tear reservoir in the fornix, the measured tear volume conceivably includes both the tear meniscus (the second compartment) and fornix reservoir (the third compartment). The diagnosis of ATD is based on the wetting length of less than 3 mm for the first two sets (10th and 20th min) for measurement of the basal tear volume. The high variability of the Schirmer test [18] is minimized by using FCT, which avoids unquantified anesthetic drop size and reduces the contact of lashes from 5 min for Schirmer I test to 1 min. Tear fluorescence measurements by FCT using the naked eyes (Fig. 14.3) correlate well with fluorophotometry [20]. The intensity of fluorescein dye fades with time under the blue light. Tear clearance is regarded normal if fluorescein becomes invisible to the naked eye after 10 min (i.e., the first pair of strips). In contrast, DTC is defined as fluorescein present on the Schirmer strips at or beyond 20 min (i.e., the second and third pair of strips). FCT can help detect clinical and subclinical DTC which has been overlooked [14].

FCT revealed low basal wetting length for 10th and 20th min on both eyes. In addition, the tear clearance that was also delayed as evidenced by the dye could still be detected by the strip taken at the 20 min interval and later (Fig. 14.2e).

How Can One Treat CCh Patients with DTC?

As DTC aggravates ocular symptoms by precipitating accumulation and prolonging the contact of intrinsic irritative stimuli in the ocular surface, elimination of such intrinsic irritative stimuli/inflammation is the first step [13]. Medicamentosa with accumulation of intrinsic toxic topical medications that contain preservatives is a common overlooked etiology for the eyes with clinically apparent inflammation. It is likely that medicamentosa can precipitate DTC, which in turn can perpetrate medicamentosa in a vicious cycle. Application of topical preservative-free steroid such as methylprednisolone or dexamethasone has shown success in tear clearance improvement by breaking the aforementioned vicious cycle [14].

Under the impression of CCh and ATD with DTC, non-preservative dexamethasone 0.1% was prescribed to control inflammation. Two weeks after treatment, symptoms were partially relieved.

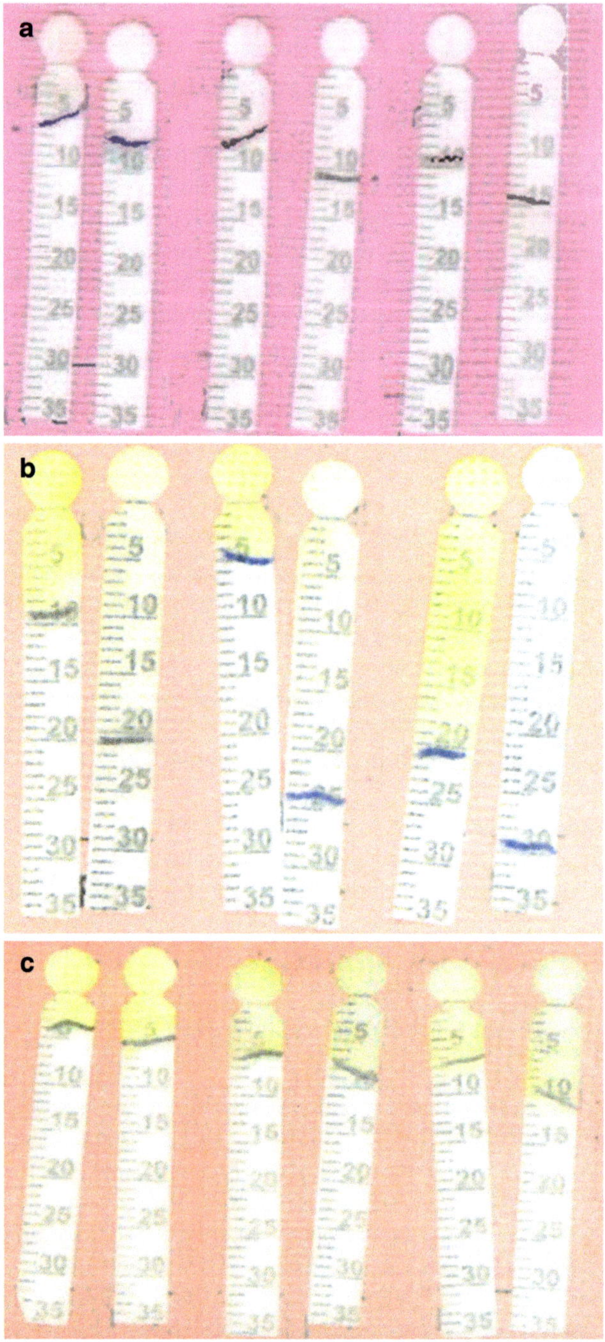

Fig. 14.3 Representative FCT Examples for different clinical diagnosis. (**a**) Normal basal tearing, clearance, and reflex tearing. Unilateral (**b**) and bilateral (**c**) delayed tear clearance as evidenced by fluorescein present in the right eye (**b**) or both eyes (**c**) beyond 20 min

What is the Pathogenesis of CCh?

Although there are conjunctival wrinkles, the underlying pathology of CCh does not reside in the conjunctiva but rather owes to dissolution of the Tenon capsule, which functions as a "carpet pad" to anchor the conjunctiva "carpet" to the underlying sclera "floor." In CCh, excessive degradation of the extracellular matrix MMPs under inflammatory cytokines results in Tenon's capsule degeneration [5, 16]. The lack of healthy Tenon's capsule hence leads to loose and wrinkled conjunctiva, prolapsed fat (Fig. 14.1c), and subconjunctival hemorrhage as the underlying blood vessels can be avulsed during conjunctival movement in the absence of the Tenon capsule.

What Will be the Next Step for Managing Symptomatic CCh After Inflammation Control?

Once ocular inflammations are controlled, restoration of fornix reservoir is the key to achieve effective tear spread for symptomatic CCh patients. Understanding of the underlying pathology of CCh helps formulate surgical procedure aimed at restoration of the fornix tear reservoir. This "reservoir restoration procedure" (Fig. 14.4) includes the following three key steps: (1) significant rearrangement of conjunctiva by recessing and anchoring it from the limbus to the fornix, (2) thorough removal of degenerated Tenon's capsule, and (3) replacement of the Tenon and the conjunctival tissue by two separate layers of cryopreserved amniotic membrane (AM) (Bio-Tissue, Miami, FL) to help prevent recurrence and expedite patient's recovery.

Because of the residual symptoms persisted despite maximal medical treatments, the patient received fornix reconstruction surgery with conjunctival recession and AM transplantation. After surgery, the epithelial defects created by the denuded AM were rapidly epithelialized within 3 weeks. Her eyes recovered smooth, non-inflamed conjunctival surface (Fig. 14.2f) with restoration of fornix reservoir and tear meniscus (Fig. 14.2g) and non-swollen puncta (Fig. 14.2h). However, she noted partial but not complete relief of symptoms including blurry vision, dryness, tearing, and conjunctival redness. Repeat FCT revealed improved tear clearance but same wetting length (Fig. 14.2i).

Why Not Just Cut Off (Resect) or Cauterize the Redundant Conjunctiva?

As of now, a number of surgical procedures have been advocated to treat CCh such as scleral fixation suture [21], crescent bulbar conjunctival excision with direct closure [7], resection combined with inferior peritomy and radial relaxing

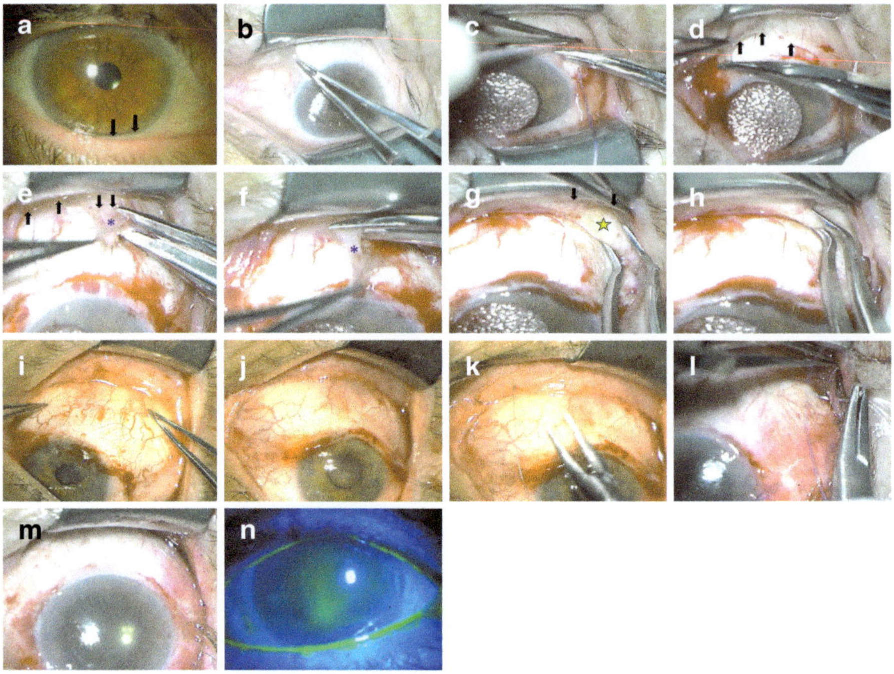

Fig. 14.4 Surgical steps of reservoir restoration procedure. Poor conjunctival adhesion to the sclera from dissolution of the Tenon capsule is noted as evidenced by easy separation of the conjunctiva from the sclera simply by forceps grabbing (**a**, *arrow*, **b**). After using several drops of epinephrine 1/1000 for hemostasis and 2% lidocaine gel for anesthesia, a traction suture made of 7-0 Vicryl is placed 2 mm posterior to the limbus at the 3 and 9 o'clock position and used to rotate the eye upward. An arc-like conjunctival peritomy is created 1–2 mm posterior to the limbus in the area of CCh (**c**) and extends to remove pinguecula, if present. Rearrangement of conjunctiva by recessing (**d**, *arrow*) from the limbus to the fornix. The abnormal Tenon's capsule (*asterisk*) that is distributed under the overlying recessed conjunctival epithelial tissue (*arrow*) and adherent over the bare sclera (**e**). The abnormal Tenon's capsule (*asterisk*) is grabbed and dissected off from the overlying conjunctival epithelial tissue and thoroughly removed by a sharp scissors (**f**). The recessed conjunctiva (*arrow*) is lifted up by a forceps to identify the prolapsed fat (*star*) that is distributed in the fornix (**g**) and cauterized to create a gap (**h**) for prevention of fat herniation through fornix. Two separate layers of cryopreserved AM are laid down to replace Tenon (**i**) and the conjunctival tissue (**j**) to help prevent recurrence and expedite patient's recovery. The conjunctival is recessed to anchor at the fornix with 8-0 Vicryl (**k**, **l**). Fornix deepening reconstruction with conjunctival recession and AM transplantation restores fornix tear reservoir (**m**) to help replenish tear meniscus and preocular surface tear film in symptomatic CCh patient (**n**)

incisions [22], excision with AM transplantation [23, 24], cauterization/laser coagulation with or without excision [25, 26], and subconjunctival fibrin sealant followed by excision [27]. Most of these procedures focus on elimination of conjunctival folds close to the tear meniscus—but do not address fornix reconstruction. While these resection procedures may be effective in many cases, reconstruction and deepening of the fornix is best done with conjunctival "recession" not "resection." In addition, complications such as scar formation and fat prolapse might be attributed to the aforementioned surgical techniques if not performed appropriately.

What is the Clinical Significance if Repeat FCT Shows No Change in the Basal Wetting Length After CCh Surgery?

Changes of basal tear volume after fornix reconstruction help discern genuine or concomitant ATD to clarify logical step in the clinical management algorithm for dry eye [9, 13]. Genuine ATD dry eye is identified by the unchanged basal wetting length despite restoration of fornix tear reservoir after CCh surgery. If there are still residual non-resolving dry eye manifestations, treatment should be directed to compositional deficiency dry eye [13]. In this regard, the conventional treatment for ATD dry eye can be managed more effectively by punctal occlusion, which remains the mainstay of managing ATD dry eye when the application of artificial tears reaches a maximum certain daily frequency. Because punctal occlusion invariably delays tear drainage/clearance, it can prolong the beneficial effect of topical artificial tears for ATD but potentially cause toxicity to the ocular surface as a result of prolonged retention of preservative-containing artificial tears. Hence, it is advised that non-preserved tear substitutes are preferred, because CCh can aggravate DTC, which is why surgical correction of CCh is performed before punctal occlusion is contemplated.

Plugs were placed in her inferior puncta (Fig. 14.2j). She noted significant complete resolution of all symptoms. Such improvement was accompanied by reduction of conjunctival hyperemia and improvement of the visual acuity of 1 Snellen line.

Case #2

A 54-year-old male noted irritation and some "collarets" in lash roots in both eyes for months. There were no associated symptoms such as photophobia, blurry vision, dryness, and tearing. Upon presentation, his vision was 20/20 with mild conjunctiva and eyelid injection (Fig. 14.5a, b). Slit lamp examination revealed cylindrical dandruffs located at the base of the lashes. Lashing sampling confirmed demodex blepharitis. There was redundant conjunctival tissue interposed between the lid margin and the eye globe. Obliterated tear meniscus was shown with fluorescein staining (Fig. 14.5c, d). FCT showed basal wetting length of 5 mm and normal tear clearance as evidenced by the disappearance of the dye in 10 min in both eyes (Fig. 14.5e).

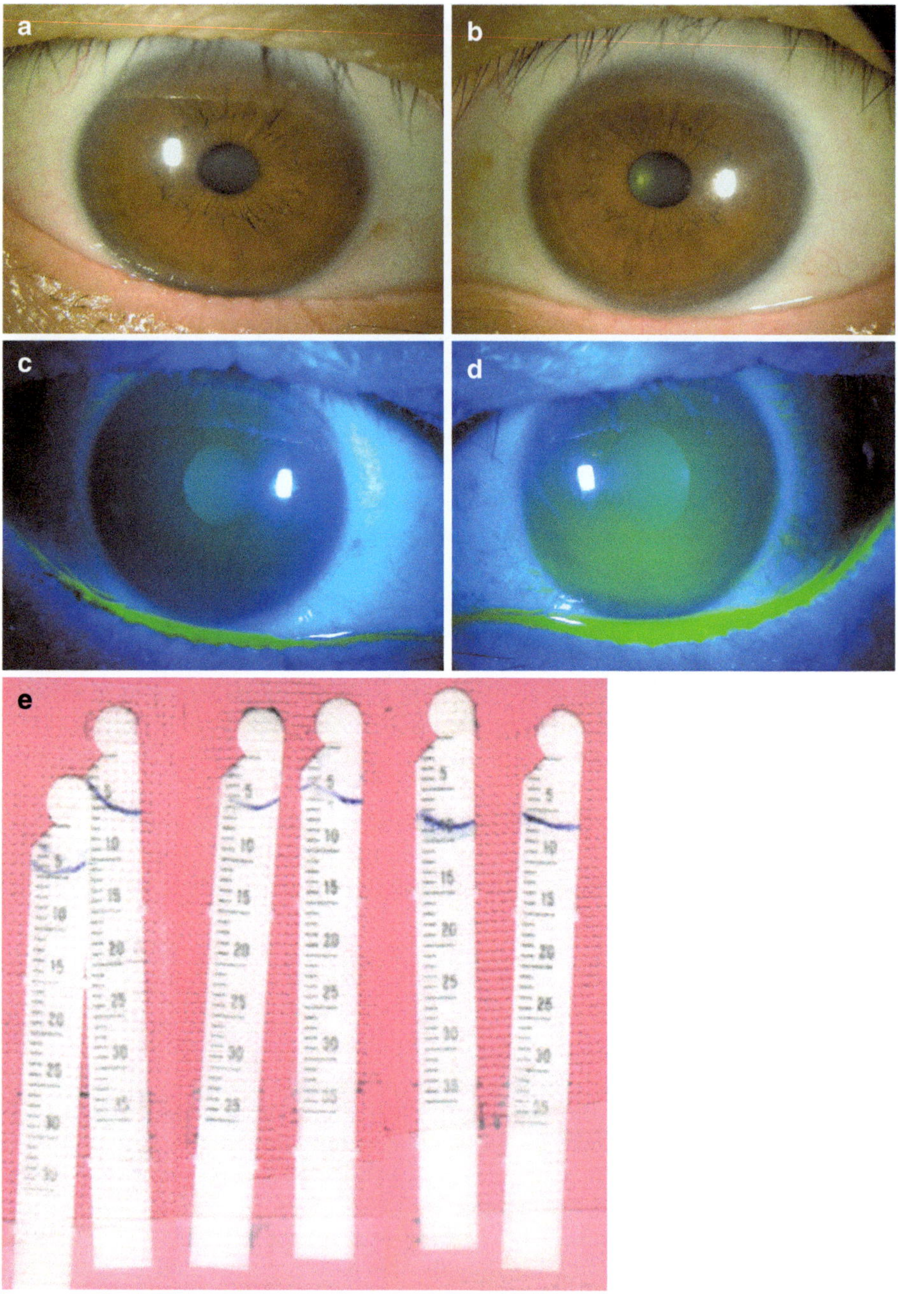

Fig. 14.5 Case #2. Bilateral mild conjunctival and eyelid injection of the right eye (**a**) and left eye (**b**) and CCh as evidenced by interference with the tear meniscus by redundant conjunctival tissue (**c, d**) in this asymptomatic patient with CCh. FCT shows the basal wetting length of 5 mm and normal tear clearance as evidenced by the disappearance of the dye in 10 min (**e**)

How Can One Discern Whether CCh is the Cause of the Said Eye Irritation?

As recently reported [10], we propose to measure the speed of recovery of the tear meniscus after depletion as a way to discern whether CCh is the cause of patient's ocular irritation. To do so, we first instill a 5 μL fluorescein drop into the inferior fornix via a pipette. [One can also do so by applying fluorescein drop by wetting a fluorescein strip with saline.] Under slit lamp examination with a blue light, the fluorescent inferior tear meniscus is then depleted by using a capillary tube. [One can also deplete it by touching with a dry Weck-Cel (Microsponge™, Alcon®).] Immediately afterward, the time in sec is measured to see the recovery of the fluorescent tear meniscus (Fig. 14.6a–c). Using this technique, we have reported that the tear reservoir in the fornix rapidly replenishes the meniscus under normal circumstances but not in CCh patients. Without eyelid blinking, the original tear meniscus

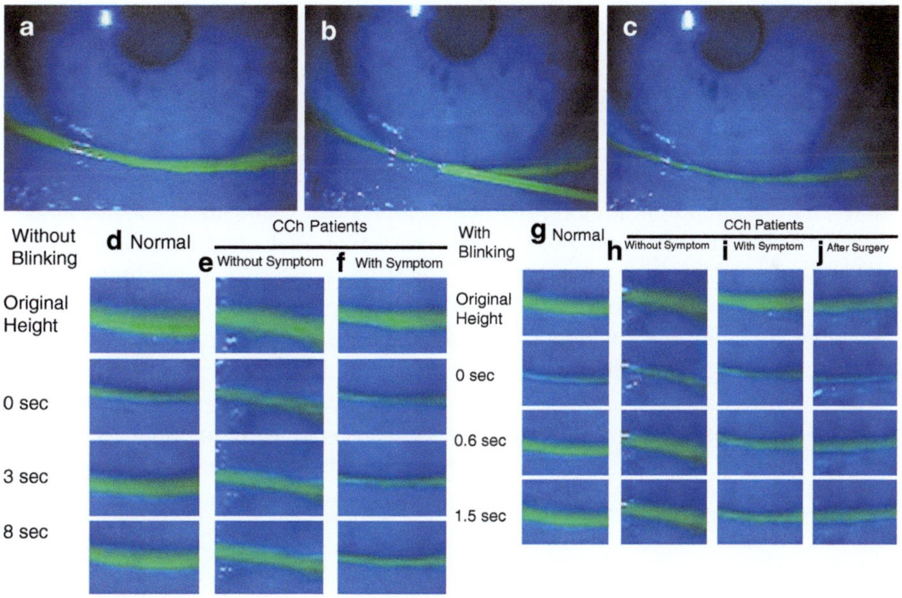

Fig. 14.6 Effect of blinking for fornix tear replenishment in asymptomatic CCh. Original tear meniscus height (**a**) is depleted by capillary tube (**b, c**). Fornix rapidly replenishes the meniscus back to normal height in normal people (**d**) but not in CCh patients regardless of whether symptoms present (**e, f**). However, one blink was sufficient to recover the tear meniscus back to normal height in asymptomatic CCh patients (**h**) as rapidly as normal subjects (**g**), whereas the tear meniscus height remained low in symptomatic CCh (**i**). CCh patients can be asymptomatic as blinking is an effective compensatory mechanism to facilitate the tear flow from the fornix to the meniscus and consequently the preocular tear film. Intriguingly, the meniscus height of symptomatic CCh after blinking could be facilitated back to normal level by restoration of fornix tear reservoir via reconstruction with conjunctival recession and AM transplantation (**j**) (Taken with permission from Huang et al. [10])

height can be recovered by fornix replenishment in <3 s in patients without CCh (Fig. 14.6d). In patients with CCh with symptoms, the meniscus recovery was significantly retarded, i.e., not recovered in 8 s (Fig. 14.6f). In patients with CCh but without symptoms, the recovery was intermediate (Fig. 14.6e). Importantly, eyelid blinking is the key compensatory mechanism to facilitate the tear flow from the fornix reservoir to the tear meniscus. Hence, upon one eyelid blinking, the meniscus recovery is significantly facilitated in patients with CCh without symptoms (asymptomatic) (back to normal tear meniscus height as in Fig. 14.6g, h) but not in CCh patients with symptoms (symptomatic) (Fig. 14.6i). Intriguingly, the meniscus height of symptomatic CCh after blinking could be facilitated back to normal level by restoration of fornix tear reservoir via reconstruction with conjunctival recession and AM transplantation (Fig. 14.6j). Collectively, blinking is an effective compensatory mechanism to distinguish CCh severity and identify asymptomatic CCh. Importantly, restoration of the tear reservoir by fornix reconstruction is an effective treatment for symptomatic CCh to ensure a continuous supply of tears from the reservoir to the tear meniscus and the preocular tear film.

Why Are some CCh Patients Asymptomatic?

The aforementioned clinical measurement of how a depleted tear meniscus is recovered after one eyelid blinking clearly demonstrates that CCh patients can be asymptomatic if the fornix tear reservoir is not completely obliterated and if the blinking remains effective in facilitating the tear flow from the fornix to the meniscus and consequently the preocular tear film. In contrast, patients with CCh can become symptomatic if the severity of CCh obliterates the fornix tear reservoir. Under this scenario, blinking although shortens the interblink interval, it still fails to replenish the already depleted tear meniscus. Given that blinking can help restore obliterated tears in the tear meniscus in asymptomatic CCh, it is also clinically important to evaluate whether some CCh patients can become symptomatic if blinking is ineffective.

Case #3

A 52-year-old male presented with ocular irritation, dryness, burning, gritty sensation, blurred vision, and photophobia in both eyes for 5 years. His past history did not disclose any associated systemic disease such as Sjögren disease, rheumatoid arthritis, or systemic lupus erythematosus. He remained symptomatic despite conventional medical therapies including topical concomitant medications (artificial tears, lubricants, steroid, and cyclosporine), bandage contact lens, or punctal occlusion. Clinical examination disclosed with ATD and CCh. The diagnosis of ATD was based on the basal wetting length of less than 3 mm at the 10th and 20th min according to FCT.

Why Did This Patient Find No Relief from Conventional Eye Drops in Dry Eye Caused by CCh?

The loose conjunctiva in CCh patients occupies the space not only in the tear meniscus but also obliterates the fornix tear reservoir to interfere tear spread from the fornix to the tear meniscus (Fig. 14.1c) [4, 7, 8, 10]. The fornix tear reservoir is the primary compartment for an eye to hold tears, i.e., estimated to be responsible for at least 50% of the total tear volume [28]. The finding that the fornix tear reservoir is obliterated by CCh [9] explains why the eye failed to hold the artificial tears. Consequently, the tears in the meniscus and the preocular tear film cannot be replenished by the fornix tear reservoir through blinking. Hence, artificial tears alone are incapable of maintaining a stable tear film.

Upon presentation, his vision was 20/30 for both eyes. His eyelids had normal blinking and closure.

What Clinical Work Up Should You Perform to Discern Whether the Eye Suffered from ATD, CCh, or Both?

The close association between CCh and ATD has been recognized [29, 30]. It has been reported that the risk of developing ATD increases with severity of CCh, suggesting that CCh itself may be a cause leading to ATD dry eye [30]. However, because both CCh and ATD dry eye are prevalent in aged populations, it is also challenging to discern ATD that may exist as an independent disease. Clinically, dry eye caused by CCh can be differentiated from dry eye caused by ATD by history taking focused on inquiring the dry eye symptoms to see if they are worsened by any specific diurnal relationship, gaze, blinking, or punctal occlusion [8]. Ocular irritation is worsen as the day progresses due to progressive exposure and desiccation in genuine ATD but tends to remain the same throughout the day in dry eye caused by CCh. CCh patients usually complain of blurry vision and pain, which are aggravated by increased conjunctival folds in downgaze during reading. On the contrary, the interpalpebral exposure zone that increases from downgaze to upgaze explains why ATD dry eye is worse in upgaze, especially when working with a computer screen. Furthermore, frequent blinking results in accumulation of conjunctival folds to the 6 o'clock position which further aggravates dry eye symptoms in CCh patients. In contrast, increasing blinking shortens the interblink interval, invariably stabilizes the tear film, and improves ATD dry eye. An additional test which is sometime helpful is that in some patients with symptomatic CCh, manually retracting the lower lid can provide some relief of their symptoms (perhaps this maneuver temporarily increases the lower fornix tear reservoir). Punctal occlusion invariably delays tear drainage and prolongs the beneficial effect of topical artificial tears for ATD. However, it further retards tear clearance in the tear meniscus and fornix that is already compromised by CCh and leads to exacerbation of CCh mimetic dry eye symptoms. The use of rose bengal may highlight ocular surface epithelial cells that exhibit a mucin-deficient state in the interpalpebral exposure zone for ATD but in the non-exposure zone for CCh. By obliterating tear meniscuses, CCh destabilizes the tear film immediately above the redundant conjunctival fold in a linear pattern of CCh area (inferior to the exposure zone).

His symptoms were worse in the morning upon awakening and remained the same throughout the day. They were aggravated with blinking and down-gaze during reading but not watching computer or television. His symptom severity was graded 25 (moderate) based on Ocular Surface Disease Index (OSDI) score. Prior maximal conventional medical treatments including artificial tears, lubricants, steroid and cyclosporine, and bandage contact lens on both eyes failed to relieve his symptoms. Symptoms persisted and were worsen with punctal occlusion. Slit lamp examination showed nasal and temporal redundant conjunctival tissue interposed between the lid margin and the eye globe impeded the formation of a proper and smooth tear meniscus (Fig. 14.7a). Fluorescein staining showed the obliterated tear meniscus but no superficial punctuate keratitis on corneal surface (Fig. 14.7b). Rose bengal staining could not be seen on the exposure zone of the central cornea. FCT revealed the basal wetting length of 2 mm (Fig. 14.7c) in both eyes.

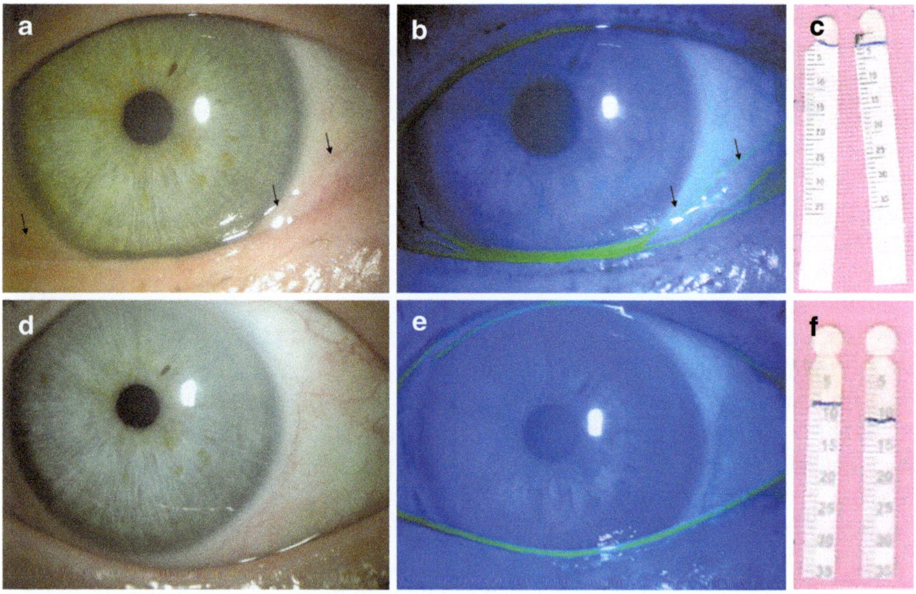

Fig. 14.7 Case #3. Redundant conjunctival folds (*arrows*) interposed between the lid margin and the eye globe obliterated the tear meniscus (**a**, **b**). FCT showed a low basal wetting length suggestive of dry eye before surgery (**c**). One month after reservoir restoration by AM transplantation, the eye regained a smooth, quiet, and non-inflamed bulbar conjunctiva (**d**) and a continuous tear meniscus (**e**). Repeat FCT showed normal basal wetting lengths (**f**), indicating that prior dry eye was secondary to CCh but not caused by ATD

Because of persistent symptoms despite the maximal medical treatments, the patient received CCh surgery with an attempt to alleviate the symptoms and restore the ocular surface health. The operative technique includes excision of mobile and degenerated Tenon's capsule, fornix deepening reconstruction with conjunctival recession, and cryopreserved AM transplantation (secured with the use of fibrin glue) under topical anesthesia (Fig. 14.4). After surgery, the patient received ofloxacin 0.3% eye drops three times daily and non-preservative dexamethasone 0.1% eye drops four times daily for 3 weeks, tapering off within 2 weeks. All epithelial defects created by the denuded AM were rapidly epithelialized within 3 weeks (Fig. 14.7d, e). Complications such as fat prolapse or scarring-induced entropion of the lower lid, retraction of the lower fornix, and restricted motility were not found. He experienced a total relief of symptoms. Furthermore, he also exhibited improved visual acuity of 1 Snellen line for both eyes. His eyes recovered smooth, wet, white, non-inflamed conjunctival surface being symptom-free in 1 month. Repeat FCT revealed increased basal wetting length from 2 to 7 and 10 mm for the right and left eye, respectively (Fig. 14.7f).

Why Did FCT Show the Improvement of Basal Wetting Length After AMT in CCh?

Under normal circumstance, the fornix tear reservoir is responsible for delivering tear fluids to the tear meniscus by blinking [10]. In CCh, the fornix tear reservoir is obliterated by loose and wrinkled conjunctiva and prolapsed fat due to degenerated Tenon's capsule [5, 9, 16]. The occupied and depleted tear reservoir conceivably results in a low basal wetting length, no different from ATD dry eye. Restoration of the fornix tear reservoir is achieved by fornix deepening reconstruction with conjunctival recession and AMT. This explains why the postsurgical basal wetting length can be improved in dry eye caused by CCh, i.e., resulting in the disappearance of ATD dry eye secondary to CCh. Using AMT to achieve reservoir restoration, we can differentiate dry eye caused primarily by ATD or secondarily by CCh [9]. Elimination of dry eye caused by CCh first by AMT also allows us to treat dry eye caused by ATD more effectively later on. That is also why we advocate AMT to restore tear reservoir prior to managing ATD dry eye as a more logical and practical management algorithm for dry eye [13].

Summary

In summary, the pathogenesis of CCh involves dissolution of the Tenon capsule that allows the conjunctiva to fold, which in turn block the tear flow into the nasolacrimal drainage system [7], interrupt the continuity of the tear meniscus [8], obliterate the fornix tear reservoir [9], and interfere with the flow or tears from the fornix tear reservoir to the tear meniscus [10]. Elimination of intrinsic irritative stimuli/inflammation by topical preservative-free dexamethansone or methylprednisolone is the initial treatment for DTC-associated CCh. After differentiating dry eye caused by CCh from that caused by ATD and determining that CCh is the cause of ocular irritation, restoration of the fornix tear reservoir by fornix reconstruction with conjunctival recession and AM transplantation is an important surgical procedure to resolve symptoms and signs in CCh. Punctal occlusion and specific management of genuine ATD dry eye take place after elimination of CCh. In conclusion, fluorescein-based testing of the tear meniscus can help distinguish symptomatic CCh from genuine ATD (independent of CCh) and allow physicians to adopt an effective treatment algorithm to restore the integrity of the ocular surface.

Acknowledgements *Financial Disclosure*: Dr. Tseng has obtained a patent for the method of preparation and clinical uses of amniotic membrane and has licensed the rights to TissueTech, Inc., which procures and processes, and to Bio-Tissue, Inc., which is a subsidiary of TissueTech, Inc., to distribute cryopreserved amniotic membrane for clinical and research uses.

Funding/Support: This study was supported in part by an unrestricted grant from Ocular Surface Research Education Foundation, Miami, FL.

References

1. Tseng SC, Tsubota K. Important concepts for treating ocular surface and tear disorders. Am J Ophthalmol. 1997;124:825–35.
2. Doane MG. Interaction of eyelids and tears in corneal wetting and the dynamics of the normal human eyeblink. Am J Ophthalmol. 1980;89:507–16.
3. Palakuru JR, Wang J, Aquavella JV. Effect of blinking on tear dynamics. Invest Ophthalmol Vis Sci. 2007;48(7):3032–7.
4. Meller D, Tseng SC. Conjunctivochalasis: literature review and possible pathophysiology. Surv Ophthalmol. 1998;43(3):225–32.
5. Li DQ, Meller D, Tseng SC. Overexpression of collagenase (MMP-1) and stromelysin (MMP-3) by cultured conjunctivochalasis fibroblasts. Invest Ophthalmol Vis Sci. 2000;41:404–10.
6. Guo P, Zhang SZ, He H, Zhu YT, Tseng SC. PTX3 controls activation of matrix metalloproteinase 1 and apoptosis in conjunctivochalasis fibroblasts. Invest Ophthalmol Vis Sci. 2012;53(14):4004.
7. Liu D. Conjunctivochalasis. A cause of tearing and its management. Ophthal Plast Reconstr Surg. 1986;2:25–8.
8. Di Pascuale MA, Espana EM, Kawakita T, Tseng SC. Clinical characteristics of conjunctivochalasis with or without aqueous tear deficiency. Br J Ophthalmol. 2004;88(3):388–92.
9. Cheng AM, Yin HY, Chen R, Tighe S, Sheha H, Zhao D, Casas V, Tseng SC. Restoration of fornix tear reservoir in conjunctivochalasis with fornix reconstruction. Cornea. 2016;35(6):736–40.
10. Huang Y, Sheha H, Tseng SC. Conjunctivochalasis interferes with tear flow from fornix to tear meniscus. Ophthalmology. 2013;120(8):1681–7.
11. Mimura T, Yamagami S, Usui T, et al. Changes of conjunctivochalasis with age in a hospital-based study. Am J Ophthalmol. 2009;147(1):171–7.
12. Hughes WL. Conjunctivochalasis. Am J Ophthalmol. 1942;25:48–51.
13. Tseng SC. A practical treatment algorithm for managing ocular surface and tear disorders. Cornea. 2011;30(Suppl 1):S8–S14.

14. Prabhasawat P, Tseng SC. Frequent association of delayed tear clearance in ocular irritation. Br J Ophthalmol. 1998;82:666–75.
15. Afonso AA, Sobrin L, Monroy DC, Selzer M, Lokeshwar B, Pflugfelder SC. Tear fluid gelatinase B activity correlates with IL-1a concentration and fluorescein clearance in ocular rosacea. Invest Ophthalmol Vis Sci. 1999;40(11):2506–12.
16. Meller D, Li DQ, Tseng SC. Regulation of collagenase, stromelysin, and gelatinase B in human conjunctival and conjunctivochalasis fibroblasts by interleukin-1b and tumor necrosis factor-a. Invest Ophthalmol Vis Sci. 2000;41:2922–9.
17. Afonso AA, Monroy D, Stern ME, Tseng SC, Pflugfelder SC. Correlation of tear fluorescein clearance and Schirmer test scores with ocular irritation symptoms. Ophthalmology. 1999;106:803–10.
18. Clinch TE, Benedetto DA, Felberg NT, Laibson PR. Schirmer's test. A closer look. Arch Ophthalmol. 1983;101:1383–6.
19. Xu KP, Yagi Y, Toda I, Tsubota K. Tear function index. A new measure of dry eye. Arch Ophthalmol. 1995;113:84–8.
20. Xu KP, Tsubota K. Correlation of tear clearance rate and fluorophotometric assessment of tear turnover. Br J Ophthalmol. 1995;79:1042–5.
21. Otaka I, Kyu N. A new surgical technique for management of conjunctivochalasis. Am J Ophthalmol. 2000;129(3):385–7.
22. Yokoi N, Komuro A, Nishii M, et al. Clinical impact of conjunctivochalasis on the ocular surface. Cornea. 2005;24(8 Suppl):S24–31.
23. Meller D, Maskin SL, Pires RT, Tseng SC. Amniotic membrane transplantation for symptomatic conjunctivochalasis refractory to medical treatments. Cornea. 2000;19(6):796–803.
24. Maskin SL. Effect of ocular surface reconstruction by using amniotic membrane transplant for symptomatic conjunctivochalasis on fluorescein clearance test results. Cornea. 2008;27(6):644–9.
25. Yang HS, Choi S. New approach for conjunctivochalasis using an argon green laser. Cornea. 2013;32(5):574–8.
26. Nakasato S, Uemoto R, Mizuki N. Thermocautery for inferior conjunctivochalasis. Cornea. 2012;31(5):514–9.
27. Doss LR, Doss EL, Doss RP. Paste-pinch-cut conjunctivoplasty: subconjunctival fibrin sealant injection in the repair of conjunctivochalasis. Cornea. 2012;31(8):959–62.
28. Mishima S, Gasset A, Klyce SDJ, Baum JL. Determination of tear volume and tear flow. Invest Ophthalmol. 1966;5:264–76.
29. Chhadva P, Alexander A, McClellan AL, McManus KT, Seiden B, Galor A. The impact of conjunctivochalasis on dry eye symptoms and signs. Invest Ophthalmol Vis Sci. 2015;56(5):2867–71.
30. Höh H, Schirra F, Kienecker C, Ruprecht KW. Lidparrallele konjunktivale Falten (LIPCOF) sind ein sicheres diagnostisches Zeichen des trockenen Auges. Ophthalmologe. 1995;92:802–8.

Chapter 15
Management of the Persistent Corneal Epithelial Defect

Nishant G. Soni, Angelique Pillar, Jordan Margo, and Bennie H. Jeng

Case #1

A 35-year-old woman underwent a pars plana vitrectomy with membrane peeling for traction retinal detachments secondary to complications from diabetic retinopathy in her left eye. Intraoperatively, her corneal epithelium was debrided.

What Risk Factors Does She Have for Developing a Non-healing Epithelial Defect?

Post vitrectomy, one of this patient's biggest risk factors for developing a non-healing epithelial defect is her underlying diabetes. Diabetic keratopathy is one manifestation of polyneuropathy seen with impaired glucose metabolism [3]. Specifically, damage to the ophthalmic division of the trigeminal nerve results in reduced corneal sensation and loss of epithelial cell integrity leading to breakdown and impaired wound healing [4]. The severity of diabetic keratopathy increases proportionally to the duration of diabetes and the degree and severity of diabetic retinopathy, which is an additional risk factor for this patient [5].

Retinal surgery, even in the absence of diabetes, has also been shown to cause neurotrophic corneal ulceration. Administration of peripheral argon laser photocoagulation, placement of encircling scleral buckles, or placement of trochars at the 3 and 9 o'clock positions can lead to damage of the long ciliary nerves as they enter the cornea and, in diabetes, can deepen already existing corneal hypoesthesia [6].

N.G. Soni, MD • A. Pillar, MD • J. Margo, MD • B.H. Jeng, MD (✉)
Department of Ophthalmology and Visual Sciences, University of Maryland School of Medicine, 419 W. Redwood Street, Suite 470, Baltimore, MD 21201, USA
e-mail: bjeng@som.umaryland.edu

A.R. Djalilian (ed.), *Ocular Surface Disease*,
https://doi.org/10.1007/978-3-319-15823-5_15

A large-diameter iatrogenic corneal abrasion is sometimes necessary for visualization during retinal surgery, and the larger the corneal abrasion, the longer the time to reepithelialization. Administration of topical medications postoperatively also can contribute to reduced corneal healing and epithelial toxicity. Topical antibiotics, intraocular pressure (IOP)-lowering agents, nonsteroidal anti-inflammatory drugs (NSAIDs), and steroids, particularly those containing preservatives, disrupt epithelial cell integrity and migration [7]. Benzalkonium chloride (BAK) is a commonly used eye drop preservative that disrupts cell walls and emulsifies membrane lipids and can lead to ocular toxicity even without underlying epithelial injury [8].

Tear surface irregularities also increase the cornea's susceptibility to poor repair. Subconjunctival hemorrhage and chemosis following intraocular surgery and reduced blink rate either from pre-existing neurotrophic changes and/or the use of a retrobulbar block lead to tear film stasis, increased tear viscosity, and poor corneal oxygenation, all of which are contributing factors to epitheliopathy and persistent epithelial defects following retinal surgery [9].

Postoperative management by the retinal service consisted of topical prednisolone acetate 1%, brimonidine, ciprofloxacin, and atropine. Artificial tears were given to help with the non-healing epithelial defect. After 7 days of non-healing epithelial defect, the patient was referred to the corneal service for further management (Fig. 15.1).

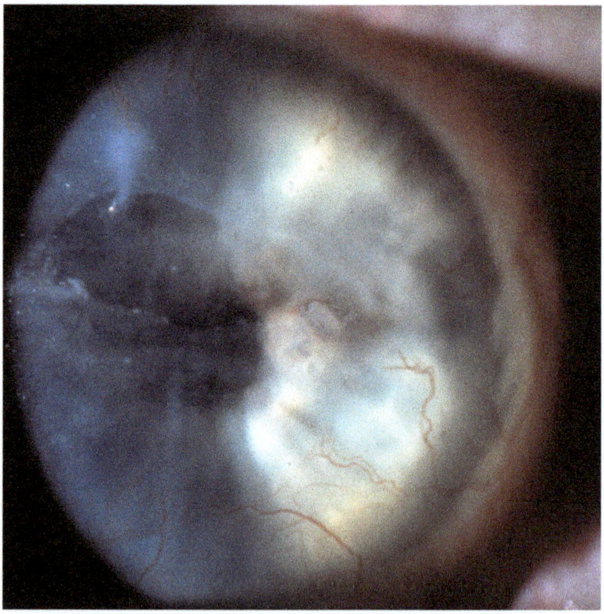

Fig. 15.1 Non-healing epithelial defect in Patient #1 after epithelial debridement during retinal surgery

What Management Strategies Should Be Considered in This Situation?

Initially, frequent application of preservative-free artificial tears every 1–2 h can be administered. However, this strategy increases eye drop burden, and the lack of compliance may be an issue. While discontinuation of additional topical drops may not be an option in the immediate postoperative setting, changing the postoperative eye drop regimen to preservative-free medications such as moxifloxacin and tafluprost or those with preservatives other than BAK such as Alphagan-P (Allergan, Irvine, CA) can help reduce corneal epithelial and limbal stem cell toxicity, especially if long-term drop use is necessary. Avoidance of common agents known to contribute to further corneal hypoesthesia such as topical anesthetics, beta-blockers, and NSAIDs is also important [10].

While the use of punctal plugs, patching, and tarsorrhaphy is frequently employed in treating persistent epithelial defects, these options should be avoided in this particular patient as plugs may intensify toxic keratitis and eyelid closure will limit retinal examination.

The use of high-oxygen permeable bandage soft contact lenses, replaced every 2–4 weeks, is an effective way to reduce tear surface irregularities and manage mechanical epithelial damage and debridement from irregular conjunctiva after surgery and blinking without obscuring the view for repeated retinal examinations. Administration of concomitant broad-spectrum topical antibiotics is required with bandage contact use.

Finally, autologous serum made from the patient's own centrifuged blood can be administered in topical eye drop form providing both lubrication and essential vitamins and growth factors and is an extremely effective agent for healing persistent epithelial defects. While the specific concentration and procedure for making serum tears have not been standardized, some groups have published protocols to optimize the composition of epitheliotropic growth factors (Table 15.1).

Autologous serum 50% was instituted starting at q2h, and the epithelial defect healed 10 days after initial presentation to the corneal service (Fig. 15.2). Unfortunately, some subepithelial haze did develop from the non-healing defect, but the patient retained an intact epithelium throughout subsequent follow-up visits.

Table 15.1 Stepwise treatment of persistent epithelial defects

1.	Minimize toxicity from eye drops:
	(a) Discontinue all nonessential topical medications (consider switching to oral medications).
	(b) Use prophylactic topical antibiotics judiciously.
2.	Improve the tear film:
	(a) Frequent lubrication with viscous non-preserved artificial tears/ointments
	(b) Punctal occlusion
3.	Enhance epithelial function:
	(a) Oral doxycycline/minocycline
	(b) Autologous serum drops/platelet-rich plasma
4.	Protect the epithelium:
	(a) Pressure patching
	(b) Bandage soft contact lens
	(c) Self-retaining amniotic membrane/amniotic membrane transplant
	(d) Scleral contact lens
	(e) Lateral tarsorrhaphy
	(f) Conjunctival flap

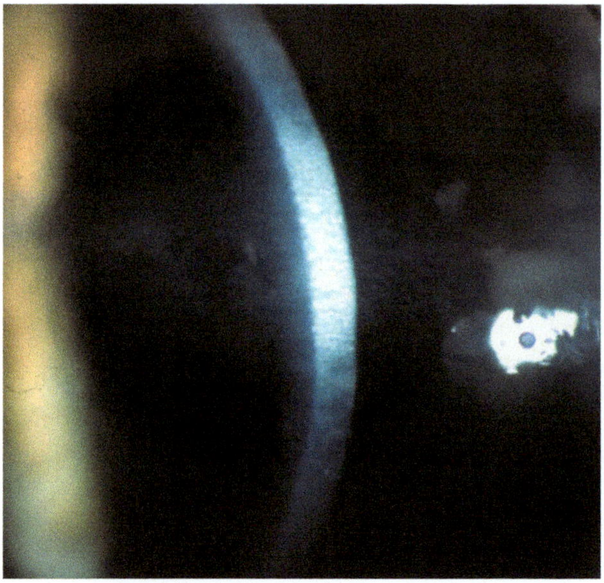

Fig. 15.2 Healed epithelial defect in Patient #1, but with subepithelial haze

Case #2

A 35-year-old woman developed a non-healing corneal epithelial defect after a bout of herpes simplex virus keratitis that was treated by her primary ophthalmologist with topical trifluridine. The patient was referred for a non-healing defect (Fig. 15.3).

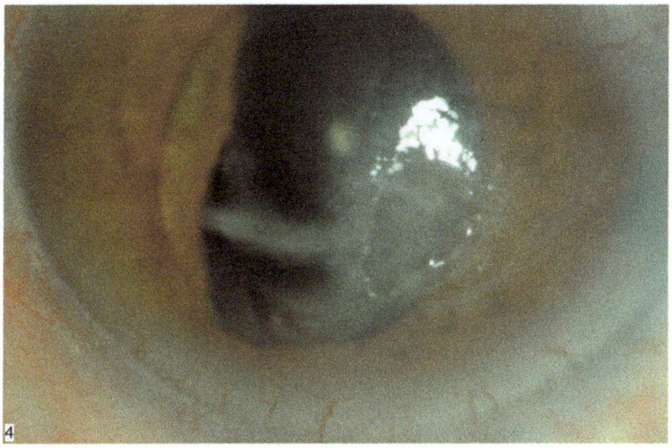

Fig. 15.3 Non-healing epithelial defect in Patient #2 secondary to herpes simplex virus keratitis

What Risk Factors Does She Have for Developing a Non-healing Epithelial Defect?

Herpes simplex virus has a predilection for the trigeminal ganglion, where the virus can lay dormant for years or actively replicate during a reactivation episode [11]. Trigeminal innervation of the corneal surface provides sensation and supplies growth factors to maintain the integrity of the corneal epithelium [12]. A herpetic eye infection can, therefore, create a neurotrophic state where damage of the corneal surface occurs by a decrease in reflex tear production, alteration of the blink response, and a lack of epitheliotropic growth factors (e.g., neuropeptides). A neurotrophic cornea is a major risk factor for the development of a non-healing epithelial defect [12].

Herpes simplex epithelial keratitis is typically treated by topical or systemic antiviral medications. All of the commonly used topical antiviral medications today, including trifluridine, acyclovir, and ganciclovir, have been shown to cause local toxicity and punctate epithelial erosions [13]. Their mechanism of action involves interfering with viral DNA replication. Trifluridine, the most commonly used topical antiviral agent in the United States, is more likely to be incorporated by host DNA and, therefore, can prevent epithelial cell proliferation along with viral replication [14]. Although topical antiviral medications can decrease the time to healing in herpes simplex epithelial keratitis, local toxicity may limit their efficacy, and oral antiviral medications may be preferred. If topical antivirals were used by the referring ophthalmologist, epithelial toxicity may have retarded the reparative process.

The length of treatment with topical antiviral medications could have also affected the chances of epithelial healing in this patient. It has been estimated that only about half of all corneal epithelial defects from herpes simplex keratitis, regardless of antiviral type and route (oral versus topical) used, heal within 1 week on treatment [15]. Therefore, typically about 2 weeks of treatment is recommended, as failure to heal after this time can reflect incomplete treatment of the viral infection. An important point is that herpetic epithelial diseases rarely need to be treated with topical antivirals more than 2 weeks (except in immune-compromised cases), and if prolonged therapy is needed, oral antivirals are the preferred method of therapy.

The patient's topical therapy was discontinued and instead was treated with oral acyclovir 400 mg 5×/day until the viral infection was thought to be completely cleared. This resulted in some healing of the corneal epithelium. However, there was still a non-healing defect afterward. Despite the use of 50 % autologous serum, the defect did not heal.

What Management Strategies Should Be Considered in This Situation?

As in all cases of neurotrophic keratitis, adequate lubrication of the ocular surface is crucial in minimizing epithelial cell loss from the mechanical trauma of eyelid blinking [12]. Preservative-free artificial tear solutions, applied frequently throughout the day, can be used as a substitute for the tear film, which is often disrupted in neurotrophic eyes for the reasons mentioned above. Punctal plugs should be used liberally in all cases of neurotrophic keratopathy. In recalcitrant cases, a lateral tarsorrhaphy is used to decrease corneal exposure and minimize blinking-related trauma to the epithelium. A lateral tarsorrhaphy that extends far enough to cover the entire epithelial defect is one of the most effective, and underutilized, treatments available for persistent epithelial defects (Table).

Amniotic membrane transplantation (as a graft or as a bandage) is effective in hastening corneal epithelial healing and has been shown to result in similar rates of epithelial defect closure to those of tarsorrhaphy and contact lens application [16]. Soft bandage contact lenses are generally not recommended for prolonged periods in neurotrophic cases not only because they can anesthetize the cornea further but also because the patients may not recognize a worsening of their condition (e.g., infectious keratitis), resulting in a potential delay in presentation [17]. On the other hand, scleral contact lenses are quite effective and may be used as an alternative to tarsorrhaphy for persistent epithelial defects; however, they require special expertise for fitting and very close follow-up.

What Is the Best Way to Use Prophylactic Antibiotics in Persistent Epithelial Defects?

Topical antibiotics are recommended in all cases of persistent epithelial defect to minimize the risk of infectious keratitis. On the other hand, the toxicity from the antibiotics and/or the preservatives can be detrimental to wound healing. Moreover, the excessive use of antibacterial medications can increase the risk of infection by fungal organisms. Therefore, topical antibiotics are used judiciously. It seems prudent to avoid medications such as aminoglycosides (tobramycin and gentamicin) which tend to be more toxic to the epithelium. Some suggested choices are fluoroquinolone or polymyxin-trimethoprim drops once or twice daily. In addition to a topical antibiotic, oral tetracyclines (doxycycline or minocycline) are often used adjunctively in persistent epithelial defects and can help promote wound healing primarily by inhibiting matrix metalloproteinases.

In this case, an amniotic membrane was sutured to the limbus using a running 8–0 Vicryl suture, and a lateral tarsorrhaphy was performed. The epithelial defect healed within 2 weeks, and this cornea has remained healed during continued follow-up.

Case #3

A 59-year-old man underwent radiation for an intracranial tumor and subsequently developed cicatrizing changes of his right lower eyelid, in addition to neovascular glaucoma. Secondary to the cicatrizing eyelid changes, the patient also developed a recurrent corneal epithelial defect.

What Other Risk Factors Does He Have for Developing a Non-healing Epithelial Defect?

The major factor leading to this patient's non-healing epithelial defect is his development of cicatrizing eyelid changes. Radiotherapy can cause contraction of soft tissues in the areas adjacent to treatment, and therefore incidental radiation involving the periocular tissues can result in exposure keratopathy. A healthy tear film cannot be maintained without good apposition of the eyelids, leading to evaporative dryness. Lagophthalmos can also result in the inability to protect the cornea from repeated external mechanical trauma. Finally, damage to the eyelid margin with resultant keratinization or misdirected eyelashes can lead to repeated microtrauma with each blink, inhibiting normal anchoring of new corneal epithelium.

Even without cicatrizing eyelid changes, radiation alone can lead to risk factors for developing a non-healing epithelial defect. Severe dry eye syndrome has been reported after external beam radiation. [18] This effect is presumably due to the unintentional radiation to the major and accessory lacrimal glands. Radiation has also been associated with neurotrophic keratitis and limbal stem cell deficiency presumably due to radiation damage to the trigeminal nerve or damage to the palisades of Vogt [19, 20].

Neovascular glaucoma due to proliferative radiation retinopathy can be associated with multiple insults on the corneal epithelium. Uncontrolled intraocular pressure from neovascular glaucoma can cause painful bullae, which may contribute to repeated corneal disruption. Finally the treatments for neovascular glaucoma can all be implicated in contributing to a non-healing defect. As mentioned previously, topical glaucoma medications containing BAK can result in epithelial injury. Intravitreal anti-VEGF has also been implicated in causing delayed epithelial healing. [21] Panretinal photocoagulation to treat retinal ischemia, as previously mentioned, can damage the long ciliary nerves resulting in a neurotrophic cornea. The long ciliary nerves can also be damaged in cyclodestructive procedures of the ciliary body such as transscleral or endoscopic cyclophotocoagulation, which is reserved for refractory glaucoma in the eyes with poor visual potential.

Despite aggressive lubrication and minimization of his topical medications, the corneal epithelial defect eventually became non-healing, and the patient was in a tremendous amount of pain.

What Management Strategies Should Be Considered in This Situation?

The management strategy in this patient is twofold: first to improve lubrication and second to minimize exposure. In addition to frequent preservative-free artificial tears every 1–2 h, moisture goggles can help to reduce evaporation of the tear film. Preservative-free lubricating ointment should be placed at bedtime or if the corneal exposure is severe, frequently during the day. Adjuvant treatment with growth factors as contained in serum tears may aid in corneal healing [22]·

In order to treat the underlying lagophthalmos, a combined oculoplastics approach with lateral tarsal strip and skin grafting may be necessary for the repair of a severe cicatricial ectropion [23]. However, for mild cicatricial changes, a temporary or permanent lateral tarsorrhaphy can reduce the amount of corneal exposure and tear evaporation. Amniotic membrane grafting can aid in healing the persistent epithelial defect prior to or combined with a tarsorrhaphy. [24] Logistically, cryopreserved (Amnion; Bio-Tissue, Inc., Miami, FL) or freeze-dried (Ambio5; IOP Ophthalmics, Costa Mesa, CA) amniotic membrane can be sutured on in the operating or minor procedure room, while the cryopreserved self-retaining amniotic membrane (e.g., Prokera, Bio-Tissue, Inc., Miami, FL) and the freeze-dried AmbioDisk (IOP Ophthalmics, Costa Mesa, CA) with a bandage soft contact lens can be placed in clinic. In general, amniotic membrane is most useful in settings where there is good likelihood of recovery of function or else if other adjunctive treatments (e.g., tarsorrhaphy) are instituted at the same time. Otherwise in advanced cases such as this, amniotic membrane alone will only be a temporary effect and will not provide any long-lasting benefit.

In a painful eye with poor visual potential and a non-healing epithelial defect resistant to medical therapy, a conjunctival flap can be the definitive strategy to manage pain. Intraocular pressure measurement, however, becomes difficult after such a procedure; therefore, a conjunctival flap should be considered after the neovascular glaucoma has been adequately addressed.

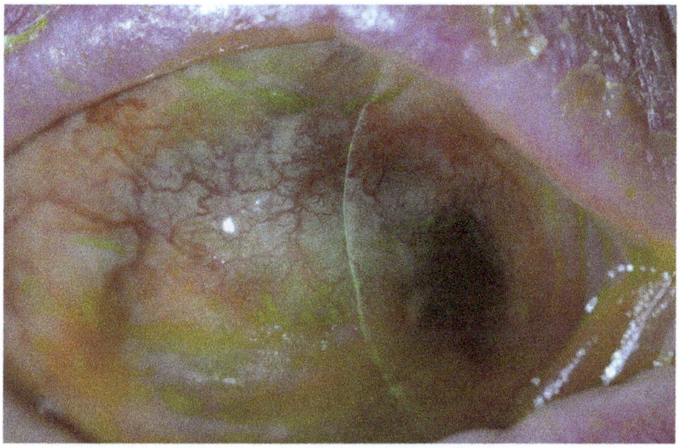

Fig. 15.4 Conjunctival flap in Patient #3

Despite a lateral tarsorrhaphy, the epithelial defect continued to recur, and as such, a conjunctival flap was performed, resulting in complete resolution of the patient's pain and discomfort (Fig. 15.4).

Discussion

The persistent corneal epithelial defects in the three cases above were all treated slightly differently, but illustrate common themes. The disruption of the tear film can lead to mechanical trauma to the epithelium from blinking, and so lubrication was a key first-line therapy in all cases. Similarly, bandage contact lenses protect the healing epithelium from being sloughed by eyelid movement, but should be used with caution in patients with neurotrophic corneas. Punctal plugs can be effective in settings with limited tear production, but may exacerbate the toxic effects of topical medications. Prevention of ocular surface exposure decreases drying of the cornea, and tarsorrhaphy is an effective treatment modality if other therapies have failed. Tarsorrhaphy can limit the retinal exam, however, so botulinum toxin A injection into the levator palpebrae superioris may be used in its place. Topical ophthalmic medication use should be decreased if possible, as both their preservative and active ingredient can cause epithelial toxicity. Reduced corneal sensation can occur from corneal nerve damage as a result of diabetic keratopathy, herpetic eye infection, and retinal surgery, leading to a decrease in reflex tear production and the delivery of growth factors to the cornea. Autologous serum tears may aid in epithelial defect closure with their combined lubricating and epitheliotropic characteristics. Amniotic membrane transplantation is also a good option for aiding the healing of an epithelial defect.

Although there are many treatment options for persistent epithelial defects, as illustrated by the three cases above, the successful management of persistent epithelial defects requires an understanding of the causative factors in that particular situation: different etiologies of the defects respond differently to the different treatment modalities that are available. With the recognition that not all persistent epithelial defects are the same and with a good understanding of the underlying mechanisms causing the epithelial defects, persistent corneal epithelial defects can be effectively treated.

Acknowledgment *Financial disclosures*: None of the authors have any relevant financial interests in the material discussed in this chapter.

References

1. Jeng BH, Dupps WJ Jr. Autologous serum 50% eyedrops in the treatment of persistent corneal epithelial defects. Cornea 2009;28(10):1104–1108.
2. Tsubota K, Goto E, Shimmura S, Shimazaki J. Treatment of persistent corneal epithelial defect by autologous serum application. Ophthalmology. 1999;106(10):1984–9.
3. Nielsen NV. Corneal sensitivity and vibratory perception in diabetes mellitus. Acta Ophthalmol. 1978;56(3):406–11.
4. Sigelman S, Friedenwald JS. Mitotic and wound-healing activities of the corneal epithelium; effect of sensory denervation. AMA Arch Ophthalmol. 1954;52(1):46–57.
5. Saito J, Enoki M, Hara M, Morishige N, Chikama T, Nishida T. Correlation of corneal sensation, but not of basal or reflex tear secretion, with the stage of diabetic retinopathy. Cornea. 2003;22(1):15–8.
6. Banerjee PJ, Chandra A, Sullivan PM, Charteris DG. Neurotrophic corneal ulceration after retinal detachment surgery with retinectomy and endolaser: a case series. JAMA Ophthalmol. 2014;132(6):750–2.
7. Hersh PS, Rice BA, Baer JC, Wells PA, Lynch SE, McGuigan LJ, Foster CS. Topical nonsteroidal agents and corneal wound healing. Arch Ophthalmol. 1990;108(4):577–83.
8. Dart J. Corneal toxicity: the epithelium and stroma in iatrogenic and factitious disease. Eye (Lond). 2003;17(8):886–92. Review
9. Gilbard JP, Rossi SR. Tear film and ocular surface changes in a rabbit model of neurotrophic keratitis. Ophthalmology. 1990;97(3):308–12.
10. Weissman SS, Asbell PA. Effects of topical timolol (0.5%) and betaxolol (0.5%) on corneal sensitivity. Br J Ophthalmol. 1990;74(7):409–12.
11. White, ML, Chodosh, J. Herpes simplex virus keratitis: a treatment guideline. Hoskins Center and Academy-approved compendium of evidence-based eye care. June 2014.
12. Sacchetti M, Lambiase A. Diagnosis and management of neurotrophic keratitis. Clin Ophthalmol. 2014;8:571–9.
13. Ching SST, Feder RS, Hindman HB, et al. Herpes simplex virus epithelial keratitis, preferred practice pattern clinical questions. Am Acad Ophthalmol. 2012:1–8.
14. Chou TY, Hong BY. Ganciclovir ophthalmic gel 0.15% for the treatment of acute herpetic keratitis: background, effectiveness, tolerability, safety, and future applications. Ther Clin Risk Manag. 2014;10:665–81.
15. Wilhelmus KR. The treatment of herpes simplex virus epithelial keratitis. Trans Am Ophthalmol Soc. 2000;98:505–32.
16. Khokhar S, Natung T, Sony P, Sharma N, Agarwal N, Vajpayee RB. Amniotic membrane transplantation in refractory neurotrophic corneal ulcers: a randomized, controlled clinical trial. Cornea. 2005;24(6):654–60.
17. Katzman LR, Jeng BH. Management strategies for persistent epithelial defects of the cornea. Saudi J Ophthalmol. 2014;28(3):168–72.

18. Bhandare N, Moiseenko V, Song WY, Morris CG, Bhatti MT, Mendenhall WM. Severe dry eye syndrome after radiotherapy for head-and-neck tumors. Int J Radiat Oncol Biol Phys. 2012;82(4):1501–8.
19. Bonini S, Rama P, Olzi D, Lambiase A. Neurotrophic keratitis. Eye (Lond). 2003;17(8):989–95. Review
20. Fujishima H, Shimazaki J, Tsubota K. Temporary corneal stem cell dysfunction after radiation therapy. Br J Ophthalmol. 1996;80(10):911–4.
21. Colombres GA, Gramajo AL, Arrambide MP, Juarez SM, Arevalo JF, Bar J, Juarez CP, Luna JD. Delayed corneal epithelial healing after intravitreal bevacizumab: a clinical and experimental study. J Ophthalmic Vis Res. 2011;6(1):18–25.
22. Young AL, Cheng AC, Ng HK, Cheng LL, Leung GY, Lam DS. The use of autologous serum tears in persistent corneal epithelial defects. Eye (Lond). 2004;18(6):609–14.
23. Tarallo M, Rizzo MI, Monarca C, Fanelli B, Parisi P, Scuderi N. Optimal care for eyelid contraction after radiotherapy: case report and literature review. J Oral Maxillofac Surg. 2012;70(10):2459–65.
24. Prabhasawat P, Tesavibul N, Komolsuradej W. Single and multilayer amniotic membrane transplantation for persistent corneal epithelial defect with and without stromal thinning and perforation. Br J Ophthalmol. 2001;85(12):1455–63.

Chapter 16
Pediatric Ocular Surface Disease

Aisha Traish

Case 1

JS is a 10-year-old Hispanic girl who was referred to you for bilateral corneal scarring with recurrent redness and infections. She presents with significant blurry vision in her left eye for the past 1 month and redness of both eyes over the past several months. She describes gradual onset of redness of both eyes and poor vision and light sensitivity in the left eye. She originally began having similar problems (intermittent redness and light sensitivity) when she was around 5 years old and it was always treated as pink eye. She is a full-time student with no other ocular disease history. She denies any recent illnesses or infectious diseases. She has no family history of eye disease.

On ophthalmic examination her best corrected vision at distance is 20/20 in the right eye and 20/400 in the left eye. She has normal ocular tensions, pupil exam, and full extraocular motility. Her funduscopic exam is unremarkable. Slit lamp examination of the anterior segment reveals eyelid inflammation with anterior blepharitis bilaterally. There is mild diffuse conjunctival injection of the right eye with fine corneal neovascularization inferiorly and corneal lipid deposition in a mid-peripheral arc at 4 o'clock. The left eye demonstrates +2 conjunctival injection with deeper nasal and temporal corneal neovascularization with a thick band of lipid deposition in the central cornea with anterior stromal corneal haze. There is no intraocular inflammation or cornea ectasia (Fig. 16.1a, b).

A. Traish, MD
University of Illinois Hospital, Chicago, IL, USA
e-mail: aisha.traish@gmail.com

A.R. Djalilian (ed.), *Ocular Surface Disease*,
https://doi.org/10.1007/978-3-319-15823-5_16

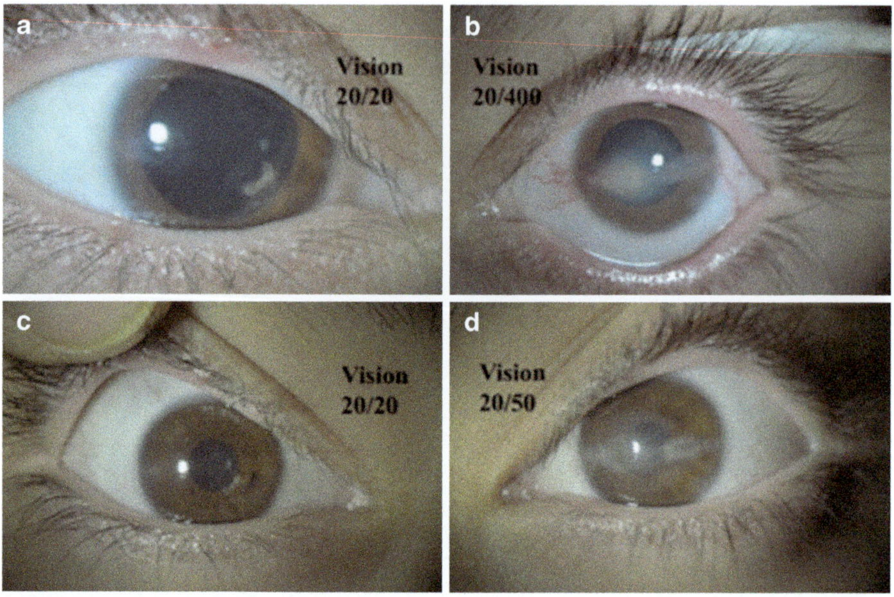

Fig. 16.1 Slit lamp images on presentation of right eye (**a**) and left eye (**b**) and on follow up of right eye (**c**) and left eye (**d**), demonstrating significant reduction in corneal neovascularization and lipid deposition primarily in the left eye over the course of 2 months

What Differential Diagnoses Do These Findings Suggest? What Additional History Would This Exam Prompt You to Obtain?

The differential diagnoses would include inflammatory and infectious causes of pediatric ocular surface disease. Infectious etiologies could include herpes simplex, although it most commonly presents unilaterally there are more severe cases with bilateral disease [1]. Allergic or immune causes include vernal keratoconjunctivitis, although vernal is more common in boys and is typically associated with giant papillae and shield ulcers [2]. From the description we know that the process is bilateral with involvement of the eyelids, conjunctivae, and corneas. The most likely diagnosis is phlyctenular keratoconjunctivitis in the setting of chronic blepharitis, which is very prevalent in children [3, 4].

There are a few more relevant historical questions to ask. You would want to know if this child has a history of oral cold sores and whether she has a history of rosacea. You would also ask if any history of contact lens wear. A history of recurrent chalazia is also consistent with the diagnosis of phlyctenulosis and frequently present.

Upon questioning her family reports that she has been diagnosed with rosacea but has no history of prior cold sores. She has never worn contact lenses.

She does have a history of multiple styes in the past. Prior to our examination, she had been initiated on oral erythromycin 400 mg by mouth twice a day and ciprofloxacin one drop every 4 h in the left eye.

What Therapeutic Plan Would You Initiate for a Child of This Age Group?

The most important element to recognize is the significant inflammation. The severe vision impairment in the left eye along with the dramatic corneal appearance of stromal haze, lipid deposition, and angry neovascularization does make one concerned for possible destructive infectious processes, but antibiotics or antivirals alone will not treat this vision-threatening condition. Anti-inflammatory activity is necessary to dampen the immune reaction that is causing lipid deposition, loss of corneal clarity, and neovascularization. The best initial approach includes topical steroids and oral anti-inflammatory and antibiotic therapy appropriate for this age group in addition to eyelid hygiene (preferably with eyelid cleansers) with warm compresses.

Due to the severe ocular inflammation, bilateral nature, and vision loss, an aggressive therapeutic approach was taken with prednisolone acetate 1% one drop every 4 h in the left eye, one drop twice a day in the right eye, and continuation of the oral erythromycin. Cyclosporine 0.05% one drop twice a day to both eyes was prescribed. The ciprofloxacin was discontinued. She was asked to return in 3 weeks, and documentation with slit lamp photography was performed.

Why Continue with Oral Erythromycin But Not Topical Ciprofloxacin?

Oral erythromycin can be an effective systemic agent for ocular surface inflammation in the pediatric age group. The macrolides' bacteriostatic properties have been found to inhibit production of pro-inflammatory cytokines and thus have been useful as an anti-inflammatory agent for the eye [5]. The challenges in compliance are tied to its requirement of multiple daily dosing.

Doxycycline, which is an inexpensive, effective option in adults and older children for ocular inflammation, has been generally contraindicated in children less than 9 years of age due to concerns of deposition of the drug in bone and teeth. However, it has been used safely in many children with manifestations of ocular rosacea with good control of their disease [6]. Due to the petite frame of this child and the other alternatives, we decided to defer the option of doxycycline for management of her disease until she is older.

Topical antibiotics are not necessary in this child because clinically her exam is consistent with inflammatory processes and there is no ulceration or epithelial breakdown to suggest ocular surface compromise with microbes. As discussed below, there may be a role for topical antibiotics to the lid (to reduce the microbial flora); however we prefer to start with systemic medications.

Initial response to the therapy was positive with significant reduction in overall ocular surface inflammation. She was unable to get the cyclosporine due to insurance coverage.

What Concerns Would You Have About Long-Term Therapy?

The goals of therapy include suppression of the ocular surface inflammation and resultant vision-threatening scars. However, one must recognize the significant side effects of the medications involved and carefully titrate to effect while also minimizing potential adverse effects. Topical steroid therapy is well known to elevate intraocular pressures, and children are more vulnerable to this problem than adults [7]. In addition, lenticular changes that can cause vision loss are also a potential concern. However, one must realize that when balancing the competing factors involved in visual preservation, corneal destruction and scarring can often be much more difficult to ultimately treat compared with the resources we have to mitigate intraocular pressure rises and cataracts. Corneal transplantation in children is fraught with challenges [8], especially in the postoperative period, and in an eye prone to inflammation the risk of graft rejection is increased.

Why Cyclosporine? What Is the Pediatric Experience?

Cyclosporine has become widely used to mediate the inflammatory component of dry eye and has been shown to increase tear production [9]. It is commercially available in a 0.05% formulation but can be compounded in a 2% formulation for more severe ocular surface disease. In a series of children with a mean age of 9 years old, the cyclosporine 2% was given four times a day for an average of 1 year with significant resolution of ocular surface inflammation. These children were selected due to poor response to topical steroids and oral antibiotics, and the topical cyclosporine was found to be well tolerated in this age group [10]. The steroid-sparing effect is clearly advantageous. Although it is not FDA approved for the treatment of phlyctenular disease in children, the literature confirms its utility for this indication as an off-label ophthalmic use.

She was not tolerating the oral erythromycin, so we switched her to oral azithromycin in addition to continuing the topical anti-inflammatory therapy. She was able to get the cyclosporine 0.05 % covered. Her vision within 2 months of treatment was improved to 20/50 in the left eye (Fig. 16.1c, d).

What Oral Antibiotics Are Safe and Effective for Children with Ocular Surface Disease and Ocular Rosacea?

As discussed earlier, doxycycline and erythromycin have been used in children when age and dose appropriate for the control of ocular surface inflammation. If these agents are poorly tolerated or contraindicated, another option that has recently been highlighted for the pediatric population is azithromycin. Oral azithromycin, dosed 5 mg/kg/day with a single daily dose, has been shown to have effective anti-inflammatory effect on the ocular surface in children with phlyctenular disease [11]. It is commonly given at that dose for approximately 1 month and then given at half dose for another month. It is well tolerated, and the once a day dosing in our experience has been great for compliance in the pediatric population.

Azithromycin has also been utilized in its topical form to treat children with this disease. One formulation studied was azithromycin topical ophthalmic solution 1.5%, and in a series of 16 children ranging in age from 4 to 16 years old who had disease poorly responsive to other typical therapies, the majority of children were found to have tolerated the eye drops (two stopped therapy due to ocular irritation), and only one child required additional therapy for disease control [12].

What Other Considerations/Treatment Approaches Would You Have if This Child Was Within the Amblyopic Age Group?

Any ocular surface disease has the potential to cause scarring or vision-threatening opacities. In the amblyopic age group, it is critical to remember that *early* intervention is the key to preservation of vision. Therefore, when a child presents with corneal scarring or severe keratitis that is primarily unilateral or asymmetric, they should be assessed for the risk of development or presence of amblyopia. Sometimes this requires early patching or more aggressive therapy than one might institute in an adult with the same findings, so as to prevent deprivational amblyopia.

She continues to have recurrent episodes of ocular inflammation (Fig. 16.2) in the left eye with deeper corneal neovascularization, despite topical and oral steroids, topical cyclosporine, and oral azithromycin.

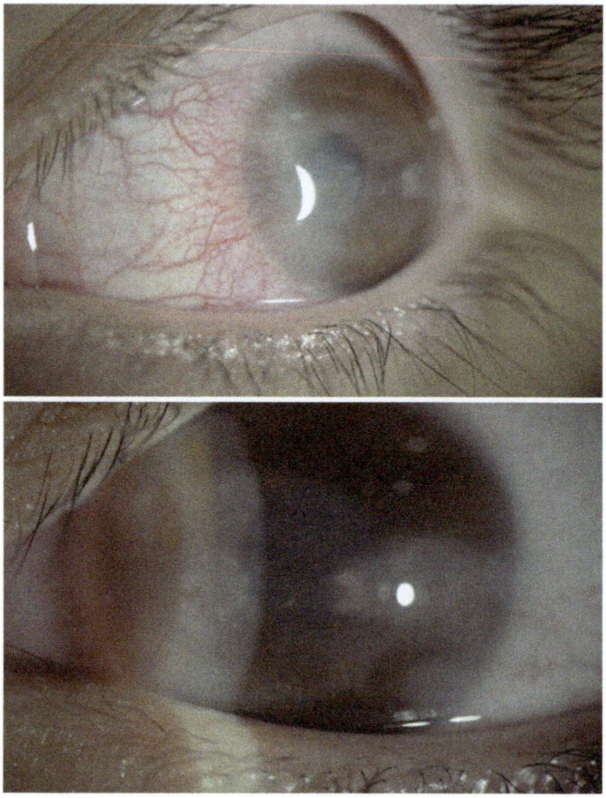

Fig. 16.2 June 2014 Slit lamp images demonstrating recurrent robust keratoconjunctivitis causing aggressive deeper stromal corneal neovascularization in the nasal region of the left eye

What Would Be Your Next Therapeutic Approach to This Challenge?

Recalcitrant phlyctenular disease can be approached using localized therapy to the eyelids, which are often the source of the inflammation. Topical tacrolimus applied to the eyelids has been proven efficacious in reduction of ocular inflammation in these more challenging cases. Tacrolimus has been shown to have a potency 30 times more than cyclosporine. The formulation evaluated in the pediatric age group for this indication is 0.03% tacrolimus ointment to the lower fornices twice daily for a few weeks with good results and was well tolerated [13].

Our patient did not initially tolerate the tacrolimus preparation available, but we recommended dilution of the ointment with artificial tear lubricating gel, and she was able to tolerate it and achieve good effect. With institution of the above alternative therapy, the robust inflammation in her left eye became quiescent, and her vision measured 20/30 (Fig. 16.3).

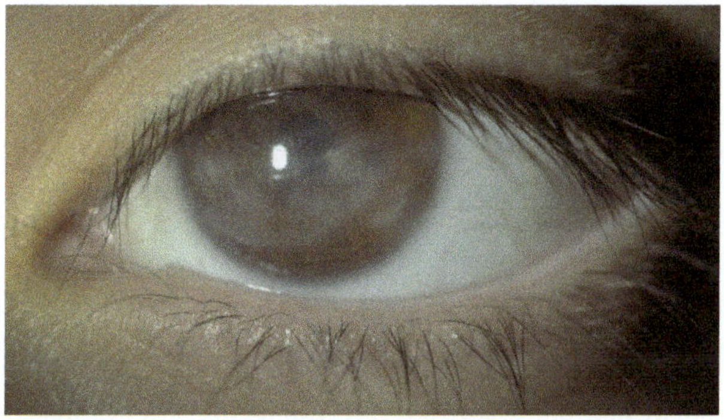

Fig. 16.3 Jan 2015: 15 months after treatment there is significant reduction of corneal haze and lipid deposition with evident control of ocular surface inflammation. Vision is 20/30 uncorrected

What Is the Underlying Cause of This Type of Ocular Surface Inflammation?

Phlyctenular keratoconjunctivitis is a common inflammatory ocular surface condition in children with many available therapies. In many literature series, the larger spectrum of blepharokeratoconjunctivitis, of which phlyctenular disease is a subset, represents the most common referral diagnosis for pediatric patients to ophthalmic referral centers. Phlyctenular disease has traditionally been associated with a hypersensitivity reaction of the ocular surface, namely, the cornea and the conjunctiva, to bacterial antigens. The most common agents implicated are tuberculosis, *Staphylococcus*, and chlamydial antigens, although other less common antigens can also trigger this disease process [14]. In patients with recalcitrant disease, it may be reasonable to check for tuberculosis (Quantiferon Gold). Phlyctenular disease can also occur in the setting of chronic eyelid inflammation, and therefore a multipronged approach to the ocular surface destruction, eyelid inflammation, and bacterial hypersensitivity is critical. Another condition that must be considered in recalcitrant disease is demodex. Diagnosis requires examining lashes under light microscope. Current treatments for demodex include eyelid scrubs with 50% tea tree oil or oral or topical ivermectin [15].

Vision-threatening and amblyogenic scarring can occur, especially since the average age of presentation of these children is reported to be around 6 years old [14–17]. Therefore, we must consider visual development in the context of therapeutic decisions and potentially involve pediatric ophthalmologists in the disease management process if the child is perhaps being managed by an internist or ophthalmic subspecialist who may not treat amblyopia as part of their daily practice.

Judy Chen, M.D.
Eric Feinstein, M.D.
Aisha Traish, M.D.

Case 2

AA is a 5-day-old infant female transferred to the neonatal ICU from an outside hospital for escalation of clinical care. You are consulted for further ophthalmic evaluation and management by the ICU team. Prenatal history is significant for poor prenatal care and alcohol abuse during pregnancy. She was born at 37 weeks without complications, but birth weight was noted to be in the third percentile (Fig. 16.4a, b).

On general examination, the patient has multiple, severe malformed features. Facial abnormalities include a sloped forehead, hypertelorism, flattened nasal bridge, macrostomia, micrognathia, deformed ear lobes, thin upper lip with long philtrum, and reduced hair of the scalp and eyebrows (Fig. 16.4a). She also has absent nipples, abnormal skin tension throughout her entire body with absence of hair or lanugo, and abnormal genitalia.

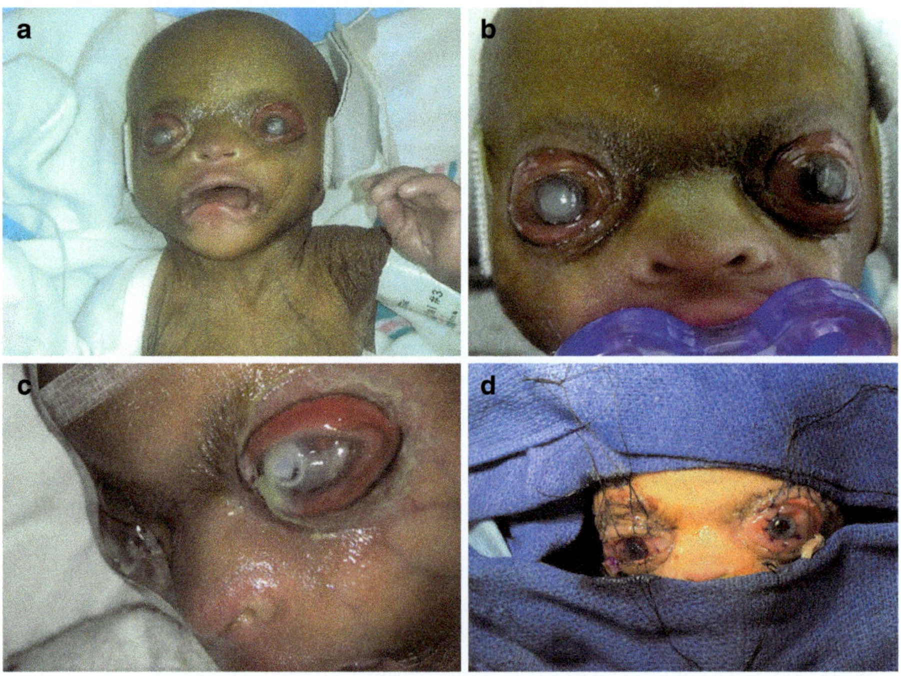

Fig. 16.4 (**a**, **b**) External photograph of 5-day-old infant with lack of eyelids, eyelashes and eyebrows. There is significant injection and chemosis OU with bilateral infiltration and ulceration of the corneas OU. Multiple anomalies can be seen on the external photograph including sloping forehead, hypertelorism, flattened nasal bridge, micrognathia, macrostomia, deformed ears, short neck, hyperpigmentation and tense and loose skin in different areas. (**c**) External photograph showing significant thinning of the cornea. (**d**) External photograph after eyelid reconstruction and bilateral penetrating keratoplasty with clear grafts

On ophthalmic examination, she is found to be averse to light in either eye. There is full extraocular motility, and intraocular pressures measured by portable Tonopen are 10 mmHg in both eyes. On external exam, there is an absence of eyelids, eyelashes, and eyebrows with scant orbicularis muscle present with retraction of the globe when blinking (Fig. 16.4b). There is marked conjunctival injection and chemosis bilaterally. The corneas are found to be opacified with infiltration and 60 % thinning bilaterally and with associated corneal epithelial defects of 5 and 6 mm in the right and left eyes, respectively. Corneal diameters are 7 mm OD and 8 mm OS. There is no view to the anterior chamber, iris, or lens. B-scan ultrasonography does not reveal any posterior abnormalities.

What Differential Diagnoses Do These Findings Suggest? What Additional History Would This Exam Prompt You to Obtain?

This patient has bilateral cloudy corneas with ulceration, infiltration, and stromal loss. In this child with multiple other congenital abnormalities, an important piece of history to gather from the outside hospital records and physicians is whether the corneas were cloudy at birth or whether they became cloudy in the postnatal period. This would be the first major branch point for diagnostic consideration.

If the corneas were noted to be cloudy at birth, the differential diagnosis would include a distinct set of congenital causes. The most common reason for congenital clouding of the cornea is congenital glaucoma. Other major causes include: sclerocornea, tears in Descemet's membrane (often caused by traumatic birth or forcep use), metabolic diseases such as Hurler Syndrome, Peters anomaly, congenital hereditary endothelial dystrophy (CHED), congenital hereditary stromal dystrophy (CSHD), and limbal dermoids. There have also been reports of children with fetal alcohol syndrome exhibiting bilateral diffusely cloudy corneas at birth, which would be an important consideration in this case given the mother's alcohol abuse during pregnancy. Other rarer cause of congenital clouding of the cornea includes congenital rubella, posterior ulcer of von Hippel, posterior keratoconus, congenital corneal staphyloma, cornea plana, corneal keloids, oculoauriculovertebral dysplasia, posterior polymorphous dystrophy, and Fryns syndrome.

However, if the corneas were noted to be clear at birth with secondary clouding, then the differential diagnosis would heavily favor an infectious, inflammatory, or exposure-related etiology. In this case, the patient's lack of eyelids predisposes the patient to developing severe exposure keratopathy. Infectious etiologies, including bacterial or fungal, cannot be ruled out in this case due to the patient's extreme presentation and exposure to pathogens in the birth canal as well as in the hospital setting. Inflammatory etiologies are much less likely in a newborn as their immature immune systems are unlikely to produce such an exuberant response.

According to outside hospital records, the corneas were essentially clear at birth but have become increasingly opacified and thinned over the past few days, and concern for corneal perforation prompted the patient's transfer to you.

What Is the Most Likely Diagnosis? What Additional Workup Would You Obtain for the Patient's Ocular Findings?

The most likely diagnosis at this point given the constellation of findings is ablepharon macrostomia syndrome (AMS), which is on the spectrum of ectodermal dysplasias. AMS is an extremely rare disorder first described by McCarthy and West in 1977, which is characterized by the absence of eyelids, sparse or absence of hair, a large fish-like mouth (macrostomia), ear and genital anomalies, and redundant coarse skin [18–21]. As of 2011, fewer than 20 cases of AMS had been reported in the literature worldwide [18].

Patients with corneal ulceration should always be worked up and empirically treated for infectious etiologies until it has been ruled out. A panculture including aerobic, anaerobic, fungal, and acid-fast cultures should be obtained. In neonates, this can be done most efficiently with topical anesthetic, calcium alginate swabs, and the aid of a portable slit lamp, if available, while an assistant holds the patient's head still; if the neonate can tolerate this bedside intervention, one can avoid unnecessary exposure to general anesthesia.

Aerobic, anaerobic, fungal, and acid-fast *Bacillus* cultures of the cornea are negative with no organisms seen on gram stain.

What are Your Next Steps in Management?

Even before knowing the culture results, the most emergent issue in this case is to stop the cycle of continued corneal ulceration and stromal loss, which is rapidly heading toward corneal perforation. The importance of diagnosing ablepharon macrostomia syndrome is to institute early treatment, starting with conservative measures such as lubrication with artificial lubricant tears, ointments, moisture chambers, etc. Ideally, these measures should be instituted as soon as the child is born and the anomalies are noted, in order to prevent progression of disease.

In cases where aggressive lubrication is inadequate or where the condition has already progressed to a severe stage upon presentation, as in our case, conservative therapies may be insufficient. There have been reports about AMS discussing the use of tarsorrhaphies [22], but these are of limited use in the severest cases where there is a complete absence of eyelids. One case report of a patient with severe exposure keratopathy and corneal desiccation due to congenital cryptophthalmos [23] described the use of an amniotic membrane to line the ocular surface and prevent further exposure. Without eyelids and associated meibomian glands, the sequelae of severe exposure keratopathy present rapidly; therefore it is important to stage treatment with both temporary (eye lubricants and amniotic membrane) and permanent solutions (eyelid reconstruction and tectonic corneal stability) to maximize visual outcomes.

Cryopreserved amniotic membranes were placed across both corneas at the bedside.

What Additional Systemic Workup Would You Recommend?

An important aspect of management for these patients is to obtain a full systemic workup in order to evaluate for life-threatening birth defects, such as congenital heart anomalies. Although cardiac anomalies are not part of the constellation of findings in ablepharon macrostomia syndrome, failure to diagnose cardiac anomalies may lead to worse overall outcomes. The management of these patients is also best approached in a team-based format, in conjunction with neonatal intensivists, pediatric otolaryngologists, and geneticists.

The vast majority of patients reported in the literature have had normal chromosomal studies [19, 20], despite observed instances of parent-to-child transmission [24, 25] suggesting an autosomal-dominant inheritance pattern. Until recently, no specific gene defect had been reported. A recent study by Marchegiani and associates at the National Institutes of Health (NIH) reported a recurrent dominant mutation in the DNA binding domain of *TWIST2* as being responsible for both AMS and Barber-Say Syndrome (BSS), an associated ectodermal dysplasia [26], although this is yet to be replicated.

Further investigation reveals no family history of maternal genetic or ocular disorders, but paternal history is significant for a prior child by a different partner with congenital heart disease and an unspecified partial absence of one arm. In our patient, an echocardiogram shows a patent foramen ovale with normal ventricles, atria, valves, and systolic and diastolic function. Ultrasounds of the abdomen (kidneys, spleen, and bladder) and head are normal. A genetic workup shows a normal standard chromosomal analysis except a normal variant of 9p12q13 mutation is observed in every cell. Chromosomal microarray and karyotype are normal.

How Would You Plan for Further Long-Term Surgical Management of This Condition?

There is a wide variety of phenotypic expression documented in the published reports of AMS. While most patients with AMS exhibit the same systemic findings such as low birth weight, sparse or absent hair, macrostomia, ear anomalies, abnormal genitalia, and redundant skin and abnormal ears [18–21], the severity of the ophthalmic findings can vary dramatically. The classic case involves complete absence of the eyelids, but many reports have documented AMS patients with variable loss of the eyelids [18, 19], leading to variable amounts of chemosis, exposure keratopathy, and subsequent vision loss. Therefore, while nearly all cases of ablepharon macrostomia syndrome will eventually require eyelid reconstruction, the necessity and timing of surgical intervention depends on the severity of the phenotype and how quickly the patient progresses with conservative measures. We typically delay surgical intervention for as long as possible, not only because of the technical challenges of operating on a neonate but also because overall cosmetic and functional outcomes are better if surgery is delayed. Approximately half of patients reported have had significant enough corneal exposure at birth to warrant early surgical intervention, involving eyelid surgery followed by skin grafting for eyelid reconstruction, within the first weeks of life [19].

There are many published techniques for four-lid reconstruction, but most are utilized in traumatic adult cases and involve some period of total visual occlusion [27, 28], which may induce amblyopia in a neonate. Price et al. described a technique of using bipedicle flaps to fill the eyelid defects in a case of ablepharon macrostomia [22]. We favor skin flaps due to surgeon familiarity with the technique and have found that flaps taken from the postauricular area tend to best mimic the texture of eyelid skin.

Despite aggressive lubrication, there is migration of the amniotic membrane followed by progressive thinning of the corneas and eventual spontaneous full thickness corneal melting bilaterally (Fig. 16.4c).

How Would You Manage This Situation?

The corneal melt and subsequent perforation make the need for surgical intervention emergent and unavoidable. One case report of spontaneous corneal perforation in the neonatal period associated with Peters anomaly described the use of a conjunctival flap sewn over the cornea in order to preserve the eye [29]. The authors advocated this approach as it restored the integrity of a compromised corneal surface while preventing progressive ulceration and secondary infection, controlled pain, eliminated the need for frequent lubrication, and improved cosmesis. However, it can be prone to flap complications, including erosion or button holes, does not allow for good visualization of the anterior chamber for monitoring, and would likely induce amblyopia, which would be undesirable in our patient since she has bilateral disease.

Full penetrating keratoplasty is another viable option; however, it would need to be undertaken in a coordinated approach with oculoplastics or plastic surgery for concurrent or staged eyelid reconstruction in order to prevent repeat corneal melting and perforation. The underlying etiology of exposure keratopathy due to the lack of adequate eyelid cover needs to be addressed at the same time in order to promote success. A penetrating keratoplasty in a neonate can often be technically difficult, and the standard equipment is often not ideal for the sizes of the trephination. We recommend the use of a dermatologic punch when small corneal trephines are not available so as to achieve a 3–5 mm uniform corneal button trephination for both the host and the donor corneas. Host corneas should also be cut in half in these situations, with half the cornea sent to pathology for analysis and half the cornea sent to microbiology for culture.

The patient is taken for immediate penetrating keratoplasty (PKP) both eyes as well as full-thickness reconstruction of the eyelids, extensive conjunctivoplasty with reconstruction of the fornices, full-thickness skin graft for upper lids from the postauricular area, and temporary tarsorrhaphies of both eyes (Fig. 16.4d). Pathology of both corneas with gram stain and giemsa staining confirms a sterile keratopathy (Fig. 16.5).

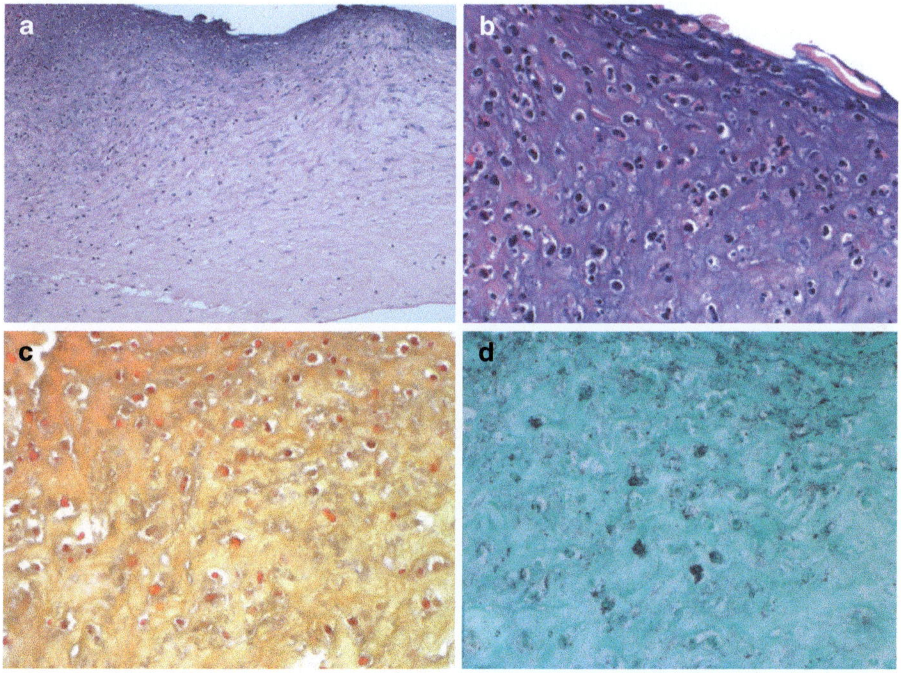

Fig. 16.5 Corneal pathology slides after full thickness penetrating keratoplasty OD. (**a**) Low power view of the right cornea with ulceration (*top*), a neutrophilic infiltrate, and stromal edema. In the *bottom right* of the image you can see Descemet's membrane with decreased corneal endothelial cells. (**b**) Higher power showing neutrophils in superficial stroma. (**c**) Gram stain which shows lack of organisms. (**d**) GMS stain negative for fungus both of which are negative (*black* areas seen on the GMS stain is non-specific background staining)

What Are Your Long-Term Goals in Management for This Patient?

The immediate goal in this patient is to stabilize the condition and prevent repeat melting of the corneal grafts to preserve her eyes. In this case, temporary tarsorrhaphies were used to encourage improved closure of the eyelids and adequate protection for the corneal grafts but still allow for adequate exposure for examination purposes. A pediatric ophthalmologist should closely monitor the patient for signs of amblyopia. As she grows, the patient will undoubtedly require additional corneal and eyelid surgeries for further visual rehabilitation, but the primary goal in her infancy is to preserve her globes so that she could have the opportunity to develop any vision in the setting of this severe condition.

Her follow-up exam at 5½ months old shows that she is able to track light binocularly OU. She has moderate haze of her right graft and significant conjunctivalization of the left graft. She also has some motility of the eyelids and globes, with an active Bell's phenomenon that is maintaining adequate lubrication of the cornea (Fig. 16.6). Systemically, the patient initially suffered from failure to thrive with weight loss but gained weight nicely with a gastric tube.

Mohsin H. Ali, M.D.
Aisha Traish, M.D.

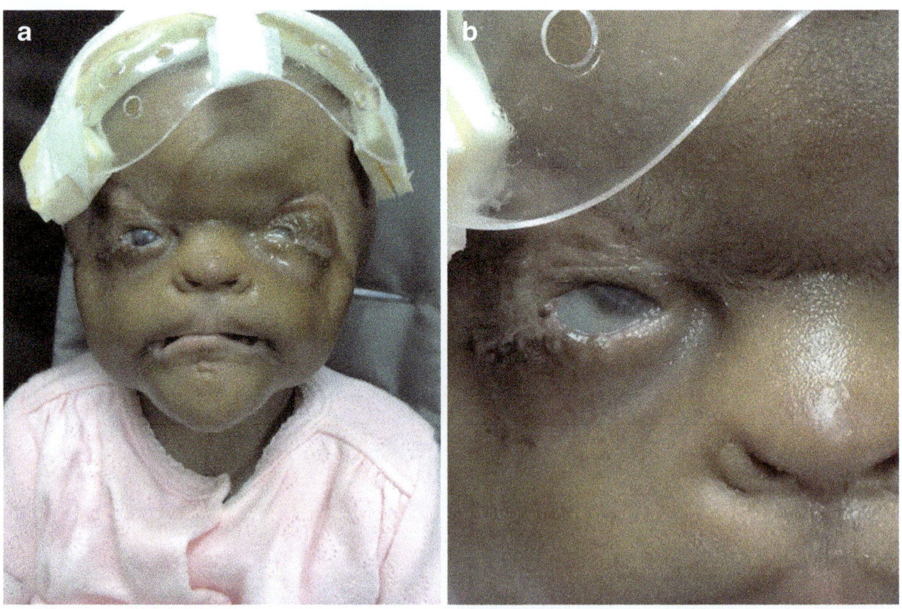

Fig. 16.6 (**a**, **b**) External photograph at exam at age of 5½ months. The patient is maintaining good lubrication of the eye with eyelid reconstruction and partial orbicularis function as well as supplemental eye drops and ointment

Case 3

A 9-year-old East Asian male with a past medical history of atopic dermatitis, allergic rhinitis, and astigmatism of the right eye (OD) for which he has been wearing eyeglasses for 3 years was referred to the pediatric cornea service for evaluation of "corneal haze" OD. His symptoms initially began 6 months prior when he was thought to have "scratched his eye" after frequent eye rubbing. Some time later, he was evaluated by a local ophthalmologist and diagnosed with stromal keratitis OD and started on topical corticosteroids. He was then referred for a second opinion to the pediatric cornea service at our institution.

At his first visit, he reported mild blurriness of his vision OD but was otherwise asymptomatic. His best-corrected visual acuity was 20/30 OD and 20/20 OS, the central corneal thickness was 434 μm OD and 456 μm OS, and the intraocular pressure was 26 mmHg OD and 17 mmHg OS. A full ophthalmologic examination was unremarkable other than an inactive-appearing, faint, central corneal haze OD. He was switched to loteprednol daily OD given his presumed steroid-induced ocular hypertension, and, correspondingly, his pressures were measured to be lower on subsequent visits.

Over the next 7 months, he was gradually tapered off of topical corticosteroids. Thereafter, he was lost to follow-up with us for the next 14 months at which time he returns to the clinic complaining of photophobia, pain, redness, and decreased vision in the right eye.

His best corrected visual acuity is 20/500 OD and 20/20 OS. His pupils, extraocular motility, and confrontation visual fields are normal. The central corneal thickness is now 802 μm OD, and the intraocular pressure is 34 mmHg OD. The anterior slit lamp examination reveals conjunctival injection and significant central corneal stromal edema OD. No epithelial defect is seen. The remainder of the examination including a dilated fundus examination and B-scan ultrasonography is normal.

What Is the Most Likely Diagnosis in This Child Given His Initial Presentation and Subsequent Disease Recurrence?

Given the patient's prior history of stromal keratitis, acutely decreased visual acuity, pain and photophobia, elevated intraocular pressure, and central corneal edema, the most likely diagnosis is recurrent herpes simplex virus (HSV) stromal keratitis. While cultures and laboratory testing may be helpful diagnostic tools for the diagnosis of HSV epithelial keratitis, they are of limited utility in cases of isolated stromal keratitis. Therefore, identification of the characteristic clinical findings, such as in this case, is essential for proper diagnosis.

In developed nations, HSV keratitis is the leading cause of corneal-related blindness [30]. Herpes simplex virus is transmitted from infected secretions (such as tears or saliva) or active lesions. Latent HSV-1 is present in the trigeminal ganglia of approximately 90% of the world's population by the age of 60, though the seroprevalence appears to be declining among both adults and adolescents in the United States [31–33]. Children from lower socioeconomic strata are more likely to be seropositive and to become so at an earlier age.

HSV keratitis can involve different layers of the cornea and may manifest as epithelial keratitis (also known as dendritic or geographic epithelial ulcer), stromal keratitis without ulceration (also known as immune stromal keratitis or interstitial keratitis), stromal keratitis with ulceration (also known as necrotizing keratitis), and endothelial keratitis (also known as disciform keratitis). If HSV keratitis recurs in a patient, it may manifest in a different layer of the cornea, for example, a patient may initially have epithelial keratitis and then later develop stromal keratitis during a recurrent HSV keratitis episode.

How Does Herpetic Eye Disease Manifest in Children as Compared to Adults?

Herpes simplex keratitis appears to manifest more aggressively in children. Children under the age of five and children aged 5 years or older may account for approximately 7% and 41%, respectively, of all primary ocular HSV keratitis cases [34]. Furthermore, recurrent episodes of HSV keratitis occur frequently in children (24–80%) [35–38]. In contrast, the Herpetic Eye Disease Study (HEDS) suggested that the recurrence rate of ocular HSV in patients age 12 years or older was 35% [39]. Children may also be more likely to develop bilateral ocular HSV (3.4–26%) [36, 37, 40, 41]. Another important risk factor present in this patient is atopy which increases the risk of ocular HSV [42] as well as the risk of bilateral and more severe involvement. Unfortunately, approximately 30% of pediatric HSV keratitis cases may be initially misdiagnosed, potentially resulting in costly delays in diagnosis and treatment [38].

How Would You Treat This patient's Acute Episode?

The pathophysiology of herpes stromal keratitis is distinct from epithelial keratitis. It is believed that the herpes stromal keratitis results from a CD4+ T cell reaction in response to viral antigens in the cornea—thereby suggesting that the primary source of damage to the cornea is the resulting inflammatory response. Therefore, the use of corticosteroids, which typically are contraindicated in the initial management of epithelial keratitis, is often necessary in the treatment of stromal keratitis (in addition, of course, to antiviral medications).

The HEDS group found a 10-week course of tapered topical prednisolone, and topical trifluridine for HSV stromal keratitis resulted in a 68% reduction in the persistence or progression of stromal inflammation as well as the duration of the episode compared to treatment with topical trifluridine and a topical placebo without corticosteroids [43]. This clearly establishes the importance of utilizing corticosteroids for this condition. Of note, the same study also suggested that delaying the use of corticosteroids, such as might seem prudent when diagnostic ambiguity or contraindications to corticosteroid use exist, may not affect the final visual outcome at 6 months.

While the HEDS group studied a 10-week treatment course, it is important to recognize that in the study evaluating treatment with topical trifluridine and topical corticosteroids and in the study evaluating treatment with topical trifluridine, topical corticosteroids, and oral acyclovir, only 33 and 25% of patients, respectively, had stable, noninflamed corneas within 6 weeks of treatment cessation [43, 44]. This suggests the importance of considering extending treatment beyond 10 weeks in patients with stromal keratitis.

Both topical antivirals, such as trifluridine or ganciclovir, and oral antivirals may be used to supplement corticosteroid treatment in HSV stromal keratitis. The choice may depend on the cost, the availability, the patient's preference for topical versus oral therapy, or the patient's other systemic conditions such as renal impairment, pregnancy, or breastfeeding. In general, however, oral antivirals may be preferable to topical antivirals in the treatment of stromal keratitis given their increased penetration into the corneal stroma, the concerns regarding ocular surface toxicity with prolonged use of topical antivirals, and the difficulty frequently encountered in appropriately administrating eye drops in children.

In summary, in both children and adults, the treatment of HSV stromal keratitis (without ulceration) requires a combination of topical corticosteroids and antivirals (preferably oral) for a duration of at least 10 weeks (though preferably longer).

What Special Considerations Must Be Made in Treating Herpetic Eye Disease in Children?

As mentioned above, HSV keratitis occurs frequently in children and adolescents, may have a more severe course than in adults, may be bilateral, and may be more difficult to diagnose given the poor cooperation many children exhibit during eye examinations—thus accounting for the high rate (up to 30%) of missed diagnoses of this condition. Therefore, when dealing with children with corneal disease, it is important to recognize that one must remain vigilant of the possibility of herpetic disease in children so as not to miss this diagnosis as well as the possibility of frequent recurrences after the correct diagnosis is made.

Children afflicted by herpetic keratitis are at risk of developing amblyopia from corneal opacification or induced refractive error. One study of children with HSV keratitis reported corneal scars in 80%, final visual acuity of 20/40 or worse in 26%, and more than 2 diopters of astigmatism in 28% [38]. Therefore, amblyopia therapy and, if necessary, comanagement of patients with pediatric ophthalmologists are essential in the management of HSV keratitis in children.

The serious risk of amblyopia highlights the importance of ensuring compliance in patients. Compliance may be aided by using oral antivirals rather than topical antivirals both because children are often averse to eye drops and the better tolerability and side effect profile of oral formulations. Some oral antivirals contain lactose which can lead to poor tolerance for certain lactose-intolerant patients. If this is a concern (e.g., if a child develops diarrhea, flatulence, bloating, or abdominal cramps), then switching to a lactose-free alternative or adding lactase supplements may be beneficial.

Acyclovir is the most commonly used oral antiviral for ocular HSV in the pediatric population, given that its safety and efficacy have been established in newborns and children. Valacyclovir may also be used in children older than age two. It is imperative that clinicians ensure that the correct weight-based dosing is being provided, especially in children who are rapidly growing, particularly during growth spurts. General guidelines for acyclovir *treatment* regimens have been previously suggested by Liu et al.: 100 mg TID for infants (up to 18 months), 200 mg TID for toddlers (18 months–3 years), 300 mg TID for young children (3–5 years), and 400 mg TID for older children (6 years or older), with a maximum daily dosage of 40–80 mg/kg/day. The general guidelines for acyclovir *prophylactic* regimens recommend these same dosages, though at a decreased frequency (twice daily instead of thrice daily).

Return to Case

The patient was advised to use a topical corticosteroid (prednisolone acetate 1%) and an oral antiviral (acyclovir). During the treatment period, his corneal edema began to resolve and vision improve. There was a constellation of central and stromal corneal opacities with associated keratitis (Fig. 16.7), which did not resolve immediately. After completing a course of treatment, his vision returned to 20/30 in the affected eye, and he was left with a faint central corneal stromal opacity. He was maintained on twice daily topical prednisolone acetate. Approximately 4 months later, he was noted to have a one-line decrease in his visual acuity (though he was otherwise asymptomatic) and slightly increased corneal stromal haze. The frequency of topical prednisolone acetate was increased to four times daily. He responded favorably, and his visual acuity returned to 20/25 OD. At this point, the clinicians and family carefully considered the role of chronic antiviral prophylaxis.

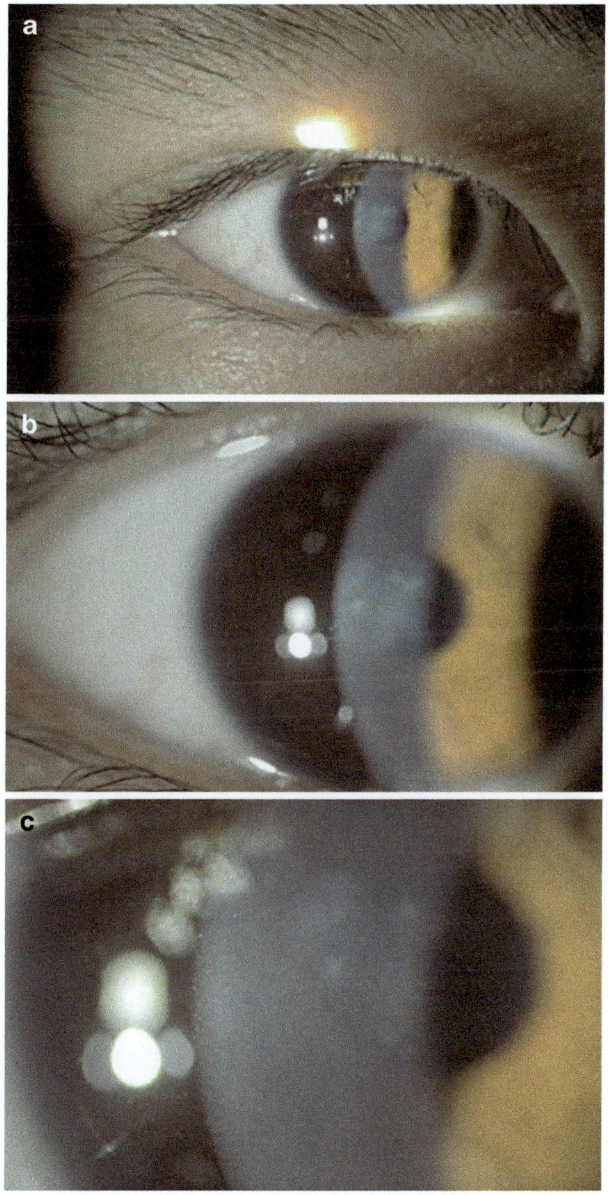

Fig. 16.7 (**a**) External photograph showing a "quiet" eye with anterior stromal keratitis. (**b**). Same slit lamp photograph with increased magnification demonstrating central constellation of stromal opacities during the keratitis flare. (**c**). Slit lamp photograph with increased magnification

Would You Place This Patient on Chronic Antiviral Prophylaxis? If so, What Medications Would You Use?

This child has had a recurrence of HSV keratitis and has a corneal opacity that is encroaching upon the visual axis. Given the high rate of recurrence in children, it would be prudent to place him on long-term antiviral prophylaxis. Patients should arguably be placed on antiviral prophylaxis for at least 1 year following their most recent episode. Afterward, a trial of a decreased prophylactic regimen or cessation of prophylaxis may be attempted. As suggested by the guidelines above, this patient was placed on oral acyclovir 400 mg twice daily for long-term prophylaxis. His pediatrician will monitor his renal and hepatic function with basic laboratory testing on an annual or semi-annual basis to ensure the medication is being well tolerated.

In addition to acyclovir, this patient also requires topical steroids to prevent recurrent stromal keratitis. A common pitfall in the setting of HSV keratitis is to taper off steroids too rapidly. It is generally recommended to taper no faster than one drop per day per month (e.g., three times a day for a month, twice a day for 1 month, once a day for a month, then every other day, etc.). In cases where there is recurrent inflammation after stopping the steroid, one tries to find the minimum dose that will prevent a flare.

References

1. Souza PM, Holland EJ, Huang AJ. Bilateral herpetic keratoconjunctivitis. Ophthalmology. 2003;110(3):493–6.
2. Bonini S, Coassin M, Aronni S, Lambiase A. Vernal keratoconjunctivitis. Eye. 2004;18:345–51.
3. Hammersmith KM. Blepharokeratoconjunctivitis in children. Curr Opin Ophthalmol. 2015;26(4):301–5.
4. Hammersmith KM, Cohen EJ, Blake TD, Laibson PR, Rapuano CJ. Blepharokeratoconjuncti vitis in children. Arch Ophthalmol. 2005;123(12):1667–70.
5. Ianaro A, Ialenti A, Maffia P, Sautebin L, Rombola L, Carnuccio R, et al. Anti-inflammatory activity of macrolides antibiotics. J Pharmacol Exp Ther. 2000;292(1):156–63.
6. Cetinkaya A, Akova YA. Pediatric ocular rosacea: long-term treatment with systemic antibiotics. Am J Ophthalmol. 2006;142(5):816–21.
7. Kwok AK, Lam DS, Fan DS, et al. Ocular hypertensive response to topical steroids in children. Ophthalmology. 1997;104(12):2112–6.
8. Huang C, O'Hara M, Mannis MJ. Primary pediatric keratoplasty: indications and outcomes. Cornea. 2009;28(9):1003–8.
9. Thomas PB, et al. Long term cyclosporine treatment improves tear production and reduces keratoconjunctivitis in rabbits with induced autoimmune dacryoadenitis. J Ocul Pharmacol Ther. 2009;25(3):285–92.
10. Doan S, Gabison E, Gatinel D, et al. Topical cyclosporine A in severe steroid-dependent childhood phlyctenular keratoconjunctivitis. Am J Ophthalmol. 2006;141:62–6.
11. Choi DS, Djalilian A. Oral azithromycin combined with topical anti-inflammatory agents for the treatment of blepharokeratoconjunctivitis in children. J AAPOS. 2013;17(1):112–3. Epub 2013 Jan 27

12. Doan S, Gabison E, Chiambaretta F, Touati M, Cochereau I. Efficacy of azithromycin 1.5% eye drops in childhood ocular rosacea with phlyctenular blepharokeratoconjunctivitis. J Ophthalmic Inflamm Infect. 2013;3(1):38.
13. Kymionis GD, Kankariya VP, Kontadakis GA. Tacrolimus ointment 0.03% for the treatment of refractory childhood phlyctenular keratoconjunctivitis. Cornea. 2012;31:950–2.
14. Gupta N, Dhawan A, Beri S, D'souza P. Clinical spectrum of pediatric blepharokeratoconjunctivitis. J AAPOS. 2010;14(6):527–9. Epub 2010 Nov 19
15. Liang L, Safran S, Gao Y, Sheha H, Raju VK, Tseng SC. Ocular demodicosis as a potential cause of pediatric blepharoconjunctivitis. Cornea. 2010;29(12):1386–91.
16. Doan S, Gabison EE, Nghiem-Buffet S, Abitbol O, Gatinel D, Hoang-Xuan T. Long-term visual outcome of childhood blepharokeratoconjunctivitis. Am J Ophthalmol. 2007;143(3):528–9. Epub 2006 Nov 9
17. Jones SM, Weinstein JM, Cumberland P, Klein N, Nischal KK. Visual outcome and corneal changes in children with chronic blepharoconjunctivitis. Ophthalmology. 2007;114(12):2271–80.
18. Kallish S, McDonald-McGinn DM, van Haelst MM, Bartlett SP, Katowitz JA, Zackai EH. Ablepharon–Macrostomia syndrome—extension of the phenotype. Am J Med Genet A. 2011;155:3060–2.
19. Stevens CA, Sargent LA. Ablepharon-Macrostomia syndrome. Am J Med Genet. 2002;107:30–7.
20. Jackson IT, Shaw KE, del Pinal Matorras F. A new feature of the ablepharon macrostomia syndrome: zygomatic arch absence. Br J Plast Surg. 1988;41:410–6.
21. McCarthy GT, West CM. Ablepheron (sic) macrostomia syndrome. Dev Med Child Neurol. 1977;19:659–72.
22. Price NJ, Pugh RE, Farndon PA, Willshaw HE. Ablepharon Macrostomia syndrome. Br J Ophthalmol. 1991;75:317–9.
23. Murthy R, Gupta H. Novel surgical technique for the management of partial cryptophthalmos. Indian J Ophthalmol. 2014;62(11):1096–8.
24. Cruz AA, Souza CA, Ferraz VE, Monteiro CA, Martins FA. Familial occurrence of ablepharon macrostomia syndrome: eyelid structure and surgical considerations. Arch Ophthalmol. 2000;118:428–30.
25. Ferraz VE, Melo DG, Hansing SE, Cruz AA, PinaNeto JM. Ablepharon-Macrostomia syndrome: first report of familial occurrence. Am J Med Genet. 2000;94:281–3.
26. Marchegiani S, Taylor D, Tessadori F, et al. Recurrent mutation sin the basic domain of TWIST2 cause Ablepharon Macrostomia and Barber-Say syndromes. Am J Hum Genet. 2015;97:99–110.
27. Mustard JC. Reconstruction of both lids. In: Mustarde JC, editor. Repair and reconstruction in the orbital region. A practical guide. 2nd ed. London: Churchill Livingstone; 1980. p. 152–4.
28. Hay D. Reconstruction of both eyelids following traumatic loss. Br J Plast Surg. 1971;24:361–4.
29. Kim M, Lee S-C, Lee S-J. Spontaneous corneal perforation in an eye with Peters' anomaly. Clin Ophthalmol. 2013;7:1535–7.
30. Liesegang TJ, Melton LJ, Daly PJ, Ilstrup DM. Epidemiology of ocular herpes simplex. Incidence in Rochester, Minn, 1950 through 1982. Arch Ophthalmol. 1989;107(8):1155–9.
31. Hill JM, Ball MJ, Neumann DM, Azcuy AM, Bhattacharjee PS, Bouhanik S, et al. The high prevalence of herpes simplex virus type 1 DNA in human trigeminal ganglia is not a function of age or gender. J Virol. 2008;82(16):8230–4.
32. Xu F, Sternberg MR, Kottiri BJ, McQuillan GM, Lee FK, Nahmias AJ, et al. Trends in herpes simplex virus type 1 and type 2 seroprevalence in the United States. JAMA. 2006;296(8):964–73.
33. Bradley H, Markowitz LE, Gibson T, McQuillan GM. Seroprevalence of herpes simplex virus types 1 and 2—United States, 1999–2010. J Infect Dis. 2014;209(3):325–33.
34. Darougar S, Wishart MS, Viswalingam ND. Epidemiological and clinical features of primary herpes simplex virus ocular infection. Br J Ophthalmol. 1985;69(1):2–6.

35. Wishart MS, Darougar S, Viswalingam ND. Recurrent herpes simplex virus ocular infection: epidemiological and clinical features. Br J Ophthalmol. 1987;71(9):669–72.
36. Beigi B, Algawi K, Foley-Nolan A, O'Keefe M. Herpes simplex keratitis in children. Br J Ophthalmol. 1994;78(6):458–60.
37. Hsiao C-H, Yeung L, Yeh L-K, Kao L-Y, Tan H-Y, Wang N-K, et al. Pediatric herpes simplex virus keratitis. Cornea. 2009;28(3):249–53.
38. Liu S, Pavan-Langston D, Colby KA. Pediatric herpes simplex of the anterior segment: characteristics, treatment, and outcomes. Ophthalmology. 2012;119(10):2003–8.
39. Herpetic Eye Disease Study Group (HEDS). Predictors of recurrent herpes simplex virus keratitis. Herpetic eye disease study group. Cornea. 2001;20(2):123–8.
40. Chong E-M, Wilhelmus KR, Matoba AY, Jones DB, Coats DK, Paysse EA. Herpes simplex virus keratitis in children. Am J Ophthalmol. 2004;138(3):474–5.
41. Poirier RH. Herpetic ocular infections of childhood. Arch Ophthalmol. 1980;98(4):704–6.
42. Prabriputaloong T, Margolis TP, Lietman TM, Wong IG, Mather R, Gritz DC. Atopic disease and herpes simplex eye disease: a population-based case-control study. Am J Ophthalmol. 2006;142(5):745–9.
43. Wilhelmus KR, Gee L, Hauck WW, Kurinij N, Dawson CR, Jones DB, et al. Herpetic eye disease study. A controlled trial of topical corticosteroids for herpes simplex stromal keratitis. Ophthalmology 1994;101(12):1883–1895; discussion 1895–6.
44. Barron BA, Gee L, Hauck WW, Kurinij N, Dawson CR, Jones DB, et al. Herpetic eye disease study. A controlled trial of oral acyclovir for herpes simplex stromal keratitis. Ophthalmology. 1994;101(12):1871–82.

Chapter 17
Oculoplastics Considerations in Ocular Surface Disease

Asim V. Farooq, Chau Pham, Pete Setabutr, and Vinay K. Aakalu

Case 1

The patient is a 5-year-old male who is referred for evaluation and possible surgical reduction of a hypertrophic buccal mucous membrane graft from the left inferior fornix. He has a history of a fireworks injury to the left eye 8 months prior. At an outside hospital, he subsequently underwent multiple examinations under anesthesia (EUAs) with removal of debris. Later he had eyelid reconstruction surgery initially with amniotic membrane alone and later with a buccal mucous membrane graft 5 months prior to presentation due to significant conjunctival scarring and symblepharon formation. His uncorrected visual acuities are 20/30 OD and 20/200 OS. Slit lamp examination is within normal limits OD, whereas there is a hypertrophic buccal mucous membrane graft in the left inferior fornix that covers the inferior half of the cornea (Fig. 17.1).

A.V. Farooq, MD
Department of Ophthalmology, University of Chicago, Chicago, IL, USA

C. Pham, MD
Department of Ophthalmology, Washington University, St. Louis, MO, USA

P. Setabutr, MD • V.K. Aakalu, MD, MPH (✉)
Department of Ophthalmology and Visual Sciences, University of Illinois at Chicago,
1855 W. Taylor St. M/C 648, Chicago, IL 60612, USA
e-mail: vaakalu@uic.edu

A.R. Djalilian (ed.), *Ocular Surface Disease*,
https://doi.org/10.1007/978-3-319-15823-5_17

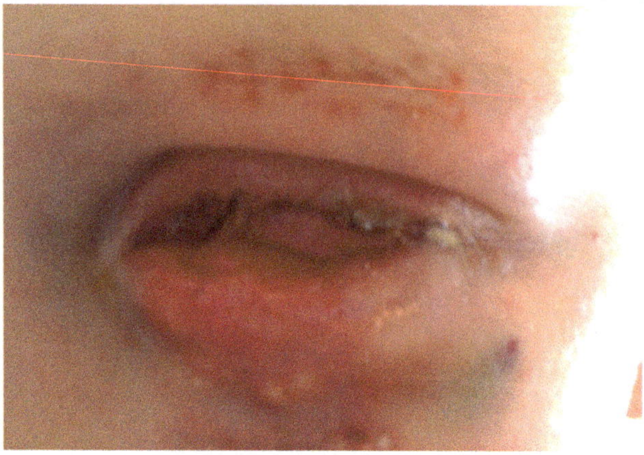

Fig. 17.1 External photograph of the left eye from Case 1. There is lower eyelid edema and ectropion as well as significant hyperemia of the eyelid margin. There is also a hypertrophic mucous membrane graft that is noted to be covering the inferior aspect of the cornea

What Were the Indications for Surgical Intervention at the Time of Referral?

In this case, there were several indications for surgical intervention. First, this child was of amblyogenic age; partial obstruction of the visual axis as well as the likely corneal astigmatism induced by the hypertrophic mucous membrane graft would have been sufficient indications for surgical reduction of the graft tissue. However, it was also noted on examination that despite the size of the graft, the inferior fornix itself was visible upon pulling the left lower eyelid inferiorly—indicating that the tissue was not in ideal position. The extension/growth of the graft onto the corneal surface coupled with altered tear film quality (buccal tissue does not contain goblet cells) created constant irritation of the corneal surface. Finally, the hypertrophic graft had resulted in poor cosmesis for this child. It is unknown at what rate mucosal graft hypertrophy occurs and there is little data in the eye literature; however, mucosal graft columnar metaplasia and hypertrophy have been reported in the urology literature and are thought to be associated with exposure of mucosal tissue to air [1].

The patient underwent excision of most of the buccal mucous membrane graft, leaving behind a small amount of tissue in the inferior fornix. He also underwent lysis of symblepharon, placement of a symblepharon ring, and a temporary suture tarsorrhaphy to keep the symblepharon ring in place. The following month, the suture tarsorrhaphy and symblepharon ring were removed, revealing a thin layer of neovascular pannus on the inferior cornea and a new area of symblepharon formation inferiorly, although the inferior fornix remained formed. Within 3 months, he developed progressive symblepharon as well as ankyloblepharon formation; he subsequently underwent a fornix reconstruction procedure with lysis of symblepharon/ankyloblepharon, application of mitomycin C (MMC), amniotic membrane transplantation (AMT), and placement of another symblepharon ring.

MMC has been found to decrease recurrence in pterygium surgery [2, 3], and Tseng et al. have reported success when using MMC in conjunction with AMT in fornix reconstruction for severe cicatrizing ocular surface disease [4].

What Is Your Preferred Method of Performing a Temporary Suture Tarsorrhaphy? What About a Permanent Tarsorrhaphy?

The placement of a temporary suture tarsorrhaphy is often required to achieve a stable ocular surface, after which it may be removed. This may be performed either in the clinic, procedure room, or operating room, depending on the situation. The eyelids should be prepped using dilute povidone-iodine solution. The eyelids are anesthetized temporally using a solution consisting of 1% lidocaine and 1:100,000 epinephrine and may be injected using a 27 or 30 gauge needle. Care should be taken to achieve adequate anesthesia, while avoiding significant distortion of the eyelid anatomy.

For a temporal, temporary tarsorrhaphy, a 5-0 double-armed nylon suture is used. A foam or silicone bolster is used for the upper and lower eyelid, and the sutures are passed through the bolster to prevent skin necrosis and irritation. After placement through a bolster, each needle is passed mattress style through the gray line of the upper eyelid (just temporal to the temporal aspect of the limbus). The suture then placed mattress style through the gray line of the lower eyelid and then tied in a 3-1-1 fashion cutting to allow a 2–3 mm tail of the suture to remain, taking care to bring the lid margins together with adequate tension but again without significant distortion of the eyelid anatomy. If for some reason a temporal tarsorrhaphy is only required for a limited period of time, an absorbable suture such a 4-0 chromic gut may be used with the same method described above, without the need for bolsters. An alternative approach that has been described is to use cyanoacrylate glue at the eyelid margin temporally. However, the duration of effect is relatively unpredictable, and exposure of the ocular surface to cyanoacrylate glue can lead to undesired irritation. Alternatively, silk suture can be used and is more tolerable to the ocular surface if the tarsorrhaphy loosens but is more irritating to the skin.

A permanent tarsorrhaphy is performed in the operating room or procedure room, with prepping and anesthetic delivery as described above. The anterior and posterior lamella of the eyelid along the length of desired tarsorrhaphy are separated using a #11 blade. The superficial 1 mm of the posterior aspect of the upper and lower eyelid margins are removed from the lateral aspect of the limbus toward the lateral canthus. A 6-0 vicryl suture is passed partial thickness, avoiding passage through the conjunctival tissue, in the posterior lamellar flap and used to affix the upper and lower eyelid. Interrupted passes are used until the posterior lamella is closed. Similarly, the anterior lamella is sutured together using an absorbable suture. Eyelashes can be removed prior to tarsorrhaphy if desired.

What Is the Role of a Symblepharon Ring in Fornix Reconstruction?

Symblepharon rings are translucent, non-sterile devices produced by multiple manufacturers and are usually made of polymethylmethacrylate (PMMA). They may be used alone or together with AMT although it has been reported that their use alone in the setting of acute Stevens-Johnson syndrome leads to more severe ocular sequelae [5]. They are used in the acute setting as well as at the time of fornix reconstruction to prevent symblepharon formation and maintain the fornices (i.e., prevent forniceal foreshortening). Other potential uses include severe chemical and thermal burns and during acute exacerbations of conditions that cause a cicatrizing conjunctivitis (e.g., rosacea keratoconjunctivitis, ocular cicatricial pemphigoid). At the time of fornix reconstruction, a symblepharon ring is often placed if there is a concern regarding reformation of symblepharon and forniceal foreshortening due to conjunctival inflammation. Even though the conjunctival surface may be quiet at the time of surgery, the lysis of symblepharon itself may lead to a significant inflammatory response. Postoperatively, we prefer to keep the ring in the eye for a minimum of 3 months (preferably longer if the patient can tolerate).

Over the course of the next year, our patient had the symblepharon ring removed, followed by a repeat fornix reconstruction procedure with symblepharon ring placement with MMC and AMT and with subsequent removal of the symblepharon ring after a few months. Unfortunately, he was found to once again develop symblepharon, as well as progressive ectropion of the left lower eyelid (Fig. 17.2). Although this patient has slowly improved with each subsequent intervention, his clinical course exemplifies the potentially difficult nature of ocular surface injuries.

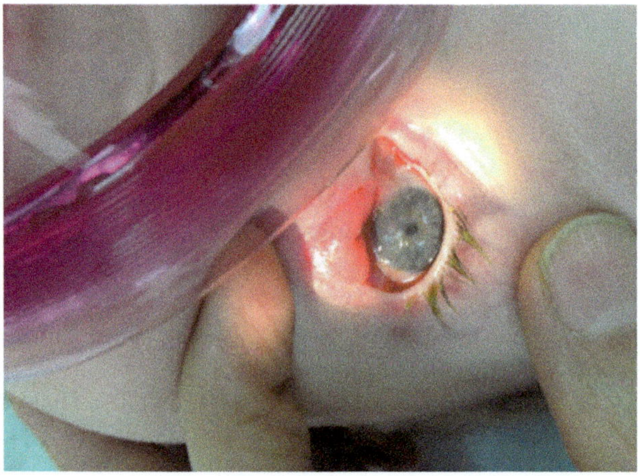

Fig. 17.2 External photograph of the left eye from Case 1 taken during an examination under anesthesia (EUA). During this examination he was noted to have lower eyelid ectropion, mucous membrane graft hypertrophy, and symblepharon

How Did You Manage Lower Eyelid Ectropion in the Presence of a Mucous Membrane Graft and Recurrent Need for a Symblepharon Ring?

We placed a 4-0 silk suture through the eyelid margin for traction and exposure. Dissection into the fornix was then performed to release the symblepharon. The buccal mucous membrane graft was debulked. A double-armed 4-0 Prolene suture was passed through the inferior section of the graft, through a number 42 retinal silicone band and then passed toward the infraorbital rim, affixing a piece of periosteum and coming out percutaneously to rotate the lid slightly toward the globe. This allowed for good draping of the palpebral portion of the buccal mucous membrane graft over the palpebral conjunctiva, reconstructing this portion of the fornix. The two arms of the suture were pulled percutaneously and tied over another section of the number 42 silicone band. After 5 months, he required another fornix reconstruction procedure using free conjunctival autograft from the superior bulbar area and this time also underwent repair of mild cicatricial entropion. The symblepharon ring was left in place for about 6 months. Following removal of the ring, the patient has done well with mild recurrence of the symblepharon. Patient does have inferior limbal stem cell deficiency which will need to be addressed in the future.

Discussion: There are several aspects of this patient's care which are worth discussing. First, starting with the initial treatment (symblepharon repair with amniotic membrane which was done prior to presentation), the timing of the surgery may have been too early. In general, it is best to wait for the inflammation from the chemical injury to subside (at least 1 year or longer if possible). In the most severe cases (e.g., Stevens-Johnson syndrome), it may be necessary to treat the patient with systemic immunosuppression for several months prior to starting surface/eyelid reconstruction. Second, when harvesting a mucous membrane graft, one may consider using a mucotome that allows for harvesting very thin tissue. Also, leaving a symblepharon ring in the eye as long as possible would also help reduce the likelihood of recurrence. We aim for a minimum of 3 months but in recurrent cases keep for up to 6 months. Finally, another adjunctive measure which was not used in this case is steroid or 5-FU injection into early recurrent lesions. Many surgeons have reported positive experiences particularly with 5-FU for stopping recurrent symblepharon. It is very well tolerated (unlike mitomycin C which has to be used with more caution).

Case 2

A 54-year-old female with advanced ocular cicatricial pemphigoid was referred for oculoplastics service evaluation in advance of a planned Boston keratoprosthesis (K-Pro) type II. She was noted to have a prior history of AMT and failed

PKP OS. On examination, her visual acuities were hand motion (HM) OD and light perception (LP) OS. There was lid margin keratinization, as well as extensive symblepharon formation, limiting extraocular movements OU. There was also a neovascular pannus over both corneas. Anterior chambers were formed and the iris was grossly within normal limits. The view to the lens was hazy in both eyes.

What Factors Require Consideration in Advance of Boston Type II K-Pro Surgery?

The first factor to consider in Boston type II K-Pro surgery is appropriate patient selection. The type II K-Pro device is generally used in patients with severe ocular surface disease in the setting of little to no tear production; these are patients in whom a type I K-Pro device would have a high risk of failure (e.g., sterile melt, infection). Patients who are selected for the type II K-Pro device have often undergone multiple prior surgeries, including penetrating keratoplasty and limbal stem cell transplantation. However, it is not necessary to have undergone prior ocular surgery, particularly if the risk of failure for any of these procedures is deemed to be sufficiently high.

It is also necessary to discuss the risks, benefits, and alternatives with the patient and often involved family members, in detail. These patients must be made aware of the cosmetic effects of the device, as the eyelids are brought together with only a small opening centrally for the protruding optic. As type II K-Pro implantation is a multiple subspecialty procedure, it is preferable for the patient to meet all of the surgeons pre-operatively. This will allow the patient to ask any questions they may have regarding the procedure, as well as allow each surgeon to assess their intended surgical approach.

What Surgical Steps Were Involved in the Oculoplastics Portion of This Patient's Boston Type II K-Pro Surgery?

The oculoplastics portion of Boston type II K-Pro surgery includes steps to rearrange the eyelid skin, tarsus, and conjunctiva to surround and support the optic of the K-Pro device. This case was performed under general anesthesia. After placement of the K-Pro device by the Cornea Service, the Oculoplastics Service was called in for reconstruction of the left upper and

lower eyelids around the optic. A small amount of local anesthetic was injected into the left upper eyelid and left lower eyelid. Examination revealed that there was absence of the left upper eyelid punctum. The left lower eyelid puncta and approximately 3 mm of the proximal canalicular system was still intact. A Colorado electrocautery needle was then advanced into the punctum and proximal canalicular system and used to cauterize and close the punctal opening.

A supersharp blade was then used to separate the lower eyelid to anterior and posterior lamellae. Hemostasis was obtained using bipolar cautery. Westcott scissors were used to excise the eyelashes along the eyelid margin. Westcott scissors were then used to recess the anterior lamella from the anterior surface of the tarsal plate. The left upper eyelid was then examined and was noted to have previously undergone anterior lamella recession with placement of an oral mucous membrane graft. A supersharp blade was then used to separate the margin into the anterior and posterior lamella. Westcott scissors were used to recess the anterior lamella and hemostasis was obtained using bipolar cautery.

A beaver blade was then used to thin the tarsal plate by approximately 50 % in the region surrounding the telescoping portion of the keratoprosthesis. A supersharp blade was used to make a relaxing incision along the temporal aspect of the left upper eyelid and the medial aspect of the left lower eyelid adjacent to the telescoping portion of the keratoprosthesis. These flaps were then used to wrap the telescoping portion of the keratoprosthesis and were sutured into position using several interrupted 6-0 vicryl sutures. A portion of the lower eyelid retractors and upper eyelid retractors were recessed. Intermarginal adhesions were then made along the length of the horizontal palpebral fissure between the posterior lamella using several interrupted 6-0 vicryl sutures.

The anterior lamella adjacent to the telescoping portion of the keratoprosthesis was then incised in a similar fashion to the underlying tarsus, and the flaps were secured into position under the flange of the keratoprosthesis using several interrupted 6-0 vicryl sutures. The anterior lamella was then sutured along the length of the horizontal palpebral fissure using several interrupted 6-0 vicryl sutures. At the conclusion of the case, a generous portion of ophthalmic ointment and a loose gauze dressing were placed over the left orbit. At postoperative day 37, significant retraction of the lower eyelid was noted, leading to partial exposure of the type II K-Pro device (Fig. 17.3). It has been reported that a significant number patients with keratoprostheses require subsequent eyelid/oculoplastic surgery, and both K-Pro type II eyes in one study required revision of blepharotomy [6].

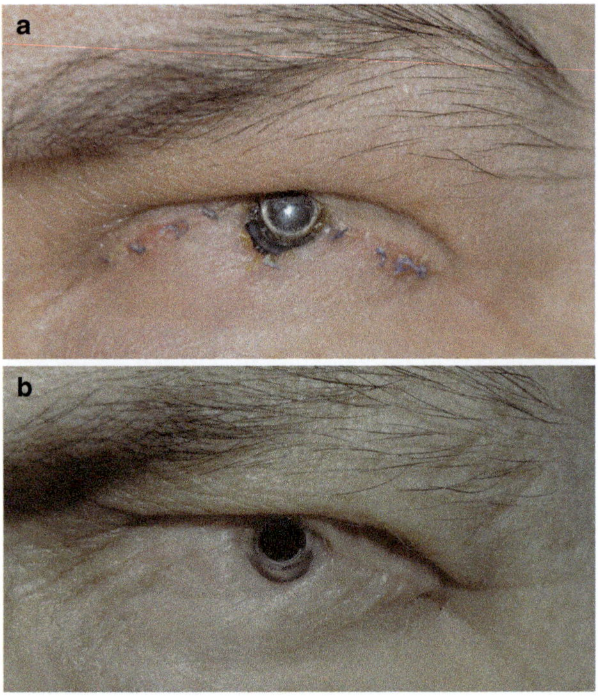

Fig. 17.3 (**a**) External photograph from Case 2 demonstrating lower eyelid retraction and K-Pro device exposure. (**b**) External photograph from Case 2 after revision with the use of a porous polyethylene spacer

How Was the Lower Eyelid Retraction and Type II K-Pro Device Exposure Managed?

A decision was made to take the patient back to the operating room to repair the eyelid retraction and K-Pro device exposure. The lower eyelid was incised adjacent to the optic and the posterior aspect of the eyelid was recessed. A 6 mm trephination blade was used to create a disc out of 0.25 mm thickness porous polyethylene material (Medpor, Stryker Craniomaxillofacial, Portage, Michigan). A 3 mm biopsy punch was used to create a slightly decentered hole within the disc, in order to fit around the optic. The disc was then fit into place, and a 6-0 prolene suture was used to tie the eyelid in a purse-string fashion circumferentially around the optic. This was the first use to our knowledge of a porous polyethylene spacer to treat eyelid retraction after type II K-Pro implantation [7].

Case 3

A 63-year-old female was referred to the Oculoplastics Service for evaluation and management of trichiasis and distichiasis. She had a history of chronic granulomatous iridocyclitis, attributed to tuberculosis (TB). Since her diagnosis

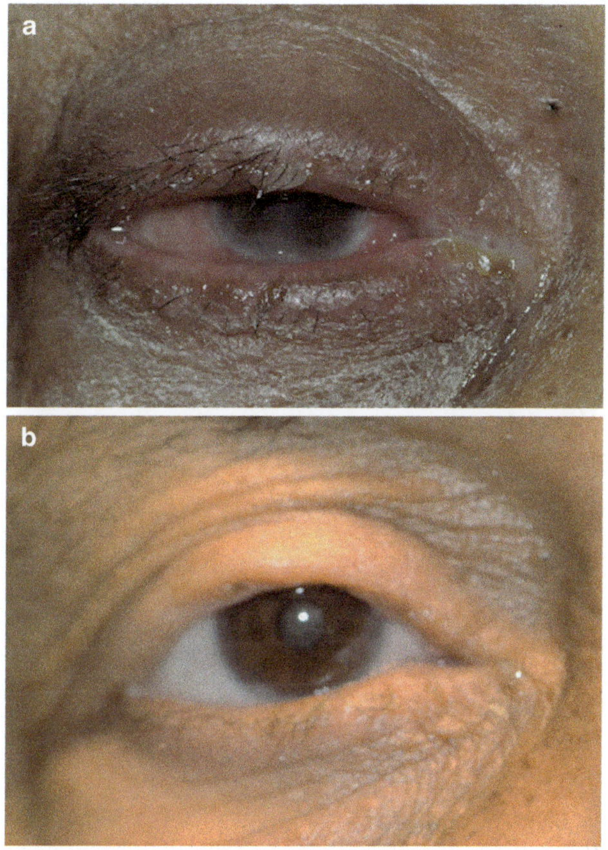

Fig. 17.4 (**a**) External photograph of the right eye from Case 3. Eyelid edema, mild ectropion, trichiasis, conjunctival injection, and mucous discharge are noted. (**b**) External photograph of the right eye from Case 3 approximately 2 years later. This patient underwent two mucous membrane graft procedures, repair of ectropion trichiasis and blepharoplasty, after which she achieved an acceptable cosmetic result and improvement in eyelid and ocular surface inflammation

of uveitis, she had been treated with courses of topical steroids, as well as oral prednisone and methotrexate. Her diagnosis of ocular TB involvement had been confirmed with a conjunctival biopsy demonstrating noncaseating granulomas. On examination, her uncorrected visual acuities were 20/30 OD and 20/100 OS pinholing to 20/50. She also had thickened eyelid margins, cicatricial ectropion, as well as trichiasis and distichiasis of both upper eyelids (Fig. 17.4a). Slit lamp examination revealed significant keratinization of the lid margins and tarsal conjunctiva. There was also noted to be 2+ conjunctival injection OU, superior corneal pannus, and diffuse punctate epithelial erosions OS > OD.

What Are Common Causes of Trichiasis and Distichiasis?

Trichiasis is an eyelid margin disorder in which the eyelashes are misdirected toward the ocular surface—usually due to chronic inflammation and scarring of the follicles. In the developing world, trachoma has remained an important cause of trichiasis. This is in contrast to the developed world, where trachoma is no longer endemic and trichiasis is more often caused by conditions associated with severe blepharitis and/or cicatrizing conjunctivitis: ocular cicatricial pemphigoid, Stevens-Johnson syndrome, ocular rosacea, atopic blepharoconjunctivitis, and chemical/thermal burns. Trichiasis may also be idiopathic. Distichiasis is characterized by an accessory row of cilia arising from behind the meibomian gland orifices and can be congenital or acquired, with many acquired cases being idiopathic. However, acquired distichiasis may also be seen in association with blepharitis and/or cicatrizing conjunctivitis. Our patient had trichiasis and distichiasis in association with ocular tuberculosis, which is a rare etiology of both of these conditions with only a few cases reported [8, 9].

What Are Treatment Options for Trichiasis and Distichiasis?

There are many treatment options for trichiasis and distichiasis and treatment goals are threefold: (1) eliminate the aberrant cilia, (2) improve the ocular surface, and (3) improve patient comfort. Temporizing measures such as the use of eye lubricants, bandage contact lens, and epilation are often used, and can be effective, in the acute setting; however, recurrence is common within 2–6 weeks. Surgical treatments tend to be more definitive and include bipolar electrolysis (best for segmental and minor trichiasis), radiofrequency ablation (less lid scarring than electrolysis), cryotherapy (effective for segmental and diffuse trichiasis), laser ablation (minor trichiasis), excision of trichiatic eyelash bulbs, full-thickness block resection, excision or repositioning of the anterior lamella, or bilamellar/posterior lamellar tarsal rotation [10]. Some authors advocate combined techniques such as addition of 0.2% MMC into the hair follicle in addition to radiofrequency ablation [11]. A 2015 Cochrane Review on the treatment of trichiasis in the setting of trachoma found that the most effective surgery required full-thickness incision of the tarsal plate and rotation of the eyelid. This same review also found that the addition of azithromycin at the time of surgery may be beneficial where postoperative trichiasis rates are low [12].

In this case, trichiasis and distichiasis were observed in the setting of cicatricial ectropion. He underwent surgical correction of the left upper and lower eyelids with eyelid margin incision, excision of aberrant lash follicles (anterior and posterior), and mucous membrane graft placement, followed by a similar procedure on the right upper eyelid. During each procedure, a crescent blade was used to separate the anterior from the posterior lamella. Westcott scissors were then used to excise the aberrant lash follicles anteriorly as well as the posterior lamella. Attention was then turned to the mouth where a graft outline was drawn with a sterile surgical marking pen on the lower lip. Exposure was achieved using two towel clips. Submucosal lidocaine with epinephrine was injected into this area and allowed to sit for approximately 5–10 min.

The oral mucosa was then incised using a #15 blade, and the graft was excised taking care to avoid resection of submucosal tissue (a typical graft size is 1 cm × 2 cm, but larger grafts can be harvested and split for multiple eyelids).

The graft was thinned as much as possible (using a mucotome can facilitate harvesting a thin graft). The graft was then placed in bacitracin irrigation solution for approximately 10 min. The bed of the donor graft was then cauterized for hemostasis using bipolar cautery, and a cold gauze soaked in local anesthetic was then placed in the mouth over the donor site. The graft was then removed from its irrigation bath and thinned by removing a minimal amount of submucosal tissue. It was then placed on the tarsal surface of the eyelid and sutured in place using several interrupted buried 7-0 chromic (or 8-0 vicryl) sutures. Once this was completed, a generous amount of ointment was placed on the ocular surface and the mouth was checked once again for hemostasis. The following year, she developed cicatricial entropion and underwent repeat bilateral mucous membrane grafts to the upper eyelids. She then underwent upper eyelid blepharoplasties 2 years later for mechanical ptosis and has achieved an acceptable anatomic result (Fig. 17.4b).

What Are Common Causes of Eyelid Margin and Tarsal Conjunctival Keratinization? What Treatment Options Are Available for This Condition?

Keratinization is the differentiation of keratinocytes from their post-germinative state to terminally differentiated, hardened cells filled with protein, creating a structurally and functionally distinct keratin-containing surface layer. Keratinization of the ocular surface can be a nonspecific metaplastic change from mucosal epithelium to stratified squamous epithelium in response to chronic irritation or inflammation or may be part of a neoplastic process. Causes of keratinization are many and include prolonged exposure; severe aqueous tear deficiency; xerosis of vitamin A deficiency; scar formation in the setting of trachoma; immune-mediated inflammatory conditions such as Stevens-Johnson syndrome, mucous membrane pemphigoid, and chronic atopic disease; and toxic exposures – either accidental or iatrogenic (e.g., blepharoconjunctivitis associated with apraclonidine usage) or as sequelae to irradiation of the ocular area. Keratinization of the ocular surface is also associated with neoplastic processes such as ocular surface squamous neoplasia or sebaceous cell carcinoma, and its presence may aid in diagnosis.

Treatment is aimed at symptomatic relief and correcting the underlying etiology. Ocular comfort can be increased by the use of eye lubricants, and topical steroids may provide relief from metaplasia-inducing inflammation. Reversal of keratinization caused by chronic exposure secondary to involutional ectropion can be achieved by surgically correcting the ectropion. If the cause is neoplastic (as in the case of ocular surface squamous neoplasia), the treatment of the neoplasm will often result in resolution of the keratinization.

In cases of persistent keratinization, superficial removal only provides temporary relief with recurrence of keratinization, while full-thickness debridement with use of mucosal grafts achieves more permanent remission [13]. Mucosal grafts can be obtained from the conjunctiva of the fellow eye, oral mucosa, or nasal mucosa and may be used in conjunction with amniotic membrane transplantation. In our case, mucous membrane grafts from the oral mucosa ultimately achieved an acceptable anatomic result and also led to resolution of lid margin keratinization.

Laznitzki showed that the addition of vitamin A could prevent keratinization of human fetal skin cultured in vivo, and since that time retinoic acid has been used therapeutically in a wide range of conditions [14]. Retinoic acid has been used in the management of intraepithelial neoplasia, Stevens-Johnson, chronic atopic keratoconjunctivitis, sarcoid-related keratoconjunctivitis sicca, and mucous membrane pemphigoid, and some authors have described the amount of keratinization to be predictive of response to treatment of retinoic acid [15, 16]. Application of topical all-trans-retinoic acid (0.01%) once daily (or every other day) at night may be used in select cases.

References

1. Ransley PG, Duffy PG, Oesch IL, Van Oyen P, Hoover D. The use of bladder mucosa and combined bladder mucosa/preputial skin grafts for urethral reconstruction. J Urol. 1987;138(4 Pt 2):1096–8.
2. Lam DS, Wong AK, Fan DS, et al. Intraoperative mitomycin C to prevent recurrence of pterygium after excision: a 30-month follow-up study. Ophthalmology. 1998;105:901–4.
3. Mastropasqua L, Carpineto P, Ciancaglini M, Giallenga P. Long term results of intraoperative mitomycin C in the treatment of recurrent pterygium. Br J Ophthalmol. 1996;80:288–91.
4. Tseng SC, Di Pascuale M, Liu DT, Gao YY, Baradaran-Rafii A. Intraoperative mitomycin C and amniotic membrane transplantation for fornix reconstruction in severe cicatricial ocular surface diseases. Ophthalmology. 2005;112(5):896–903.
5. Hsu M, Jayaram A, Verner R, Lin A, Bouchard C. Indications and outcomes of amniotic membrane transplantation in the management of acute stevens-johnson syndrome and toxic epidermal necrolysis: a case-control study. Cornea. 2012;31(12):1394–402.
6. Baker MS, Krakauer M, Gupta S, de la Cruz J, Cortina MS, Kitzmann AS, Goins KM, Allen RC, Setabutr P. Eyelid procedures in patients who have undergone Boston keratoprostesis surgery. Ophthal Plast Reconstr Surg. 2012;28(4):286–8.
7. Sivaraman KR, Aakalu VK, Sajja K, Cortina MS, de la Cruz J, Setabutr P. Use of a porous polyethylene lid spacer for management of eyelid retraction in patients with Boston type II keratoprosthesis. Orbit. 2013;32(4):247–9.
8. Seo Y, Choi M, Park CK, Yoon JS. A case of paradoxical reaction after treatment of eyelid tuberculosis. Korean J Ophthalmol. 2014;28(6):493–5.
9. Salam T, Uddin JM, Collin JRO, Verity DH, Beaconsfield M, Rose GE. Periocular tuberculous disease: experience from a UK eye hospital. Br J Ophthalmol. 2015;99:582–5.
10. Ferreira IS, Bernardes TF, Bonfioli AA. Trichiasis. Semin Ophthalmol. 2010;25(3):66–71.
11. Kim GN, Yoo WS, Kim SJ, Han YS, Chung IY, Park JM, Yoo JM, Seo SW. The effect of 0.02% mitomycin C injection into the hair follicle with radiofrequency ablation in trichiasis patients. Korean J Ophthalmol. 2014;28(1):12–8.
12. Burton M, Habtamu E, Ho D, Gower EW. Interventions for trachoma trichiasis. Cochrane Database Syst Rev. 2015;11:CD004008.
13. Maumenee AE. Keratinization of the conjunctiva. Trans Am Ophthalmol Soc. 1979;77:133–43.

14. Lasnitzki I. Effect of carcinogens, hormones, and vitamins on organ cultures. Int Rev Cytol. 1958;70:79–121.
15. Wright P. Topical retinoic acid therapy for disorders of the outer eye. Trans Ophthalmol Soc U K. 1985;104(8):869–74.
16. Herbort CP, Weissman SS, Ostler B, Cevallos A, Char DH. Ocular surface keratinization as a predictor of response to topical retinoic acid therapy. Arch Ophthalmol. 1989;107(9):1275–6.

Chapter 18
Effective Use of Amniotic Membrane in Ocular Surface Disease

Asim V. Farooq and Andrew J.W. Huang

Case 1

Patient SN is a 76-year-old male who presents for follow-up of radiation keratopathy OS. He has a history of basal cell carcinoma of the left upper eyelid, status post-surgical excision with eyelid and forehead reconstruction about 1 year prior. He has also undergone several sessions of external beam radiation treatment, which were concluded about 6 months prior. Since radiation treatment, he was found to develop left-sided madarosis, lid margin keratinization, exposure keratopathy, and neurotrophic keratopathy. These eventually led to a persistent epithelial defect, with stromal thinning and a focal corneal perforation that has required corneal gluing × 2. His uncorrected visual acuity OS on the day of follow-up is counting fingers (CF) at one foot. Slit lamp examination is relatively stable, demonstrating glue in place paracentrally within an area of stromal thinning. There is also an epithelial defect measuring 3.5 mm high × 7.0 mm wide.

What Is the Risk of Keratopathy in Patients Undergoing Radiation Treatment to the Eye/Orbit?

Although patients have been treated with radiation to the eye and orbit for many years, there is a dearth of information in the published literature regarding the risk factors for and management of radiation keratopathy; by comparison, there is a

---

A.V. Farooq, MD • A.J.W Huang, MD, MPH (✉)
Department of Ophthalmology and Visual Sciences, Washington University in St. Louis, 4921 Parkview Place Suite 12B, St. Louis, MO 63110, USA
e-mail: HuangA@vision.wustl.edu

A.R. Djalilian (ed.), *Ocular Surface Disease*,
https://doi.org/10.1007/978-3-319-15823-5_18

much greater body of literature on radiation retinopathy and optic neuropathy, perhaps in part due to the advent of plaque brachytherapy in the treatment of uveal melanomas. Nonetheless, among patients receiving any form of radiation treatment around the eye, there appears to be a dose-dependent effect on the ocular surface and cornea [1].

Eyelid skin inflammation and necrosis, madarosis, ocular surface keratinization, and limbal stem cell dysfunction or deficiency are among the changes that may be seen in association with radiation keratopathy [1–3]. Corneal changes may range from a mild, reversible punctate epithelial keratopathy to corneal melting and perforation. A study of 88 eyes that received external beam radiation to the orbit showed that severe radiation keratopathy developed in 32 patients, with a mean time to development of 15 months [1]. The reported rate was 0% in those receiving less than 59 Gy and 100% in those receiving more than 70 Gy. Among patients receiving between 59 and 70 Gy, there was a higher risk of keratopathy in those treated without the use of a lacrimal shield. It should be noted that these patients were all being treated for nasopharyngeal carcinoma, some of which may have had trigeminal nerve involvement.

What Is Your Method for Gluing in Patients Presenting with a Corneal Perforation?

First, we should mention that there are some important considerations in deciding whether to perform corneal gluing. For example, if a patient presents with a perforation in the setting of infectious keratitis, one must carefully consider the clinical course; if the infection is fulminant, then gluing may be a short-lived, temporizing measure in advance of an urgent patch graft or therapeutic penetrating keratoplasty [4]. Corneal gluing may also make it more difficult to assess for the development or progression of infectious keratitis [5]. Cultures should be carefully performed if an infectious cause is suspected, with the use of frequent topical antibiotics after the gluing procedure. In the setting of a neurotrophic ulcer and corneal melt (e.g., in the setting of radiation keratopathy), there may often be a lifelong risk of keratolysis [6]. These patients may therefore require multiple corneal gluing procedures. In many cases, there are advantages of corneal gluing over surgical intervention in the acute setting: corneal scarring will occur over time, and the glue (followed by an underlying scar) often allows for deepening of the anterior chamber and normalization of the intraocular pressure. Surgery can then be performed at a later time with a lower risk of intraoperative and postoperative complications, particularly if the ocular surface can be rehabilitated to some extent [4]. A caveat is that the size of the perforation should be small enough to allow for closure with a gluing technique.

Our preferred method of corneal gluing employs the use of a sterile disc and cyanoacrylate glue. The discs are prepared out of sterile drape material with disposable punch biopsy instruments in 2, 3, and 4 mm sizes and are kept in our clinic as part of a gluing kit. We place a small amount of antibiotic ointment onto a sterile platform, such as the wooden end of a cotton-tipped applicator. Using Jewelers forceps, the appropriate size disc is then placed onto the platform, which is now semi-adhesive due to the ointment. A single drop of cyanoacrylate glue is then placed onto the disc. Topical anesthetic and antibiotic (e.g., ofloxacin) drops are placed onto the ocular surface, and the ocular surface is gently dried with either a Weck-cel sponge or a cotton-tipped applicator. At the slit lamp, the disc is then delivered to the area of perforation using the platform. This method is highly reproducible and allows for successful closure of larger perforations, depending on the size of the disc. A bandage contact lens is often placed and the patient is started on a topical antibiotic. Depending on the mechanism and suspected duration of perforation, an oral antibiotic (e.g., moxifloxacin) may be added.

What Are Important Considerations in the Assessment of a Persistent Epithelial Defect?

A persistent epithelial defect is most often seen in the setting of neurotrophic keratopathy, which can occur secondary to herpes simplex virus, herpes zoster virus, uncontrolled diabetes, or radiation treatment, among other causes [6]. Collagen vascular diseases, tumors, toxic keratoconjunctivitis, ocular graft versus host disease, and ocular cicatricial pemphigoid are important considerations in the differential diagnosis; a complete medical history is very important in these cases. Clinical examination should be comprehensive, including an assessment of motility, confrontation visual fields, lids and lashes (assessing for entropion, ectropion, trichiasis, and lagophthalmos), and a detailed evaluation of the ocular surface (assessing for conjunctival scarring, size/location of epithelial defect, extent of underlying stromal thinning, and corneal sensation). Intraocular examination should focus on signs of current or prior inflammation.

What Is Your Approach for Treating Neurotrophic Keratopathy, Specifically in the Presence of a Persistent Epithelial Defect or Ulcer?

Frequent lubrication with non-preserved artificial tears and ointment, topical cyclosporine, and punctal occlusion may be used initially. In the presence of lid margin keratinization, vitamin A ointment should be applied, usually twice per week, to prevent repetitive trauma to the ocular surface. In many cases, additional therapies may need to be considered, such as serum tears, a rigid scleral contact lens, patching, tarsorrhaphy, or amniotic membrane transplantation (AMT), to help resolve a persistent epithelial defect [7–10]. Among these, we most often employ patching/tarsorrhaphy or AMT, depending on individual patient considerations. Some have advocated for the use of multiple layers of amniotic membrane for deep neurotrophic ulcers, with some studies demonstrating integration into and thickening of the underlying corneal stroma over time [11–14]. If using serum tears, the patient should be informed of the likely need for multiple blood draws. Similarly, a motivated patient is required for the daily insertion and removal of a scleral contact lens.

In this patient we decided that a dry amniotic membrane graft (BioDOptix, Cordova, Tennessee) would aid in healing of the persistent epithelial defect, as well as provide additional support in the area of severe stromal thinning. A bandage contact lens (Extreme H20, Sarasota, Florida) was placed over the amniotic membrane graft. He was continued on a regimen of prednisolone acetate 1% BID OS, ofloxacin 0.3% QID OS, and vitamin A 0.01% ointment 2×/week. At his subsequent follow-up visits, the glue was no longer visualized—however, the area of perforation had been sealed, and the epithelial defect resolved within 3 weeks. The following month, the epithelium remained intact, although there was significant thinning noted over the area of previous perforation. Corneal gluing was performed prophylactically using the method described above, and a tarsorrhaphy was placed (Figs. 18.1 and 18.2). He continues to be followed closely.

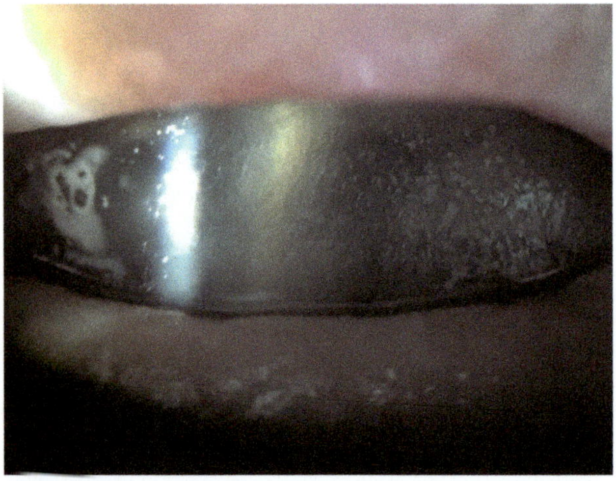

Fig. 18.1 Slit lamp photograph of the left eye from Case 1. There is near-complete madarosis, and on the ocular surface there is glue with an overlying clear disc, a faint outline of which can be seen temporally. The anterior chamber is deep centrally, as indicated by the posterior slit beam. There is ointment on the ocular surface. Not visualized in this image is a temporal suture tarsorrhaphy (see Fig. 18.2).

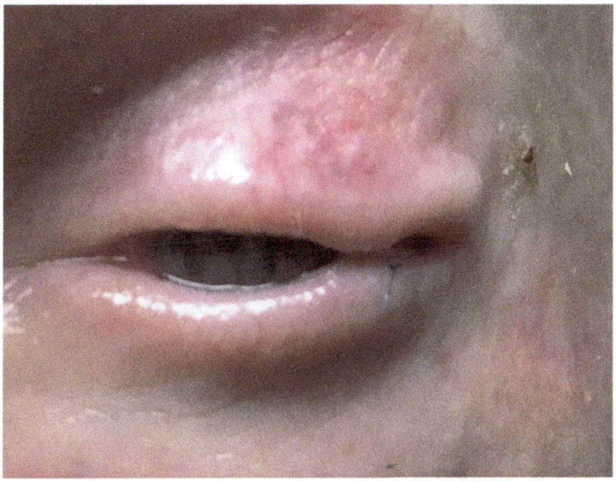

Fig. 18.2 External photograph of the left eye from Case 1. This once again demonstrates near-complete madarosis and in this image a suture tarsorrhaphy is noted temporally. After placement of amniotic membrane, followed by corneal gluing and a suture tarsorrhaphy, the ocular surface stabilized

Why Was a Dry Amniotic Membrane Graft Used in This Patient?

Amniotic membrane is harvested at the time of elective Cesarean delivery from consenting donors. The tissue can be freeze-dried by a commercial processor, after which it may be stored at room temperature in your clinic and applied directly to the ocular surface followed by the placement of a bandage contact lens. This is known as a dry (or dehydrated) amniotic membrane graft. An alternative method of processing involves immersion in glycerol and cryopreservation (the actual procedure is proprietary). This is known as a wet amniotic membrane graft and can come in several forms including as a flat sheet on a cardboard bed (e.g., AmnioGraft, manufactured by Biotissue, Doral, Florida) or attached to a ring (Prokera, Biotissue). In this patient we used a dry amniotic membrane graft largely due to ease of use (we have a supply stored at room temperature in our clinic) and ease of application (it can be handled and placed on the ocular surface relatively easily). The AmnioGraft should ideally be secured with either glue or sutures, and our patient was not an ideal candidate for ProKera due to significant eyelid scarring that may have prevented the device from staying in place.

Case 2

A 69-year-old female presented for annual follow-up of bilateral pterygia and Salzmann nodular degeneration. She noted that over the prior year her quality of vision had deteriorated, and she had been noticing occasional glare in bright lights. Her best-corrected visual acuity was 20/40 OD and 20/30 OS, with a decrease to 20/70 OD and 20/60 OS with brightness acuity testing. Slit lamp examination revealed a nasal and temporal pterygium with surrounding

Salzmann changes OD, and a temporal pterygium and nasal Salzmann changes OS. She also had 2+ nuclear sclerosis OU. After an extensive discussion, the patient decided to proceed with pterygium excision and superficial keratectomy OD with both nasal and temporal amniotic membrane transplantation and with plans for cataract surgery in the future.

How Is Your Management of Pterygium or Salzmann Nodular Degeneration Affected by Lens Status?

In these cases, the lens status is an important consideration. If cataract surgery is in the near future, then ocular surface irregularities that may affect the corneal curvature (and, therefore, intraocular lens calculations) should be addressed first. In the case of pterygium, some studies have attempted to determine the predictability of its impact on K measurements and use this information for combined pterygium and cataract removal [15]. At this time, there appears to be less than optimal predictability based on available regression formulas, particularly for larger lesions. We take into consideration clinical examination findings, refraction, and corneal topography in determining whether a pterygium is visually significant and warrants excision prior to cataract surgery. The same principles apply for Salzmann nodular degeneration. Typically, we will obtain measurements for cataract surgery no sooner than 4–6 weeks after surgery for pterygium or Salzmann nodular degeneration.

If the patient does not have a visually significant cataract, then there may be more time to observe or pursue medical treatments, unless the patient is symptomatic or has disease that threatens involvement of the visual axis. For Salzmann nodular degeneration, any associated underlying conditions (e.g., blepharitis, ocular surface disease, interstitial keratitis) are treated aggressively, often with some form of local immunosuppression such as a topical steroid or cyclosporine. In patients with visual impairment and a lack of improvement with conservative treatments, surgical intervention is then recommended.

What Is Your Method of Choice for Surgical Excision of Pterygium? What About Salzmann Nodular Degeneration?

For pterygium excision, a conjunctival autograft is often a reasonable consideration, provided that the ocular surface is otherwise healthy and there are no signs of limbal stem cell deficiency. However, in the presence of ocular surface disease, conjunctival scarring or a double-headed pterygium, we prefer amniotic membrane transplantation over the area of excised conjunctiva. The graft may be secured in placed with fibrin glue, sutures, or both. We typically reserve the use of mitomycin C for recurrences or cases that are at high risk for recurrence (e.g., younger age). A recent study found that mitomycin C in conjunction with either AMT or conjunctival autograft resulted in a similar rate of success [16]. In the case of Salzmann nodular degeneration, the role of amniotic membrane is dependent on the extent of involvement; if a large superficial keratectomy is required, then an amniotic membrane graft over the area of excision can reduce the risk of recurrence while improving the rate of epithelial healing [17]. The patient should be made aware that the amniotic membrane graft will cause visual blurring if placed over the visual axis.

This patient had a visually significant cataract OD greater than OS, and therefore we recommended surgical intervention for the right eye. Intraoperatively, the nasal and temporal pterygia were excised and a superficial keratectomy was performed using a 57 blade and non-toothed forceps. A larger conjunctival excision was performed nasally than temporally, and eraser tip cautery was used to achieve hemostasis. The nasal and temporal amniotic membrane grafts were sequentially secured in place with fibrin glue as well as 9-0 vicryl sutures on the limbal side and 8-0 vicryl sutures on the conjunctival side. Postoperatively, the patient was treated with prednisolone acetate 1% and ofloxacin 0.3% drops, both QID. She initially noted foreign body sensation and photophobia with a drop in visual acuity to 20/500 on postoperative day one; however, these symptoms improved significantly over the first week with vision returning to baseline. The ocular surface was noted to heal well, and there was a small amount of residual anterior stromal scarring nasally (Fig. 18.3).

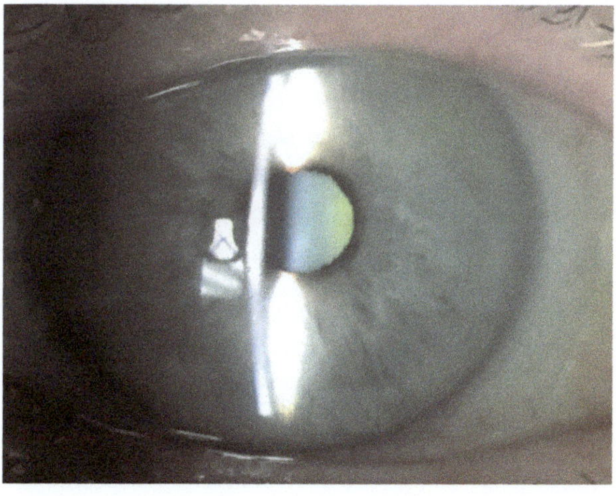

Fig. 18.3 Slit lamp photograph of the right eye from Case 2, 1 month after nasal and temporal pterygium excision, superficial keratectomy for Salzmann nodular degeneration, and AMT. There was a faint residual anterior stromal scar noted nasally. There is a bandage contact lens in place

Why Did You Choose a Wet Amniotic Membrane Graft in This Patient?

In this particular case, there was both a nasal and temporal conjunctival excision as well as a superficial keratectomy performed. Given the location and extent of involvement, neither a dry amniotic membrane disc nor a ProKera would have provided adequate coverage. Therefore, we used two sheets of amniotic membrane (AmnioGraft) over the involved areas, which we secured in place with both glue and sutures. Although it requires more delicate handling than the other two products, the AmnioGraft can be cut to the appropriate size and shape based on anatomical considerations.

Case 3

The patient is a 60-year-old male who presents for follow-up of rosacea blepharitis. The patient notes that since his last visit 20 months ago the vision in his left eye has been decreasing. He also notes significant redness, irritation, and photophobia in both eyes. His uncorrected visual acuities on the day of follow-up are 20/200 OD and hand motion (HM) OS. Slit lamp examination demonstrates significant eyelid margin hyperemia and vascular telangiectasias, meibomian gland dysfunction, and 2+ conjunctival injection in both eyes. There is corneal pannus superiorly and inferiorly in both eyes. The right cornea has an area of mild stromal thinning temporally, while the left cornea has an area of severe thinning to less than 10% of normal stromal thickness with underlying endothelial pigment, suggesting a possible micro-perforation in the past. He also has 2+ nuclear sclerosis OD and 3+ nuclear sclerosis OS.

How Did You Arrive at the Diagnosis of Ocular Rosacea?

In this case, the diagnosis of ocular rosacea was straightforward. The patient had numerous facial telangiectasias, skin papules, rhinophyma, and the ocular findings described above (Fig. 18.4). The findings in ocular rosacea can range from only mild meibomian gland dysfunction and vascular telangiectasias at the eyelid margin to severe ocular surface disease with chronic conjunctival injection, symblepharon formation, corneal neovascularization, and corneal melt. The diagnosis may be challenging when facial skin changes are subtle or when ocular rosacea precedes extraocular changes; the symptoms of ocular rosacea (e.g., redness, irritation, foreign body sensation) are also relatively nonspecific [18]. Some patients with ocular rosacea have chronic blepharitis and ocular surface disease, whereas others have

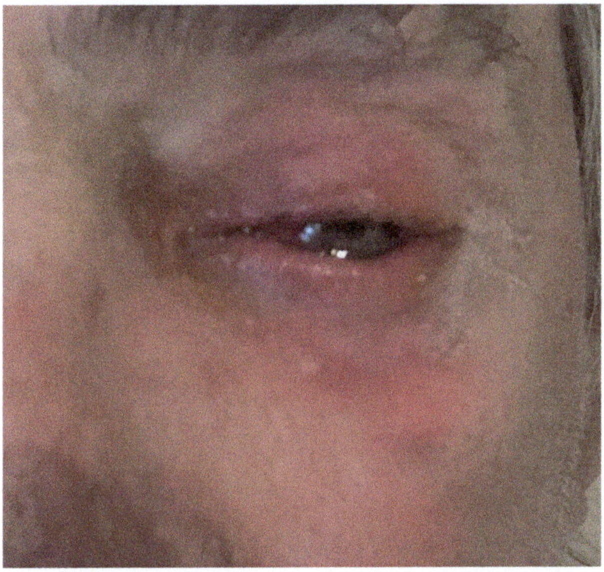

Fig. 18.4 External photograph from Case 3 demonstrating significant periocular and eyelid hyperemia and crusting. There were also rhinophyma and facial telangiectasias noted on gross external examination, consistent with the diagnosis of rosacea. Slit lamp examination revealed significant meibomian gland dysfunction, eyelid margin telangiectasias, conjunctival injection, and corneal thinning

more of a relapsing remitting course. The differential diagnosis in severe cases includes graft versus host disease, atopic keratoconjunctivitis, ocular cicatricial pemphigoid, Stevens-Johnson syndrome, and chemical burn. In the absence of characteristic clinical features of rosacea, a thorough history and potentially a conjunctival biopsy may be indicated.

What Is the Proposed Pathophysiology of Ocular Rosacea, and How Does This Shape Your Management of This Condition?

The pathophysiology of ocular rosacea remains unclear at the present time, although it is thought to represent an inflammatory condition affecting the facial skin, eyelids, and ocular surface. Increased levels of inflammatory mediators including matrix metalloproteinase-9 (MMP-9) have been detected from the tear film of patients with rosacea, and treatment with topical steroids and medications that inhibit MMP-9 (such as doxycycline) tend to be beneficial [19, 20]. The inflammation appears to be in part induced by the microbial flora. There is much more information regarding the management of rosacea in the dermatology literature, and some of the ophthalmic treatments that are commonly employed were first used by dermatologists for management of facial skin changes [21]. Management of severe ocular rosacea often requires a combination of therapies targeted at the inflammatory cascade, controlling the microbial flora and optimization of the ocular surface.

In our patient we decided that a dry amniotic membrane graft (BioDOptix, Cordova, Tennessee) would provide support in the area of severe stromal thinning in the left eye. A bandage contact lens was placed over the amniotic membrane graft. He was also started on a regimen of loteprednol etabonate 0.5% QID OU, ofloxacin 0.3% QID OS, and oral doxycycline 100 mg PO BID. At his follow-up visit 2 weeks later, he noted some improvement in symptoms. He also noted good compliance with his topical medication regimen but was unable to start doxycycline due to insurance issues. His visual acuities had improved to 20/60 OD and 20/200 OS. The area of severe stromal thinning in the left eye had improved to 20% of normal stromal thickness. He was continued on his topical medication regimen. At his subsequent follow-up visit one month later, his visual acuity was stable in the right eye and improved to 20/150 in the left eye, while his symptoms and eyelid margin/ocular surface inflammation had significantly improved.

What Was the Role of Amniotic Membrane in This Case?

When we saw this patient for follow-up after 20 months, we were concerned about evidence of a prior perforation in the left eye in an area of severe thinning. We decided to use an AmnioDisc to prevent what may have been an impending perforation in the setting of uncontrolled ocular surface inflammation. Fortunately, with the use of amniotic membrane as an acute intervention while initiating chronic treatment with a topical steroid, the area of severe thinning quickly improved and the inflammation gradually decreased over several weeks. As mentioned earlier, this is some evidence for integration of amniotic membrane into the host corneal stroma with thickening of underlying tissue, particularly with the use of multilayered amniotic membrane [12]. This effect on corneal tissue volume may also be supported by the presence of numerous growth factors and cytokines within amnion [22, 23]. Some have demonstrated an anti-inflammatory effect of amniotic membrane transplantation; Shimmura et al. showed that samples retrieved from patients revealed sequestration and apoptosis of inflammatory cells on the amniotic membrane surface [24]. Therefore, the role of amniotic membrane in our case may have been to allow for thickening of the underlying stroma as well as to reduce ocular surface inflammation. It is unclear to what extent the AMT graft may have incorporated into the cornea, versus the facilitation of corneal remodeling and eventual stromal thickening.

Similar to our first case, we used a dry amniotic membrane graft largely due to ease of use and ease of application. The patient could also have been treated with a ProKera device. However, in that circumstance, we may have also considered a temporary suture tarsorrhaphy at the time of ProKera placement in order to help keep the device in place; patient comfort was a consideration, as he had noted significant foreign body sensation at the time of evaluation. The ProKera device has been reported to be used successfully in a number of conditions, including non-healing epithelial defects (e.g., neurotrophic keratopathy), acute chemical injury, and Stevens-Johnson syndrome. We feel that the device itself may help to prevent symblepharon formation when used in the acute setting or when combined with an ocular surface reconstruction procedure. We have occasionally used the device at the time of high-risk corneal transplantation surgery in order to promote ocular surface rehabilitation.

What Is Your Long-Term Management Plan for This Patient?

It should be noted that the effect of amniotic membrane transplantation is transient, and as demonstrated in this case, it often needs to be used in combination with other therapies to achieve stability of the ocular surface. Long-term management in this case will include topical steroids and a systemic tetracycline, if the patient is able to obtain and tolerate these medications; given the risks of glaucoma and cataract progression, topical steroids may be reduced over an extended duration, as long as his blepharitis and ocular surface disease remain controlled. Additional interventions to consider include non-preserved artificial tears, topical cyclosporine (or tacrolimus) as a steroid-sparing agent, and topical metronidazole gel to the eyelid margin [25, 26]. Visual rehabilitation may require a rigid gas permeable contact lens given his irregular astigmatism, as well as cataract extraction once the ocular surface is stable for some time. A scleral lens may be useful as a therapeutic agent as well as for visual rehabilitation.

References

1. Kwok SK, Ho PC, Leung SF, Gandhi S, Lee VW, Lam DS, et al. An analysis of the incidence and risk factors of developing severe keratopathy in eyes after megavoltage external beam irradiation. Ophthalmology. 1998;105(11):2051–5.
2. Macfaul PA, Bedford MA. Ocular complications after therapeutic irradiation. Br J Ophthalmol. 1970;54(4):237–47.
3. Fujishima H, Shimazaki J, Tsubota K. Temporary corneal stem cell dysfunction after radiation therapy. Br J Ophthalmol. 1996;80(10):911–4.
4. Jhanji V, Young AL, Mehta JS, Sharma N, Agarwal T, Vajpayee RB. Management of corneal perforation. Surv Ophthalmol. 2011;56(6):522–38.
5. Cavanaugh TB, Gottsch JD. Infectious keratitis and cyanoacrylate adhesive. Am J Ophthalmol. 1991;111(4):466–72.
6. Bonini S, Rama P, Olzi D, Lambiase A. Neurotrophic keratitis. Eye (Lond). 2003;17(8):989–95.
7. Cosar CB, Cohen EJ, Rapuano CJ, Maus M, Penne RP, Flanagan JC, et al. Tarsorrhaphy: clinical experience from a cornea practice. Cornea. 2001;20(8):787–91.
8. Soni NG, Jeng BH. Blood-derived topical therapy for ocular surface diseases. Br J Ophthalmol. 2016;100(1):22–7.
9. Sacchetti M, Lambiase A. Diagnosis and management of neurotrophic keratitis. Clin Ophthalmol. 2014;8:571–9.
10. Khokhar S, Natung T, Sony P, Sharma N, Agarwal N, Vajpayee RB. Amniotic membrane transplantation in refractory neurotrophic corneal ulcers: a randomized, controlled clinical trial. Cornea. 2005;24(6):654–60.

11. Kruse FE, Rohrschneider K, Volcker HE. Multilayer amniotic membrane transplantation for reconstruction of deep corneal ulcers. Ophthalmology. 1999;106(8):1504–10. discussion 1511
12. Nubile M, Dua HS, Lanzini M, Ciancaglini M, Calienno R, Said DG, et al. In vivo analysis of stromal integration of multilayer amniotic membrane transplantation in corneal ulcers. Am J Ophthalmol. 2011;151(5):809–22.
13. Seitz B, Resch MD, Schlotzer-Schrehardt U, Hofmann-Rummelt C, Sauer R, Kruse FE. Histopathology and ultrastructure of human corneas after amniotic membrane transplantation. Arch Ophthalmol. 2006;124(10):1487–90.
14. Resch MD, Schlotzer-Schrehardt U, Hofmann-Rummelt C, Sauer R, Kruse FE, Beckmann MW, et al. Integration patterns of cryopreserved amniotic membranes into the human cornea. Ophthalmology. 2006;113(11):1927–35.
15. Kim SW, Park S, Im CY, Seo KY, Kim EK. Prediction of mean corneal power change after pterygium excision. Cornea. 2014;33(2):148–53.
16. Katircioglu YA, Altiparmak U, Engur Goktas S, Cakir B, Singar E, Ornek F. Comparison of two techniques for the treatment of recurrent pterygium: amniotic membrane vs conjunctival autograft combined with Mitomycin C. Semin Ophthalmol. 2015;30(5-6):321–7.
17. Rao A, Sridhar U, Gupta AK. Amniotic membrane transplant with superficial keratectomy in superficial corneal degenerations: efficacy in a rural population of north India. Indian J Ophthalmol. 2008;56(4):297–302.
18. Vieira AC, Mannis MJ. Ocular rosacea: common and commonly missed. J Am Acad Dermatol. 2013;69(6 Suppl 1):S36–41.
19. Sobolewska B, Doycheva D, Deuter C, Pfeffer I, Schaller M, Zierhut M. Treatment of ocular rosacea with once-daily low-dose doxycycline. Cornea. 2014;33(3):257–60.
20. Sobrin L, Liu Z, Monroy DC, Solomon A, Selzer MG, Lokeshwar BL, et al. Regulation of MMP-9 activity in human tear fluid and corneal epithelial culture supernatant. Invest Ophthalmol Vis Sci. 2000;41(7):1703–9.
21. Weinkle AP, Doktor V, Emer J. Update on the management of rosacea. Clin Cosmet Investig Dermatol. 2015;8:159–77.
22. Choi JA, Jin H-J, Jung S, Yang E, Choi J-S, Chung S-H, et al. Effects of amniotic membrane suspension in human corneal wound healing in vitro. Mol Vis. 2009;15:2230–8.
23. Bomfim Pereira MG, Pereira Gomes JA, Rizzo LV, Cristovam PC, Silveira LC. Cytokine dosage in fresh and preserved human amniotic membrane. Cornea. 2016;35(1):89–94.
24. Shimmura S, Shimazaki J, Ohashi Y, Tsubota K. Antiinflammatory effects of amniotic membrane transplantation in ocular surface disorders. Cornea. 2001;20(4):408–13.
25. Donnenfeld E, Pflugfelder SC. Topical ophthalmic cyclosporine: pharmacology and clinical uses. Surv Ophthalmol. 2009;54(3):321–38.
26. Barnhorst DAJ, Foster JA, Chern KC, Meisler DM. The efficacy of topical metronidazole in the treatment of ocular rosacea. Ophthalmology. 1996;103(11):1880–3.

Chapter 19
Management of Limbal Stem Cell Deficiency

Elham Ghahari, Duaa Sharfi, Edward J. Holland, and Ali R. Djalilian

Case 1: Contact Lens-Induced Limbal Stem Cell Deficiency

A 55-year-old male was referred for corneal changes and decreased vision in the right eye for 16 months. He had a history of soft contact lens wear for 36 years. Patient also reported photophobia, foreign body sensation, and reduced contrast. His medications include artificial tears every hour in both eyes, fluorometholone daily in the right eye, and cyclosporine 0.05% QID in the right and BID in the left eye. Patient had previously undergone a superficial keratectomy in the right eye which cleared his vision for a while, but gradually the blurriness has returned.

On examination, the visual acuity was 20/50 OD and 20/20 OS. His slit lamp exam was remarkable for significant Meibomian gland plugging and lid margin telangiectasia in both eyes. The right cornea demonstrated an opaque epithelial sheet extending from the superior limbus toward the central cornea. This opaque epithelium stained with fluorescein in a whorl pattern (Fig. 19.1a, b). The inferior cornea in both eyes demonstrated punctate epithelial staining consistent with tear film issues.

E. Ghahari, MD • D. Sharfi, MD • A.R. Djalilian, MD (✉)
Department of Ophthalmology and Visual Sciences, Illinois Eye and Ear Infirmary, University of Illinois at Chicago, Chicago, IL 60607, USA
e-mail: adjalili@uic.edu

E.J. Holland, MD
Cincinnati Eye Institute, University of Cincinnati, Cincinnati, OH 45220, USA

A.R. Djalilian (ed.), *Ocular Surface Disease*,
https://doi.org/10.1007/978-3-319-15823-5_19

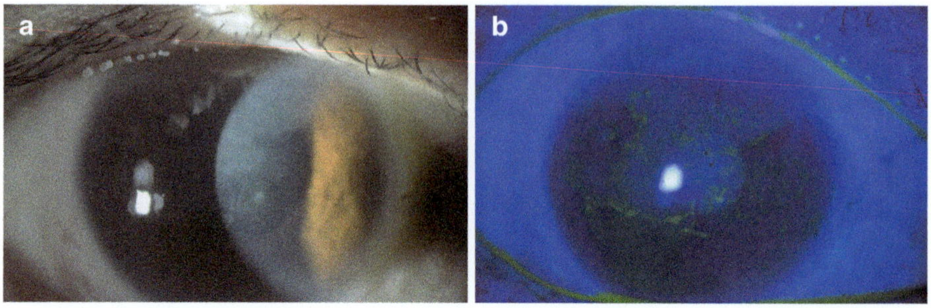

Fig. 19.1 Contact lens induced limbal stem cell deficiency (patent described in this chapter). Note the opaque epithelial sheet extending from superior limbus into visual axis (**a**) which stains with fluorescein in a whorl pattern (**b**). Taken with permission [3]

What Is the Diagnosis?

Limbal stem cell deficiency (LSCD) is a state of insufficiency or functional impairment of the limbal stem cells leading to conjunctivalization of the cornea. The presence of conjunctival epithelium over the cornea leads to chronic inflammation, recurrent/persistent epithelial defects, neovascularization, scarring, and loss of vision. Clinically, patients present with decreased vision, photophobia with or without discomfort. The most common etiologies of LSCD are listed in Box 19.1.

In this case, the patient has contact lens-induced LSCD. A retrospective review of 591 soft contact lens (SCL) wearers reported that focal LSCD associated with SCL wear was found in 2.4% of patients [1]. Only 28.6% of them reported symptoms associated with these findings; most were found to have these findings incidentally on routine examination. This supports the fact that LSCD associated with SCL wear may be more common than previously reported. All SCL wearers should be cautioned about this potential complication of SCL wear, and slit lamp examination with special attention to the superior cornea is warranted on an annual basis.

Box 19.1 Etiologies of Limbal Stem Cell Deficiency

Etiologies of Limbal Stem Cell Deficiency

Congenital

Aniridia (PAX6 related)

Ectodermal Dysplasia

Inflammatory

Stevens-Johnson Syndrome/TEN

Mucous Membrane Pemphigoid

Atopic/vernal Keratoconjunctivitis

Superior limbic keratoconjunctivitis

Severe limbal inflammation

Traumatic/Toxic
Chemical/Thermal injuries
Limbal surgeries, Mitomycin C
Contact lens wear
Chronic topical medications

What Causes LSCD in Contact Lens Wearers?

Contact lens-induced LSCD almost always has been reported in SCL wearers (it is rare with rigid gas permeable lenses). It is multifactorial and can result from the mechanical friction on the limbus, toxicity from preservatives in contact lens disinfecting solutions, and perhaps hypoxia [2]. It almost always occurs in the setting of dry eyes including Meibomian gland disease.

What Are the Characteristic Signs of LSCD in Contact Lens Wearers?

The superior limbus, which likely sustains more mechanical rubbing from the SCL, is the most common site of involvement. Findings leading to the diagnosis included whorl-like epitheliopathy, corneal conjunctivalization, and late fluorescein staining of the involved epithelium. The earliest sign of the disease is punctate staining in the superior cornea. Some patients may present with 360 disease; these are the patients who are most at risk for total stem cell failure.

What Are the Medical Management Options of LSCD in Contact Lens Wearers?

The first and most important treatment is to ask the patient to completely stop contact lens wear (no part-time wear). Preservative-free artificial tears must be used frequently along with lid hygiene and doxycycline if there is associated Meibomian gland disease. If there is minimal/no improvement after conservative therapy for 2 months, then we start anti-inflammatory therapy, particularly topical corticosteroid drops—if available, preservative free. In most cases, we see a significant response to steroids and continue this therapy as long as there is improvement. Patients are later switched to topical cyclosporine as steroids are tapered. Other treatments which can be used alongside anti-inflammatory therapy include vitamin A ointment 0.01% and autologous serum tears 20% [3].

The patient was asked to discontinue CL wear (which he had done already) and use frequent non-preserved artificial tears, fluorometholone was changed to topical

methylprednisolone 1% (preservative free) four times daily along with lid hygiene and doxycycline 100 mg twice daily for Meibomian gland disease. After 2 months, there was some reduction in the density of the conjunctivalized epithelium; however, it was still within the visual axis. The steroids had to be changed to loteprednol 0.5% given elevation in the IOP. Topical vitamin A 0.01% qhs was added along with autologous serum tears 20% q2h. After 2 months there was slight improvement in the appearance of the cornea, but the patient was still symptomatic.

What Are the Treatment Options for Recalcitrant Contact Lens-Induced LSCD?

Before considering any surgical options, it is important to maximize the health of the ocular surface and tear film, as was done in this case. The next reasonable option is mechanical debridement of the conjunctival-type epithelium. However, as noted in this case, there can be recurrence, especially if it is done too soon (before properly controlling the inflammation and maximizing the health of the tear film) or if there is extensive disease. A more advanced option is to combine the superficial keratectomy with a peritomy and conjunctival recession in the involved area and then using fibrin glue to secure an amniotic membrane over the involved limbus and de-epithelialized cornea.

Another treatment, which may seem counterintuitive, is scleral lenses, particularly the larger diameter ones that can vault over the limbus. The scleral lens can potentially protect the limbus from lid trauma (from blinking) while providing a more stable tear film. We have had success particularly in patients with recurrent disease after a superficial keratectomy.

A repeat superficial keratectomy was performed to remove the irregular epithelium superiorly. This was done at the slit lamp using a Weck-Cel sponge (conjunctival epithelium that grows over the cornea is very loosely adherent and can be removed by gentle scraping with a sponge, while corneal epithelium is much more adherent and can be left intact). The patient was followed daily and any recurrent conjunctival growth from superior cornea was scraped again ("sequential superficial corneal epithelialectomy," SSCE as described by Dua). Patient noted definite improvement; however by 3 months, the conjunctival-type epithelium had recurred and was obstructing the visual axis.

The patient was referred for scleral lens fitting in both eyes.

What Are the Limbal Transplantation Options for Advanced CL-Induced LSCD?

In patients whose vision is compromised from the disease, limbal transplantation is considered as a last resort option. Harvesting limbal stem cells from the fellow eye of a patient with bilateral contact lens wear is contraindicated given that the other eye, despite looking normal, almost always has compromised limbal stem cells and harvesting a donor graft can induce LSCD. Alternatively, one option which may be considered in patients who have some remaining healthy limbus is an ipsilateral limbal autograft (e.g., from inferior limbus to superior limbus). Although we have not yet tried this procedure in a SCL-related case, we have used it successfully in cases with iatrogenic LSCD (multiple superior limbal surgeries, mitomycin C).

Allograft limbal transplantation is an option for bilateral extensive disease whose vision is significantly compromised. Our preferred option, when a suitable donor is available, is a living related graft and often two pieces of two clock hours (four clock hours total) is enough to restore a healthy corneal epithelium. If a donor is not available, then standard keratolimbal allograft may be performed. As explained later in this chapter, the success of allograft procedures is highly dependent on the proper use of systemic immunosuppression.

The patient was successfully fitted with scleral lenses in both eyes which improved his vision to 20/20 in the right (and left) eye. The appearance of the epithelium did not change significantly and he continued to have evidence of conjunctival-type epithelium in the superior cornea extending into visual axis (spectacle corrected vision was still 20/50 in right eye). A recommendation was made for him to undergo superficial keratectomy, peritomy, and an ipsilateral limbal transplant (CLAU or SLET) from inferior to superior cornea; however, given that he could see 20/20 with the scleral lens, he has deferred this option for now.

Can a Patient with CL-Induced LSCD Go Back to Wearing Contact Lenses?

It is very unlikely that a patient with SCL-induced LSCD could ever go back to wearing SCLs since the disease will recur. However, hard (RGP) lenses may be an option. Given that these patients frequently also have dry eyes, scleral lenses are actually a great option and as mentioned above may actually have a therapeutic role if they are large enough to vault over the limbus. Another option for patients who prefer not to wear spectacles is refractive surgery and both LASIK and surface ablation (especially if there is any stromal haze) have been used successfully in patients with treated LSCD.

In conclusion, LSCD associated with SCL wear can present with varying manifestations and early changes can be asymptomatic. These changes can occur from 1 year to 30 years after SCL wear, so patients who chose to wear SCL must be instructed to follow-up for routine slit lamp examination on an annual basis. Early identification of this process with subsequent cessation of wear is of utmost importance to proper treatment. Additional measures are aimed at restoring a healthy limbal niche using anti-inflammatory therapy and tear film optimization. Scleral lenses may provide a therapeutic effect, while surgical options are considered as last resort.

Case 2: Limbal Stem Cell Deficiency in Aniridia

37-year-old female with a history of congenital aniridia presented with progressive decreased vision in both eyes. She was frustrated with the use of contact lenses, which although helpful for her vision, frequently caused her to develop abrasions/ulcers. Her past ocular history included bilateral cataract extraction at age 19. Besides artificial tears she did not use any other medications. Multiple family members all had aniridia.

On examination, her best corrected visual acuity was 20/300 in both eyes. The intraocular pressure was 31 in her right and 18 in her left eye. Slit lamp exam of the right eye was remarkable for opaque/grayish epithelium extending into the visual axis from the limbus in all quadrants. There were no palisades of Vogt, and there was superficial neovascularization and Salzmann's like nodules in the periphery (Fig. 19.2a). The left eye had a similar appearance, although there were a few small remaining pockets of clearer epithelium. The more opaque epithelium demonstrated whorl pattern on fluorescein staining. Fundus exam was remarkable for foveal hypoplasia.

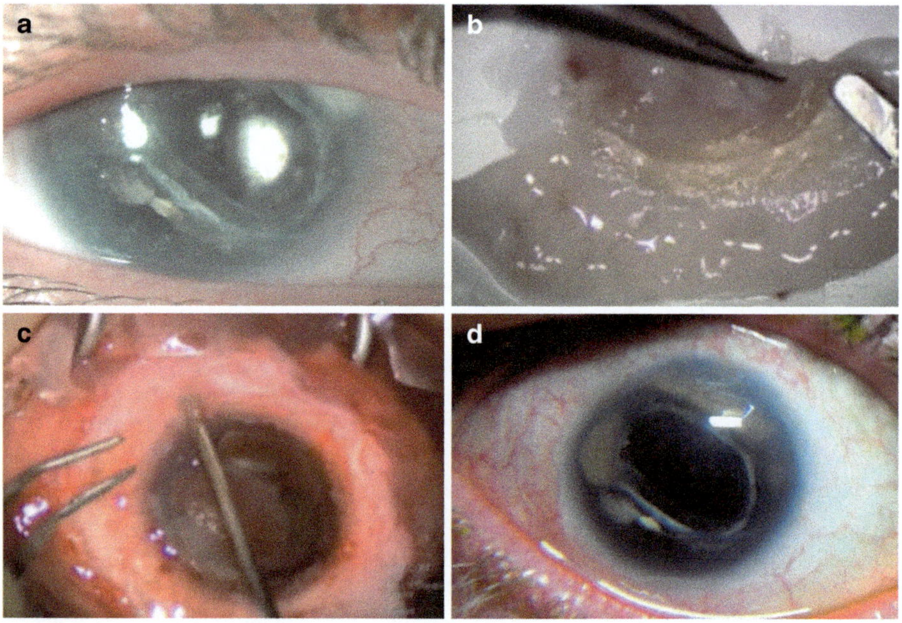

Fig. 19.2 Keratolimbal allograft for aniridia (patient described in this chapter). Pre-operatively, the cornea demonstrates a clear stroma but opaque epithelium extending into visual axis with areas of Salzmann's nodule like changes (not easily seen in this photo) (**a**). Intra-operatively, the limbal stem graft is dissected from one piece of 180° cadaver tissue that has been fixed in place using cyanoacrylate glue (**b**). Three pieces of 180° grafts are secured to the recipient eye using fibrin glue (**c**). The recipient eye (right eye) at 2.5 years after surgery demonstrating a corneal type epithelium (**d**)

Why Is This Patient Experiencing a Decline in Her Vision?

Aniridia is a bilateral, panocular disorder presenting with abnormalities in the cornea, anterior chamber angle, iris, lens, optic nerve, macula, and retina. All patients with congenital aniridia have foveal hypoplasia which leads to various degrees of nystagmus and reduced visual acuity; however this is fixed and does not lead to progressive loss of vision. The most common causes of progressive visual decline in aniridic patients are cataracts, LSCD and glaucoma. Most patients have a visual potential in the 20/100 to 20/200 range. In this case, the main reason for the progressive visual changes is LSCD. This is based on the characteristic opaque late staining conjunctival epithelium extending into the visual axis.

What Is Aniridic Keratopathy?

Aniridic keratopathy (AK) is actually a manifestation of LSCD and can be observed in about half of aniridia patients under age 10, but reaches nearly 100% in adulthood. AK/LSCD is caused by a combination of factors: developmental abnormalities and progressive loss of the limbal stem cell niche with subsequent conjunctivalization of the cornea. AK is highly variable and asymmetric. Signs of keratopathy appear in the first decade of life, with peripheral superficial opacity (e.g., conjunctival epithelium). However over the years, it slowly progresses and involves the central cornea. The peak age for the development of near total LSCD is 30–40, but some may be sooner and some later. Clinically, we suspect that prolonged use of eye drops, namely, glaucoma medications, may lead to faster progression of the epithelial disease in aniridia.

Holland et al. described the progression of AK to LSCD in five distinct stages [4]. Neovascularization may be present at any point during disease development and is not a sensitive indication for severity or prognosis:

- Stage I is characterized by abnormal peripheral corneal epithelium. This change is reflected in the increased uptake of fluorescein (late staining).
- Stage II is observed once centripetal extension of epithelial changes is noted.
- Stage III is characterized by central corneal epithelial changes and peripheral superficial neovascularization.
- Stage IV involves the entire cornea with abnormal epithelium in addition to subepithelial fibrosis.
- Stage V involves Stage IV accompanied by deep and permanent stromal scarring.

Staging of the disease is important in determining progression and timing of intervention. Stromal scarring which begins in Stage IV highlights the potential of these changes becoming permanent. If the patient develops stromal scarring, then they may no longer qualify for a limbal stem cell transplant alone and thus require additional procedures for therapeutic restoration of the corneal clarity.

How Does PAX6 Mutation/Deletion Affect the Disease?

About two-thirds of aniridia cases are inherited while the rest are sporadic. Most aniridia cases are due to a heterozygous mutation in the PAX6 gene (all sporadic cases should be screened at birth for gene deletions which if present will require screening for Wilms' tumor in the first 5 years of life). The PAX6 gene plays a vital role in the regulation of genes/proteins that are crucial during eye development as well as normal tissue homeostasis. Previous studies have not found a significant correlation with the type of mutation (or deletion) in the progression of the disease since most of them lead to loss of function. The issue is likely a dosage effect, where having only one functional copy of PAX6 leads to reduced level of PAX6 protein which leads to abnormal development and function of the limbal niche.

It is worth noting that aniridic keratopathy may present in the absence of other classic stigmata of aniridia and be associated with minimally affected irides. These patients often have mutations in PAX6 and once identified can be counseled appropriately [5]. Previously, this condition used to be called by names such as autosomal dominant keratitis, but a more appropriate and encompassing name is PAX6-related keratopathy [5].

What are the Treatment Measures for AK?

Management of mild AK (Stage I) includes mainly preservative-free lubricants. In moderate keratopathy (Stage II), measures that can improve the health of the epithelium include topical steroids, autologous serum drops, and amniotic membrane transplant. Most of these measures are aimed at improving the health of the ocular surface and enhancing the survival and expansion of surviving limbal stem cells; however, they are temporary and not a long-term solution. Another temporizing measure which can help improve the visual function is RGP/scleral lenses, which help correct the optical irregularities on the surface.

In more advanced disease (Stage III or later), limbal stem cell transplant is recommended. Penetrating keratoplasty as a primary procedure is contraindicated given the inevitable recurrence of LSCD in the graft. Finally another option is keratoprosthesis. It is best not to wait until Stage V since that would necessitate a keratoplasty as well.

How Does One Decide Which Surgical Procedure Is Most Appropriate for Advanced LSCD in Aniridia?

There are several issues that need to be considered: First, is whether the patient is a candidate for systemic immunosuppression. At the time of presentation of total LSCD, most aniridics tend to be younger and healthy and thus are good candidates for immunosuppression. Older patients (above 60), or those with systemic comorbidities such as diabetes may not be good candidates. A patient who is not a candidate for immunosuppression is best managed with keratoprosthesis. In patients who are good candidates for immunosuppression, limbal allograft is the most reasonable first choice. Previously, we used cadaveric tissue (KLAL) for all such patients; however, in recent years we consider lr-CLAL to be the first choice—given the lower risk of rejection—and cadaveric tissue is used only when a first-degree relative is not available.

Another issue that must be considered is whether the eye has had previous transplant surgeries. It is not uncommon that an aniridic patient may have previously undergone a penetrating keratoplasty in the past which has subsequently failed due to recurrent LSCD and/or rejection. In these cases, since the eye has already been sensitized immunologically, the risk of future rejection is significantly higher and therefore our preference is to use a keratoprosthesis, namely, Boston type I.

Another issue is the severity of the glaucoma. A patient with very advanced glaucoma that requires close monitoring of IOP is not a very good candidate for keratoprosthesis since the IOP cannot be measured accurately.

The final issue that must be considered is the status of the stroma and endothelium. When conjunctivalization is not accompanied by deep stromal scarring and fibrosis, then a limbal transplant (as a non-penetrating procedure) is definitely the most appropriate choice since it avoids the need for more invasive interventions. In the case of stromal scarring, a limbal transplant followed by anterior lamellar keratoplasty is also preferred over Kpro. However, in the case of endothelial compensation, especially due to a tube shunt, going straight to Kpro may be more appropriate given the high likelihood of subsequent endothelial failure after keratoplasty.

The patient has minimal stromal scarring; therefore a limbal transplant is the first choice. She has a strong familial history of aniridia, consequently a living related donor was not available and KLAL was recommended. The patient was referred to her primary care physician where she underwent a complete history and physical as well as age-appropriate screening for any malignancy. Laboratory evaluation included CBC, comprehensive metabolic panel (including kidney and liver function tests), Hepatitis B and C screening, QuantiFERON Gold (tuberculosis), and HIV.

What Is the Surgical Technique for KLAL?

First, it is important to specifically request KLAL tissue from the eye bank. We ask for tissue that is from a donor younger than 50, that is less than 5 days old, and has at least 3 mm of conjunctival skirt. We punch the tissue with a 7.5–8 mm trephine—leaving at least 1.5 mm of peripheral cornea. The tissue must then be thinned before it can be transplanted. Our preferred technique for thinning the tissue is to make a single cut in the limbal ring and then using a few drops of medical-grade cyanoacrylate glue to secure the graft to a flat surface (epithelial side up). Once the tissue is secure, we perform a controlled lamellar dissection (using a crescent knife) starting from the conjunctival side (Fig. 19.2b). The last part of the dissection is carried out with a Vannas scissor. The resulting tissue can be secured to the host limbal area with fibrin glue alone (after 360 peritomy and superficial keratectomy). Because the tissue is thin, there is no need to create a "bed," and also there is minimal step off. Dr. Holland's technique is similar except that he uses three pieces of 180° grafts that are secured at the anterior corneas with interrupted 10-0 nylon sutures, while the posterior aspects of the graft are secured to the sclera with fibrin glue.

She underwent a right KLAL involving 3 × 180 pieces, which were secured using fibrin glue only (Fig. 19.2b, c). She was prescribed prednisolone acetate 1% QID, gatifloxacin, and Restasis while continuing her current drops (latanoprost, brimonidine). She was started on systemic immunosuppressive medications on the day of surgery: prednisolone (1 mg/kg), mycophenolate (1000 mg BID), and tacrolimus (4 mg BID). Patient was not started on any systemic antimicrobial prophylaxis given her low-risk status. Patient noted improved vision and by 1 month demonstrated clear cornea and grafts with resolving post-op inflammation and hemorrhage.

What Is the Current Immunosuppression Protocol in KLAL Patients?

The most widely used protocol is the one developed in Cincinnati (EJH). Management of systemic immunosuppression is best done in collaboration with an organ transplant team given their familiarity with prescribing and monitoring of the medications. The Cincinnati protocol is summarized in Fig. 19.3 and consists of:

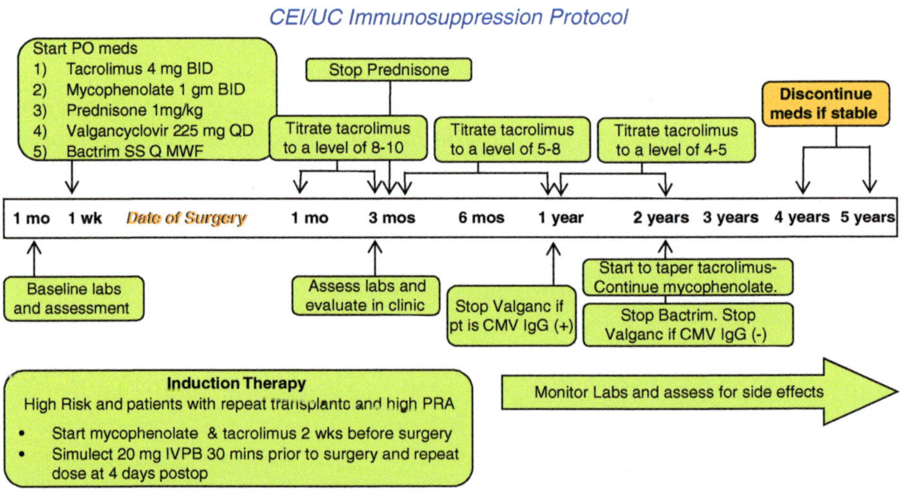

Fig. 19.3 The Cincinnati systemic immunosuppression protocol after limbal allograft transplantation (with permission) [4]

1. Steroids—oral prednisone tapered off by 2–3 months.
2. T-cell inhibitor—cyclosporine or tacrolimus for 2 years.
3. Antiproliferative/antimetabolite agent—azathioprine, mycophenolate mofetil, or rapamycin for 3–5 years (or longer).
4. Infection prophylaxis individualized to patient risk.

While the level and duration of systemic therapy is individualized, for most patients at minimum 3 years, it is necessary. Most often it can be tapered off successfully in patients with noninflammatory diseases such as aniridia, while in patients with inflammatory disease such as Stevens-Johnson syndrome, it often has to be used indefinitely to maximize graft survival.

In general, patients with limbal transplant are at very low risk for developing opportunistic infections; however, in order to minimize risk even further, prophylactic treatment can be given to prevent CMV and Pneumocystis carinii with the use of valganciclovir and sulfamethoxazole/trimethoprim, respectively.

What Is the Recommended Topical Therapy after KLAL?

In addition to frequent non-preserved lubricants, topical therapy includes a combination of corticosteroids and cyclosporine (or tacrolimus). The preferred topical steroids for the first year are the potent agents such as difluprednate acetate 0.05% (four times a day) or Pred Forte 1% (four to six times a day) titrated to the level of inflammation. IOP is monitored closely, and in the event of elevation, topical agents are used to lower the pressure. After the first year, loteprednol or fluorometholone may be used if there are still IOP issues. An important point is that topical steroids must be used indefinitely— as demonstrated later in this patient. Topical cyclosporine (prefer 0.05% given the availability) is also used indefinitely; however, its use may not as essential in the first 1–2 years and is probably most helpful after systemic therapy has been discontinued (topical tacrolimus may be used alternatively).

Another adjunctive topical therapy is autologous serum tears. This is typically not necessary in patients with aniridia after limbal transplant, given that the rest of the ocular surface is relatively healthy; however, it can be beneficial in patients with significant dry eyes such as SJS or severe chemical injuries.

What Are the Risks with Systemic Immunosuppression?

There is significant misconception about the risks of immunosuppression in this patient population. With proper patient selection and appropriate monitoring, the risk is quite low mainly because patients undergoing limbal transplant are younger and relatively healthy. Typically, patients with advanced age (above 65) or associated comorbidities such as diabetes are considered poor candidates for immunosuppression and is best to consider keratoprosthesis first. The largest study that confirms the safety of immunosuppression in this population is by the Holland and colleagues from Cincinnati [6]. They reported 136 patients, mean age of 43.6 years (range, 9–80 years) who received immunosuppression for an average of 42.1 months (range, 3.6–128 months). There were three severe adverse events in two patients (1.5%): myocardial infarctions and pulmonary embolus—both of which are unusual and not typically associated with immunosuppression—and 21 minor adverse events in 19 patients (14.0%) (hypertension, elevated glucose, liver enzyme changes, etc.), all of which resolved/were treated. They concluded that "with appropriate long-term monitoring the risk of irreversible toxicity is minimal" and the risks are more than outweighed by the significant visual gain and improved quality of life offered by limbal allograft transplantation.

The patient was monitored closely by monthly laboratory testing. The tacrolimus level was maintained at 8–10 for the first 3 months and then 5–8 afterwards. Prednisone was tapered off by 4 months. Following surgery, however, she continued to exhibit high intraocular pressures (IOP) particularly in the right eye (OD 34, OS 28). Timolol-dorzolamide was added to both eyes and prednisolone eye drops were changed to loteprednol. After a month, IOP was 22 in both eyes. At 1 year after the first surgery, KLAL was performed in OS at which time she was placed back on oral prednisone for 3 months. The technique for this eye involved one 360 graft secured with fibrin glue.

Two years after the surgery in the left eye, the grafts remained clear, but the IOP continued to be an issue in the left eye and was consistently in the 30s on maximal drops. Oral methazolamide was added but had to be discontinued after she developed an allergic rash. She was offered the option of undergoing a tube shunt which she declined, and therefore she underwent a diode cyclophotocoagulation (360°) in the left eye. Patient was treated with a 3-week course of oral steroids and frequent topical steroids to control the inflammation.

What Is the Best Way to Manage Co-existing Glaucoma in Aniridia Patients Undergoing Limbal Transplant?

It is well known that aniridia patients have a high likelihood of developing glaucoma due to anatomical and developmental anomalies of their angles. In our experience, any patient who comes in on IOP lowering drops before limbal transplant has a very high likelihood of requiring glaucoma surgery after limbal transplant as a result of the topical steroids—as evident by the course of this patient. Therefore, we feel quite confident in recommending glaucoma surgery before limbal transplant (even when the IOP is controlled with drops). A preferred surgical procedure is a tube shunt in the sulcus, away from the cornea. While this patient elected to undergo a cyclodestructive procedure (which turned out OK), we do not favor this procedure

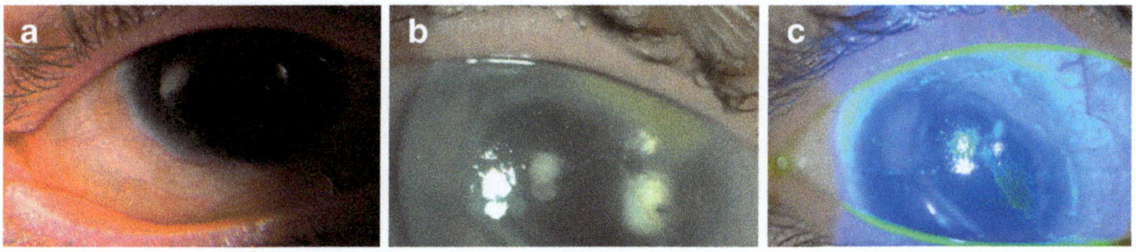

Fig. 19.4 Clinical forms of rejection after KLAL. Injection of the limbal graft without an epithelial rejection line (**a**). Severe rejection with an epithelial rejection line (**b**, **c**)

as the first choice given that it induces significant inflammation and occasionally can precipitate aniridia fibrosis syndrome. Based on these experiences, our management of the glaucoma in this patient would have been different if they presented to us for the first time today. In particular, we would first recommend that she undergo a tube shunt in the sulcus before performing limbal transplantation. Doing the glaucoma procedure before ocular surface surgery is advantageous because it not only avoids any disturbance to the grafts but also reduces the burden of the glaucoma drops on the ocular surface and limbal transplants.

At 6 month follow-up after diode, the patient was incidentally noted to have 1+ conjunctival injection and more engorgement of the grafts (Fig. 19.4a). We changed loteprednol QID to prednisolone and increased her immunosuppressive dosage including mycophenolate. A month later, there was less conjunctival injection.

Two and a half years after the right eye surgery, the vision was near her best potential at 20/200 OD and 20/100 OS with a healthy corneal epithelium (Fig. 19.2d). We began to taper off her oral tacrolimus over the course of 6 months. She was maintained on mycophenolate for another year and half and at 4.5 years after the right eye surgery (3.5 years after the left eye) her systemic immunosuppression was discontinued.

One year later (5.5 years after initial surgery), the patient ran out of her steroid drops and did not immediately seek a refill. Within 1 month she developed severe pain and decreased vision in the right eye. On exam an epithelial rejection line was noted (Fig. 19.4b, c). She was diagnosed as severe rejection and treated with frequent topical steroids and restarting oral mycophenolate (she declined oral steroids). She went on to develop sectoral failure and superior limbal stem cell deficiency in the right eye.

What Factors Increase the Risk of Limbal Allograft Rejection?

Immune rejection is the most commonly observed complication following limbal allograft transplantation. It is reported to occur in 20–30% of ocular transplant surgeries despite treatment with systemic immunosuppression [7]. The source of tissue, the underlying disease, the age of the patient, and the level of immunosuppression are the main factors that affect the risk of rejection. Patients with inflammatory diseases such as Stevens-Johnson syndrome have a significantly higher risk of rejection compared to noninflammatory diseases such as aniridia. History of previous transplant failure (e.g., keratoplasty) or previous limbal transplant also raises the risk for rejection given that the eye and immune system is already sensitized. Younger age of the patient is likewise associated with higher chance of rejection. Finally, non-compliance or inadequate systemic immunosuppression can both increase the likelihood of rejection. Obviously, KLAL carries a higher risk of rejection compared to lr-CLAL.

How Does Rejection Manifest in a Patient after KLAL, and How Is It Treated?

Limbal allograft rejection can be acute or chronic. Most cases of acute rejection occur within the first year, but it has been reported to occur up to 8 years after the surgery. Signs and symptoms of acute stem cell rejection can vary between mild and severe rejections. The most common signs and symptoms include the following:

- Severe (discomfort):
  - Graft edema and intense injection
  - Epithelial rejection line
  - Subconjunctival hemorrhage
- Mild (asymptomatic):
  - Mild limbal and graft injection
  - +/– Epithelial rejection line

In our experience, mild rejection can be easily overlooked since the patient is typically asymptomatic. Mild acute rejection is treated by increasing topical steroids and systemic immunosuppression. Severe rejection is treated by intense topical steroids (q1h), oral steroids, and increasing systemic immunosuppression. Subconjunctival injection of steroids may also be considered.

Chronic rejection is less obvious on exam and is manifested mainly by chronic conjunctival/graft injection. It is best treated by increasing the level of systemic immunosuppression.

She was offered a repeat sectoral KLAL in her right eye; however, given that vision was still good in the left eye, the patient declined any intervention particularly since it would require her to go back on more systemic immunosuppression. At 6 years after the surgery in the right eye, the pressure in the right was consistently in the 30s on maximal drops, and therefore she underwent a diode cyclophotocoagulation (360°) in the right eye as well. She has been maintained on low-dose mycophenolate. IOP continues to be an issue in the left eye requiring multiple drops to stay marginally under control (low 20s). Her graft in the left eye remains stable (no recurrence of LSCD) at 8 years after initial surgery with BCVA of 20/100, while right eye is at 20/400 due to the sectoral superior limbal stem cell deficiency.

How Long Does a Limbal Transplant (Donor Stem Cells) Survive?

There have been a number of studies looking at this question. We previously reported donor tissue survival at least up to 3.5 years using DNA evidence [8]. More recently, in a series of patients with late acute graft rejection, we have found indirect evidence for the survival of donor cells at least up to 8 years [9]. Likewise, the patient presented in here also demonstrated acute graft rejection after 5.5 years. In contrast, there have been a few studies that have failed to find donor cells beyond the first year, arguing that donor cells do not survive in the long run and simply help to restore the environment that allows the host stem cells to "come back." While we agree with the idea that host cells can come back when the environment is improved, in most patients with true total LSCD, as in aniridia, there aren't many host stem cells to come back, and therefore it is the transplanted donor stem cells which remain the main source for regenerating the epithelium. The implication is that immunosuppressive therapy is necessary in order to help keep the donor cells avoid rejection. In some patients with aniridia, we have clinically observed survival of donor grafts beyond 15 years. This is contrast to inflammatory diseases such as SJS (illustrated by case 3) where repeat limbal grafting may be necessary after 5 years given the more hostile ocular surface environment.

What Are the Latest Trends in the Treatment of Aniridic Keratopathy?

In general, we try to limit the exposure of the ocular surface to drops with potential toxicity and recommend using preservative-free (or non-BAK) agents. In early disease (Stage II, encroaching on visual axis but no stromal scarring) a temporizing measure that may improve the vision is topical steroids (FML, loteprednol)— while watching the IOP—with or without autologous serum. This can help "buy some time" before needing limbal transplant. Likewise, the use of RGP/scleral lenses can significantly help the visual function in patient with early disease.

In patients requiring limbal transplantation, we now insist that all patients using two or more drops to first have a tube shunt placed in the sulcus and postpose limbal grafting until after the IOP is stable without drops. In terms of donor tissue, we now prefer lr-CLAL over KLAL and our experience is showing that two pieces of two clock hours each seems to be enough for aniridia patients (Fig. 19.5)—KLAL is used when a suitable donor is not available. We typically place a large bandage lens (e.g., Kontur) either at the end of surgery or on post-op day 1 and keep it in place for a few weeks until the epithelium is healed. Postoperatively we continue to follow the Cincinnati protocol for systemic therapy, and whenever possible, we use topical difluprednate which is more potent and less toxic compared to other steroids. For younger aniridic patients (under 50), we use tacrolimus for a full 2 years and typically continue low-dose mycophenolate typically up to 5 years (or longer as in this case). Overall, the most important factor in the success of limbal transplant in aniridia remains proper use of systemic immunosuppression.

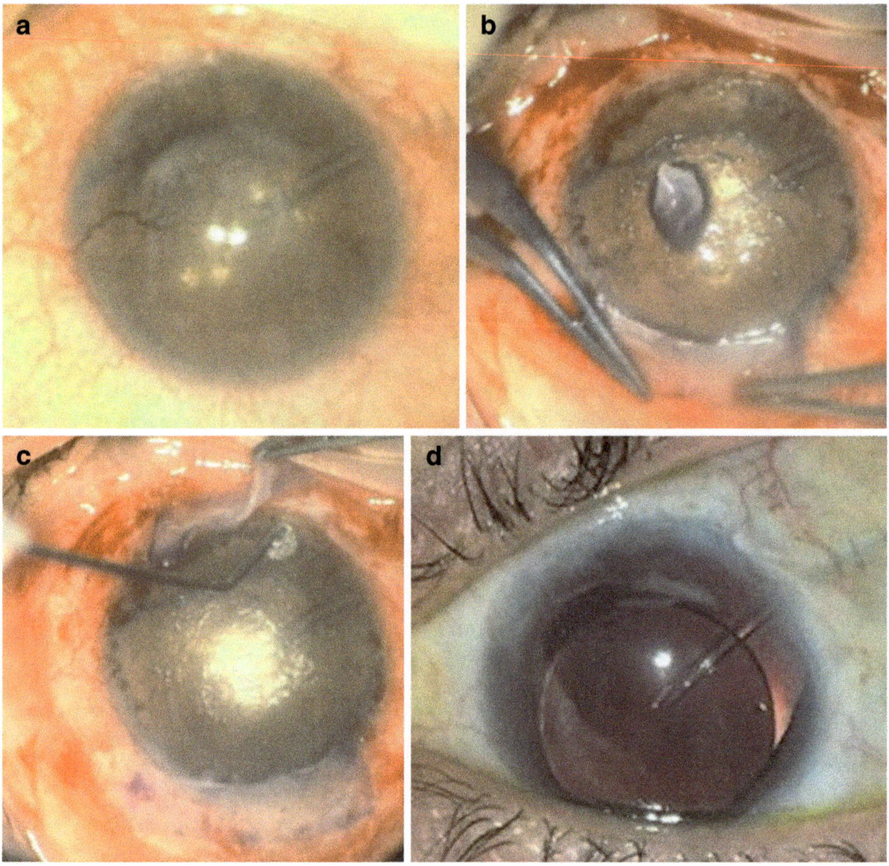

Fig. 19.5 Living related conjunctival limbal allograft in aniridia (a different patient than the one described in this chapter). Pre-operative photo demonstrating limbal stem cell deficiency (the patient had previously been referred to Dr. Ahmad Aref for a tube shunt since she was requiring two different drops to control her IOP) (**a**). Two pieces of limbal grafts (two clock hours each) were harvested from the patient's sister and secured to the inferior (**b**) and superior (**c**) limbus using fibrin glue. Postoperative photo demonstrates a healthy corneal epithelium at 6 months (**d**)

Case 3: Limbal Stem Cell Deficiency in Chronic Stevens-Johnson Syndrome

The patient is a 31-year-old female with a history of Stevens-Johnson Syndrome (SJS) at age 6 who presents with progressive decline in vision of the left eye. She had undergone a corneal transplant in her right eye within 1 year of her SJS diagnosis. Although the corneal transplant ultimately failed in the right, she was able to function quite well with her left eye. In the last few years, she has experienced a gradual decline in her vision particularly within the last few

months. Her ocular history includes multiple oculoplastic surgeries for trichiasis. Her past medical history includes a petit mal seizure disorder and a cervical laminectomy for Chiari Malformation. She is currently taking escitalopram, clonazepam, cyclobenzaprine, omeprazole, and birth control pills. Her ocular medications include artificial drops and topical antibiotic used frequently in her left eye. She has taken Restasis in the past but discontinued due to discomfort.

On examination, the visual acuity was light perception in her right eye and 20/300 in her left eye. In left eye, lid margin irregularities (left lower lid margin had been completely excised) with fornix shortening inferiorly and symblepharon superiorly was noted.

Slit lamp examination of the right eye showed diffuse corneal opacification and vascularization. Anterior segment details could not be assessed. In the left eye, the conjunctiva was uninflamed, and there appeared to be LSCD with vascularization superiorly with paracentral subepithelial fibrosis (Fig. 19.6a). The inferior epithelium appeared to be more corneal-type epithelium. The intraocular pressures were 12 on the right and 13 in the left.

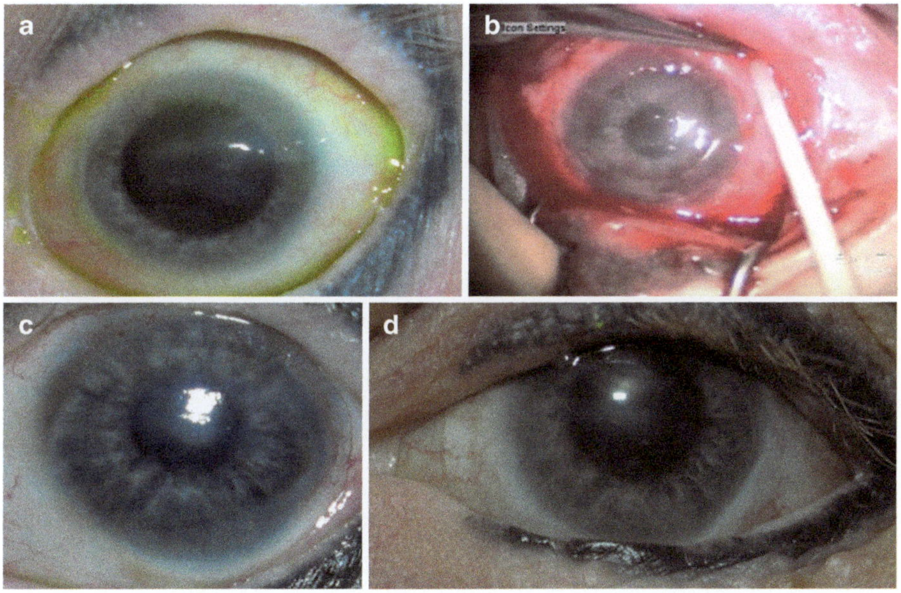

Fig. 19.6 Limbal transplantation in the SJS patient described in this chapter. Pre-operative photo demonstrating superior limbal stem cell deficiency (**a**). Intra-operative photo demonstrating a 360° limbal graft being secured to the eye using fibrin glue (**b**). Postoperative photo at 3 months (**c**) and 3 years (**d**)

What Are the Ocular Manifestations of Chronic Stevens-Johnson Syndrome?

The ocular surface represents one of the major targets in acute SJS. Acute ocular involvement is reported to occur in 50–90% of SJS cases (the presentation and management of acute SJS is discussed in another chapter). Up to 50% of patients with acute SJS will go on to develop chronic ocular sequelae, including progressive symblephara, lid margin keratinization, trichiasis, entropion, Meibomian gland atrophy, dry eye syndrome, and limbal stem cell deficiency [10, 11].

Is It Possible to Limit the Progression of the Ocular Surface Disease in Chronic SJS?

There are several strategies for potentially preventing progression in chronic SJS:

Controlling inflammation—The development of progressive ocular surface fibrosis in chronic SJS in many ways mimics other cicatricial diseases such as mucous membrane pemphigoid. Therefore, patients with ongoing active inflammation, especially in the first few months to years after the acute attack, may benefit from immunosuppressive therapy. Both topical and systemic corticosteroids are effective but cannot be continued at high doses for long term. In addition to low-dose topical steroids, we typically start with a course of oral steroids while at the same time starting a steroid-sparing systemic agent. Reported treatments include cyclosporine, azathioprine, cyclophosphamide, methotrexate, mycophenolate, and infliximab. Our preferred starting agent is oral mycophenolate 1000 mg BID, but in more severe cases, we get the best results from monthly intravenous cyclophosphamide (or daily PO). Close monitoring by rheumatology or hematology/oncology is necessary for cyclophosphamide [12].

Preventing ocular surface damage from lashes—Misdirected and distichiatic lashes can mechanically abrade the corneal epithelium, leading to recurrent corneal epithelial defects, infections, and stromal melting/scarring. The best immediate treatment is to protect the ocular surface with a soft bandage contact lens. Given the compromised ocular defenses, we use antibiotic prophylaxis in all SJS patients wearing long-term bandage lenses. Long-term eyelid surgery offers the more definitive treatment, but is best done when inflammation is under control.

Managing eyelid margin keratinization—Eyelid margin ulceration in the acute phase of SJS destroys the mucocutaneous junction and Meibomian glands with resultant overgrowth of the keratinized epithelium onto the tarsal conjunctiva. It is present in nearly very chronic SJS patient. Repetitive friction from the keratinized inner eyelid during blinking leads to recurrent corneal microtrauma and is a major cause of pain and photophobia. The resultant epitheliopathy predisposes these eyes to persistent epithelial defects, infection, stromal melting, and perforation, while also leading to LSCD and conjunctivalization of the cornea. Thus, early intervention for eyelid margin keratinization is crucial to stabilize the ocular surface and prevent end-stage corneal blindness.

Treatment of lid margin keratinization in SJS can include topical vitamin A 0.01% ointment (for milder cases) while more extensive disease may require mucous membrane grafting. Another option to prevent corneal damage from lid margin keratinization in SJS is chronic use of a soft bandage lens or better yet a large diameter, rigid gas permeable contact lens such as PROSE (Prosthetic Replacement of the Ocular Surface Ecosystem, Boston Foundation for Sight, Needham, MA). Scleral lenses have been shown to significantly improve visual acuity and comfort and reduce corneal epitheliopathy in chronic SJS. Fornix reconstruction may be necessary prior to lens fitting.

The clinical impression at this point was that the patient has superior LSCD in the left eye. This patient has an acceptable tear function; therefore, she is a good candidate for OS reconstruction. The right eye was felt to be prephthisical. There was no sign of active inflammation, consistent with the fact that her SJS attack was more than 25 years ago. The plan was to release symblepharon in order to get a scleral lens to fit but also see if the LSCD could possibly be addressed with amniotic membrane alone. Another adjunctive treatment that was not considered in this case but could have also been useful was autologous serum drops.

What Is the Surgical Approach for Reconstructing the Ocular Surface in Chronic SJS?

Before starting ocular surface reconstruction in SJS patients, we first make sure the inflammation is well controlled. We try to avoid doing surgery in the first year or two after the acute attack and quiet the eyes with systemic agents instead (as described above).

Reconstruction begins by first addressing the eyelid and conjunctival disease. Amniotic membrane alone is useful only in localized symblepharon without extensive conjunctival deficiency; otherwise a mucous membrane graft is necessary in every severe SJS case. A mucous membrane graft (from oral or nasal mucosa) to the palpebral surface of the eyelid is one the most useful procedures in SJS and addresses entropion, symblepharon/ankyloblepharon, lid margin keratinization, and conjunctival deficiency. Mitomycin C is used intraoperatively in the fornix for severely scarred eyes, while oral steroids are used perioperatively to limit inflammation (Fig. 19.7).

The next step is to address the limbal stem cell disease. In SJS, living related limbal tissue offers the great advantage of providing both conjunctiva and limbus. Therefore, when harvesting a limbal graft from the relative donor we bring a large conjunctival skirt. When there is total LSCD, we typically use both lr-CLAL and KLAL tissue to cover the entire limbal areas (i.e. Cincinnati procedure) [13]. During the limbal transplant procedure, we sometimes do not scrape the recipient epithelium/

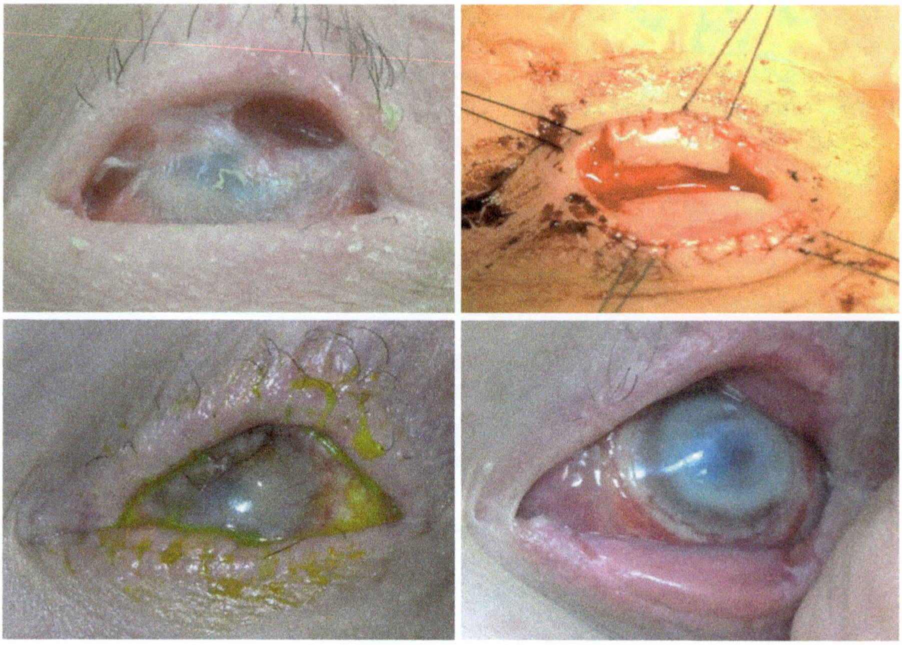

Fig. 19.7 An SJS patient (not the patient described in this chapter) with severe keratinization and ankyloblepharon who underwent oral with mucous membrane grafts to the upper and lower palpebral as well as bulbar surfaces along with a KLAL. At last follow-up the patient demonstrates a mucosal phenotype on the ocular surface (Courtesy of Dr. Charles Bouchard)

pannus in the central cornea to avoid creating a persistent epithelial defect (allow the donor cells to gradually replace the host). Likewise, we almost never do any dissection to remove scarring from the cornea, since the stroma is frequently thin in SJS patients. Systemic immunosuppression is necessary to reduce the risk of rejection.

Patients with extensive surface keratinization are generally poor candidates for ocular surface reconstruction and may be considered for other options such as type II Kpro or OOKP. Nonetheless, rehabilitation of the surface can be achieved in select cases with mucous membrane graft [14].

Since the patient had a limited symblepharon without extensive conjunctival deficiency, she underwent conjunctival peritomy, release of symblepharon with wide excision of Tenon's, mitomycin C in the fornix, superficial keratectomy of the superior (conjunctivalized) cornea with amniotic membrane transplant over the corneal, and conjunctival defect using fibrin glue. She was started on oral prednisone which was tapered over the course of 1 month. Postoperatively, a bandage lens was used for a few weeks until she was stable enough to be referred for scleral lens fitting.

In the months following the surgery, she noted improvement in her vision. Slit lamp examination, however, demonstrated gradual recurrence of conjunctivalization and neovascularization in the superior quadrant. In order to provide a new supply of limbal stem cells she underwent a KLAL procedure (one 360 graft) along with systemic immunosuppression (Fig. 19.6b). Three months later, her vision was 20/60 in the left eye, and the cornea demonstrated a healthy epithelium with minimal conjunctival injection (Fig. 19.6c).

As mentioned, lr-CLAL would have been a better choice; however, since a suitable donor was not available at that time, she underwent a KLAL.

Patient was maintained on topical steroids and systemic tacrolimus and mycophenolate. She experienced a number of side effects including migraines, stomach ache, and generalized body aches particularly in the arms and calves, which was attributed in part to the tacrolimus. At some point it was thought that she may have had a seizure and tacrolimus was abruptly stopped at an outside hospital. Within a few weeks, the patient presented with acute rejection which was treated with oral and topical steroids. Rapamycin was added as a substitute for tacrolimus.

Although this patient was young and healthy, given her seizure disorder and other systemic medications, the standard immunosuppression was not very well tolerated. Nonetheless, she was maintained on lower doses of medications along with more potent topical steroids.

Over the next few years, the patient maintained a vision in the 20/50–20/60 range (with scleral lens) (Fig. 19.6d). She also developed elevated intraocular pressure and IOP lowering drops were added. Her corneal epithelium demonstrated a mixed corneal and conjunctival phenotype. As a result of chronic steroids, her posterior subcapsular cataract slowly progressed reducing her vision to CF at 2 m. Therefore, she underwent phacoemulsification and intraocular lens implantation in the left eye improving her VA to 20/70 with a scleral lens.

Two years later, her LSCD had continued to progress and she was developing recurrent epithelial defects. Visual acuity was reduced to count finger. She was scheduled for living related conjunctival-limbal allograft from her son. The donor was screened for hepatitis B and C, HIV, HTLV-1, and syphilis. Given that the patient had more severe disease superiorly, the donor tissues were placed in the temporal and nasal quadrants but decentered superiorly. Postoperatively, the patient noted improved vision to 20/100 (20/50 with scleral lens) with healthy corneal epithelium covering most of the cornea (some conjunctival-type epithelium inferiorly). She continues to take mycophenolate 1000 mg twice daily and rapamycin 2 mg daily.

This patient's vision could be improved further with a keratoplasty; however, we have elected to keep her own cornea in part since keratoplasty could make the cornea more prone to wound healing issues.

As this case demonstrates, the management of chronic SJS can be challenging. This patient did not have extensive keratinization or scarring and the main problem was LSCD which made them a good candidate for surface reconstruction. Nonetheless, it is not uncommon that these patients have to undergo repeat limbal transplants every few years. Given that SJS patients have compromised defense mechanisms on the ocular surface, they seem to be more prone to infectious complications, and therefore in general, for SJS patients we do not recommend Kpro except in cases where functional vision cannot be maintained using tissue transplants.

Case 4: Simple Limbal Epithelial Transplantation

The patient is a 43-year-old male with a history of unilateral acid injury in the left eye. His past ocular history was remarkable for a history of LASIK 10 years earlier. At the time of his injury, his severity level was considered to be a Dua grade 4 with total corneal and conjunctival epithelial defect. His LASIK flap was found to be necrotic and was amputated. He was managed in a standard fashion with frequent topical steroids (q1–2 h initially, tapered after a few weeks), oral doxycycline, oral vitamin C, as well as topical IOP lowering medications. His course was remarkable for a persistent epithelial defect that took 5 months to heal only after he underwent a tarsorrhaphy.

At 7 months after his injury, he was evaluated for a possible autologous limbal transplantation. His medications at the time included autologous serum and topical steroids to reduce inflammation. His visual acuity in the affected eye was 20/600 (PH to 20/400), IOP was 18. The exam revealed 360° of limbal stem cell deficiency with superficial neovascularization and anterior stromal haze (Fig. 19.8a).

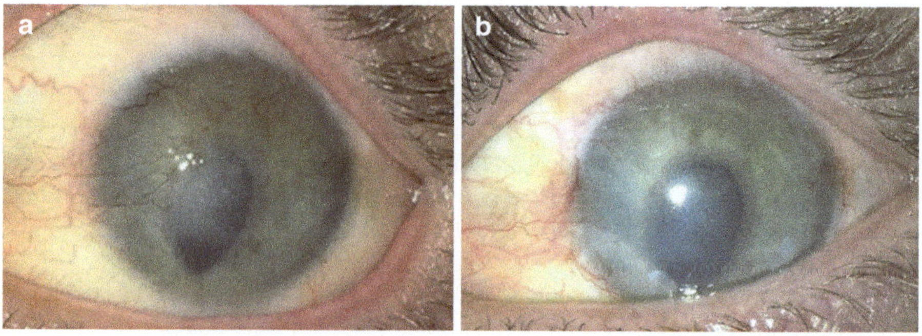

Fig. 19.8 Pre-operative appearance of the cornea demonstrated total limbal stem cell deficiency (**a**). Postoperative appearance at 12 weeks (**b**) demonstrating a healthy corneal-type epithelium. The limbal pieces are becoming less apparent with time

When Is the Best Time to Do Limbal Transplantation in a Patient with Chemical Injury?

The most important issue is to delay surgery until the ocular surface becomes more suitable for the new limbal grafts, in particular, to wait until the inflammation from the acute injury has subsided. Typically, this takes a minimum of 6 months, but it is preferred to wait up to 1 year (or longer). In patients with ongoing inflammation several months after the injury, we continue topical steroids (assuming there is no persistent epithelial defect and IOP is controlled) and also add a systemic agent such as mycophenolate. Other measures that may be considered for improving the ocular surface include punctal occlusion and serum tears.

What Are the Surgical Options in a Patient with Unilateral LSCD due to Chemical Injury?

The first step is to make sure that the injury was definitely unilateral and that the other eye is completely healthy. This can be ascertained by asking the patient to recall if the injury affected the other eye and by closely examining the unaffected eye for signs of limbal damage. The most effective surgical procedure with the longest track record is a conjunctival-limbal autograft (CLAU). This involves taking two pieces of two clock hours each from the inferior and superior limbal area of the healthy donor eye and transplanting to the same location in the recipient eye. The tissue can be secured using fibrin glue only. The risk of inducing limbal stem cell deficiency from harvesting the grafts [in a completely healthy donor eye] is essentially zero given that the procedure has been performed hundreds of times worldwide and there is only one report of inducing limbal stem cell deficiency—in a donor eye that had subclinical disease due to contact lens wear. The other two options are simple limbal epithelial transplantation (SLET) and cultivated limbal epithelial transplantation (CLET)—described further below.

What is SLET, and What Are Its Advantages over CLET?

SLET is a procedure where a very small piece of limbus (one clock hour) is harvested from a healthy limbus and split into very small pieces and glued to an amniotic membrane that is glued over the diseased cornea. The donor limbus is often the contralateral eye but can also be ipsilateral eye if there is enough healthy limbus remaining. It is very analogous to CLET in which a similar size limbal tissue is harvested and expanded in the laboratory typically on an amniotic membrane substrate then a few weeks later the cultured epithelial sheet is transplanted to the patient. The main advantages of SLET are that it avoids the major cost and technical resources needed for CLET to expand the cells in culture. SLET only involves one procedure while CLET requires two procedures. Based on the midterm results published by the group in LV Prasad, the results of SLET seem to be very comparable to CLET [15].

How Do You Decide Between CLAU and SLET?

There is no easy answer to this question since there is no head-to-head comparison between these two procedures. However, if a patient has extensive conjunctival deficiency then a CLAU may be preferred since the graft can be harvested in a way to include a large conjunctival piece which can be used to reconstruct the conjunctiva. Also, if there is a high likelihood that the patient will need a keratoplasty in the near future due to extensive corneal thinning or scarring, then we prefer CLAU (given the concern that a keratoplasty after SLET may end up removing many of the limbal tissue pieces during the trephination of the host). In a patient with extensive pannus where the corneal stromal depth and extent of scarring cannot be assessed at the slit lamp an anterior segment OCT preoperatively can help with surgical decision-making.

The patient underwent a SLET procedure where the recipient eye first underwent a 360 peritomy with removal of the pannus. Next, one clock hour of limbal tissue was removed from the other eye and split into seven pieces (four relatively larger pieces and three small pieces) and secured to the contralateral side using fibrin glue. At the conclusion of the surgery, a 20 mm Kontur lens was placed in the eye.

Postoperatively, one of the larger grafts and two of the smaller grafts fell off in the first few weeks, but the remaining pieces remained adherent. The bandage contact lens was kept on the eye for 6 weeks (longer than really needed).

What Are Some Pearls for a Successful SLET Procedure?

Given that most surgeons have limited experience with this procedure, we consulted with Drs. Sangwan, Basu, and Amescua who are pioneers and experts in this procedure. Here are some of their pearls for success with this procedure:

- Preoperatively, one can use OCT to assess the corneal thickness. Lamellar dissection to remove any stromal scarring should be minimized particularly since stromal scarring often reduces significantly after SLET.
- One or two drops of brimonidine 0.2% prior to surgery help to minimize bleeding intraoperatively in both donor and recipient eye.
- Prior to gluing the amniotic membrane onto the cornea and exposed sclera, good hemostasis is essential (to minimize the likelihood of hemorrhage under the

membrane). Freeze dried/dehydrated amniotic membrane is generally not preferred since it has a lower adherence rate.
- When harvesting the limbal tissue, one can use the adjacent conjunctiva as a handle to facilitate the dissection (by avoiding the need to grab/crush the limbal tissue). This excess conjunctiva is trimmed off and if large enough can be glued back to cover the conjunctival defect at the donor site.
- The idea size for harvested limbal tissue is 1–1.5 clock hours (3–4 mm). It should be cut into 8–10 pieces of which 6–8 are placed peripherally and 2–3 paracentrally (sparing the central 3–4 mm).
- A small drop of fibrin glue is placed over each piece (not too much to cause the pieces to float).
- A bandage contact lens is absolutely critical and a larger lens that is less likely to fall out may be preferred. If there is any doubt, a temporary tarsorrhaphy can be used. The bandage lens is left in place for at least 2 weeks after which it is removed to assess epithelialization. It can be placed back if not completely healed.

At 3 (Fig. 19.8b) and 6 months after surgery, the patient continues to display a corneal-type epithelium over 100% of the cornea with visual acuity of 20/60 (limited by the residual stromal haze).

What Are Some New Thoughts in the Management of Acute Chemical Injuries?

The management of acute chemical injury has been reviewed recently [16]. It is well known that the most severe injuries carry a poor prognosis. Amniotic membrane as a graft or as a sutureless device is now used commonly after chemical injuries and appears to accelerate healing in the lower-grade injuries. However, for the most severe cases, amniotic membrane does not appear to alter the course, and thus many patients go on to have persistent epithelial defects that lead to stromal melting or ultimately perforation. At this time, there is no specific treatment that can alter the course of such cases. One new proposed treatment for a severe chemical injury is an allo-SLET (SLET using allograft tissue). Although the tissue is expected to be rejected over time, it can potentially promote re-epithelialization and help to stabilize the surface to hopefully prevent more serious complications such as melting and perforation. Another similar treatment proposed by Dua is the use of a free conjunctival autograft from fellow eye (not including any limbus) placed over the cornea in the acute stage. This provides a source of live cells given that in the most severe injuries there are no viable cells after the injury. More recently, we have observed promising results with the use of mesenchymal stem cells in experimental models.

References

1. Martin R. Corneal conjunctivalisation in long-standing contact lens wearers. Clin Exp Optom. 2007;90(1):26–30.
2. Rossen J, Amram A, Milani B, Park D, Harthan J, Joslin C, McMahon T, Djalilian A. Contact lens-induced limbal stem cell deficiency. Ocul Surf. 2016;14(4):419–34.
3. Kim BY, Riaz KM, Bakhtiari P, Chan CC, Welder JD, Holland EJ, Basti S, Djalilian AR. Medically reversible limbal stem cell disease: clinical features and management strategies. Ophthalmology. 2014;121(10):2053–8.
4. Mayer KL, Nordlund ML, Schwartz GS, Holland EJ. Keratopathy in congenital aniridia. Ocul Surf. 2003;1(2):74–9.
5. Skeens HM, Brooks BP, Holland EJ. Congenital aniridia variant: minimally abnormal irides with severe limbal stem cell deficiency. Ophthalmology. 2011;118(7):1260–4.
6. Holland EJ, Mogilishetty G, Skeens HM, Hair DB, Neff KD, Biber JM, Chan CC. Systemic immunosuppression in ocular surface stem cell transplantation: results of a 10-year experience. Cornea. 2012;31(6):655–61.
7. Ang AY, Chan CC, Biber JM, Holland EJ. Ocular surface stem cell transplantation rejection: incidence, characteristics, and outcomes. Cornea. 2013;32(3):229–36.
8. Djalilian AR, Mahesh SP, Koch CA, Nussenblatt RB, Shen D, Zhuang Z, Holland EJ, Chan CC. Survival of donor epithelial cells after limbal stem cell transplantation. Invest Ophthalmol Vis Sci. 2005;46(3):803–7.
9. Eslani M, Haq Z, Movahedan A, Moss A, Baradaran-Rafii A, Mogilishetty G, Holland EJ, Djalilian AR. Late acute rejection after allograft limbal stem cell transplantation: evidence for long-term donor survival. Cornea. 2016;36(1):26–31.
10. Kohanim S, Palioura S, Saeed HN, et al. Stevens-Johnson syndrome/toxic epidermal necrolysis—a comprehensive review and guide to therapy. I. Systemic disease. Ocul Surf. 2016;14(1):2–19.
11. Kohanim S, Palioura S, Saeed HN, et al. Acute and chronic ophthalmic involvement in Stevens-Johnson syndrome/toxic epidermal necrolysis—a comprehensive review and guide to therapy. II. Ophthalmic disease. Ocul Surf. 2016;14(2):168–88.
12. De Rojas MV, Dart JK, Saw VP. The natural history of Stevens Johnson syndrome: patterns of chronic ocular disease and the role of systemic immunosuppressive therapy. Br J Ophthalmol. 2007;91(8):1048–53.
13. Biber JM, Skeens HM, Neff KD, Holland EJ. The cincinnati procedure: technique and outcomes of combined living-related conjunctival limbal allografts and keratolimbal allografts in severe ocular surface failure. Cornea. 2011;30(7):765–71.
14. Nordlund ML, Holland EJ, Kersten RC. Ocular surface reconstruction in a patient with complete ankyloblepharon resulting from Stevens-Johnson syndrome. Arch Ophthalmol. 2004;122(6):934–5.
15. Basu S, Sureka SP, Shanbhag SS, Kethiri AR, Singh V, Sangwan VS. Simple limbal epithelial transplantation: long-term clinical outcomes in 125 cases of unilateral chronic ocular surface burns. Ophthalmology. 2016;123(5):1000–10.
16. Baradaran-Rafii A, Eslani M, Haq Z, Shirzadeh E, Huvard MJ, Djalilian AR. Current and upcoming therapies for ocular surface chemical injuries. Ocul Surf. 2016;15(1):48–64. pii: S1542-0124(16)30172-0.

Chapter 20
Surgical Management of Pterygium

Mehran Zarei-Ghanavati and Hamed Ghassemi

Case 1: Primary Pterygium

S.H.H. is a 45-year-old male with gradually decreasing vision and irritation in the right eye for the last 3 years. He has also noticed a reddish triangular growth onto his cornea from the nasal side. Patient is a farmer and works with direct exposure to the sunlight several months a year. Otherwise, he is healthy and takes no other systemic medications.

On examination, his refraction was:

$$\mathrm{OD}: +2.50 - 4.00 \times 170 \quad \mathrm{CDVA}: 20/50$$

$$\mathrm{OS}: +0.50 - 0.50 \times 090 \quad \mathrm{CDVA}: 20/20$$

On slit lamp examination, there is significant meibomian gland dysfunction (MGD) and a fleshy fibrovascular tissue advancing 4 mm onto his right cornea (Fig. 20.1). The remainder of the exam was unremarkable.

What Treatment Options Would You Recommend?

Because of his decreased vision and high amounts of astigmatism, an elective surgery is recommended—after at least 3 months of treating his MGD. In patients with any level of MGD, even minimal surgical manipulation of the ocular surface can result in refractory annoying symptoms. Based on this fact, we treat all MGD patients before any type of ocular surface surgery. Dry eyes, either due to evaporative or aqueous deficient dry eye, is present in nearly all patients with pterygium.

M. Zarei-Ghanavati, MD (✉) • H. Ghassemi, MD
Farabi Eye Hospital, Tehran University, Tehran, Iran
e-mail: Mehran_zarei@yahoo.com

A.R. Djalilian (ed.), *Ocular Surface Disease*,
https://doi.org/10.1007/978-3-319-15823-5_20

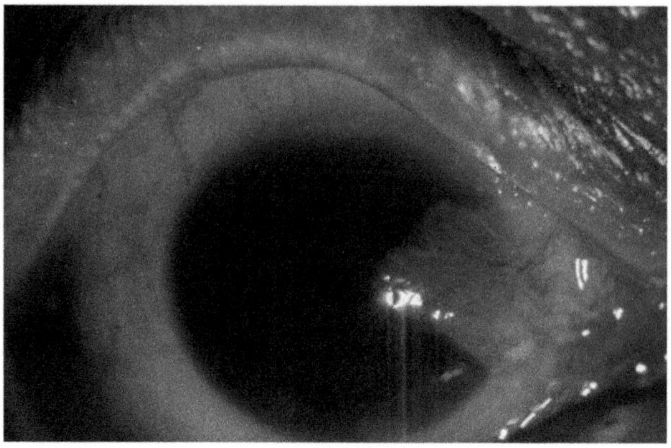

Fig. 20.1 A primary pterygium near the visual axis

What Is Your Preferred Technique for Pterygium Excision?

It is usually possible to perform surgery in primary pterygium with topical + subconjunctival anesthesia, although peribulbar anesthesia may be preferred in more pain-sensitive patients. For better exposure of the surgical site, we use a limbal or episcleal traction suture at the 6 and 12 o'clock position. The upper and lower borders of pterygium must be marked as well as the nasal border. After infiltrating the pterygium with lidocaine with epinephrine, scissors are used to cut into the pterygium along the nasal border which is extended to the upper and lower borders.

We propose a simple technique for cutting the firm attachment between pterygium and cornea. As we know the cornea is a multilamellar tissue and fibrovascular tissue of pterygium attaches to the cornea in different depths (deeper in periphery and more superficial in central area). If we attempt to avulse the pterygium as a whole from the cornea, deep centrally located intact corneal lamella must be sacrificed simultaneously with peripheral deep fibrovascular tissue, and this can result in thinning of the central cornea and a flattening effect in 180° meridian and high amounts of with-the-rule astigmatism. In our technique named "multiple rhexis" method, we grasp the fibrovascular tissue superficially as much as possible and try to separate one plane of fibrovascular tissue by capsulorhexis-like movements. This fibrovascular rhexis must be repeated plane by plane until all of fibrous tissue is separated from cornea. Afterwards any stromal irregularity must be smoothened with a rotary burr.

How Much Fibrovascular Tissue Should Be Excised from Free Borders of Conjunctiva?

Many authors believe that activated fibroblasts at the free borders of excised conjunctiva play a major role in the pathogenesis of recurrence. Therefore, all fibrovascular tissue should be excised with extension of at least 1–2 mm under the conjunctival free edge. The end point of this step is obtaining 1–2 mm of transparent conjunctiva at all free margins.

How and When Are Antifibrotic Agents Used?

Antimetabolite such as mitomycin C suppresses the activated fibroblasts that lead to the recurrence. Antifibrotic agents can be used in different ways. Many surgeons prefer to use them intraoperatively. In this method many pieces of soaked sponges with 0.02% mitomycin C will be placed for 1–2 min in the subconjunctival area near the free conjunctival rim. It is important not to use mitomycin C directly on the bare episclera as it can prevent remodeling of episcleral tissue after surgery and increase the risk of thinning and perforation, especially if cautery has been applied. In primary pterygium, we typically use mitomycin C only in cases that we use amniotic membrane and otherwise in cases where a conjunctival autograft is used mitomycin C is usually not necessary (except in younger patients with very inflamed Tenon's where we believe there is a higher risk of recurrence).

What Is the Preferred Technique for Closing/Covering the Defect?

Almost always after excising the pterygium, the defect area should be covered. Simple closure, conjunctival grafts, conjunctival flaps, and amniotic membrane all can be used for this purpose [1]. Simple closure can be used only in small pterygia with minimal defects and judicious dissection and separation of conjunctiva from underlying Tenon's capsule (the tractional forces can sever the sutures and cause the defect to open postoperatively). Conjunctival graft is the gold standard for defect management in pterygium surgery with the lowest recurrence rate and good cosmetic appearance. Attention should be paid not to include Tenon's in the graft. Conjunctival flap also can be used with recurrence rates comparable to conjunctival grafting. The cosmetic results with a flap may be inferior to an autograft. Amniotic membrane grafting is another option for covering defects where conjunctival autograft is not used [2]. If the conjunctival defect is very large, it is advisable to perform a temporary medial tarsorrhaphy at the end of surgery. Likewise, inferior punctal cautery may be performed at the end of the case.

We prefer to use fibrin glue to secure the graft (autograft or amniotic membrane). It decreases the operative time, improves patient comfort postoperatively, and reduces postoperative inflammation compared to suturing. Theoretically, recurrence rate with fibrin glue may be lower than suturing because of reduction of inflammation.

What Is the Postoperative Management of a Patient After Pterygium Surgery?

The two important points after pterygium excision are to decrease inflammation and to promote reepithelialization. Subconjunctival steroid at the end of surgery and frequent topical steroid in the early period after surgery are vital for reducing inflammation. Steroids are typically used for 3–4 months on a tapering dose. We prefer potent steroid drop such as betamethasone or prednisolone acetate 1% for 1 month after surgery and after that exchange it with a low-potent one such as fluorometholone. We often use a bandage contact lens to help promote epithelialization. Antibiotics are used while contact lens is in place. To promote reepithelialization, aggressive nonpreserved lubrication and nighttime ointment (after removal of contact lens) are used.

Lid hygiene and warm compress were recommended to the patient. Systemic azithromycin was also prescribed. Three months later he underwent pterygium excision with application of mitomycin C 0.02% for 1 1/2 min. Amniotic membrane was attached to conjunctival defect with fibrin glue and subconjunctival long-acting steroid was injected. Postoperatively, he was maintained on a tapering dose of steroids up to 3 months. At 12-month follow-up, the patient's best spectacle-corrected visual acuity had improved to 20/20 with minimal residual astigmatism.

Case 2: Recurrent Pterygium

The slit lamp photograph belongs to a 34-year-old man with history of pterygium surgery 4 years ago. The operation was done with mitomycin C application and amniotic membrane (AM) transplantation. Refraction is +2.0-6.0@175 with BCVA 20/20. He complains of decreased vision and eye redness (Fig. 20.2).

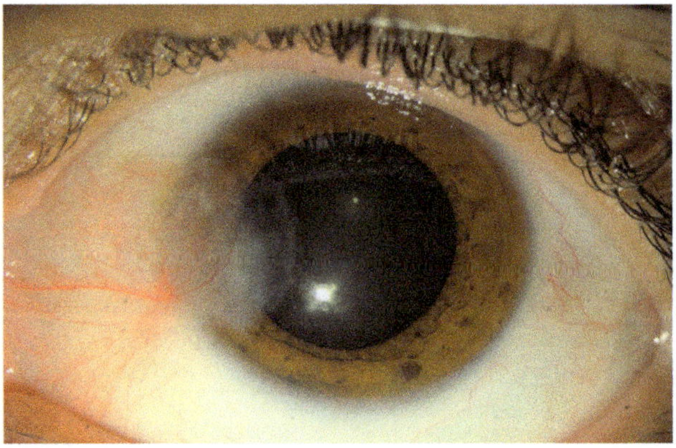

Fig. 20.2 Photograph of a large pterygium recurrence with induced corneal horizontal flattening, compatible with decreased vision and with-the-rule astigmatism

What Are the Important Issues That Must Be Considered When Planning Surgery for Recurrent Pterygium?

Since the specifics of the prior surgical procedure(s) may not be available, one should be ready for the worst-case scenario. One may encounter significant complicating factors such as corneal thinning, medial rectus fibrosis, contracture, severe conjunctival deficiency, and symblepharon. A preoperative OCT is helpful to determine the residual corneal thickness below the pterygium.

How Do You Explain the Prognosis to the Patient?

The patient should understand that the operation will be more challenging than the primary surgery. The chances of recurrence are higher and the visual outcomes; especially postoperative astigmatism are unpredictable [3]. The astigmatism (regular and irregular) will usually decrease after surgery, but more often than not, there will be visually significant residual astigmatism. If the pterygium involves the more central aspect of the cornea, the stromal haze will likely persist after surgery and affect the final visual outcome. Postoperatively, the patient will require closer follow-up and likely need topical medications, especially steroids, for several months, thus increasing the risk of increased intraocular pressure.

What Is the Preferred Method for Anesthesia?

Anesthesia will be very important in these cases. Topical or subconjunctival lidocaine is usually insufficient for recurrent pterygium surgery. Subenon's or peribulbar injection with good sedation is advisable. General anesthesia may be even necessary.

What Are the Key Steps in the Dissection of the Recurrent Pterygium?

Limbal tractional sutures are very helpful for exposure. The starting point for the pterygium excision can be either corneal or the limbal. While some surgeons recommend starting from the cornea in order to save more conjunctiva, particularly for patients with more contracture, we generally prefer starting near the limbus by finding an area where the conjunctiva is not fused to the sclera. This will help the surgeon dissect in the right plane; otherwise, it can sometimes be difficult to find the normal anatomical plane and one can inadvertently end up dissecting into sclera which has become fused with the fibrovascular tissue.

Meticulous removal of the fibrovascular tissue is one of the most important steps in preventing recurrence. The fibrovascular tissue is often bulky and becomes mixed with fat as one carries the dissection further back (in general, one tries to limit excision of the periorbital fat). Fibrotic tissue over medial rectus can be dissected more safely by first hooking medical rectus muscle. If medial rectus is not involved and no scar tissue is detected, muscle hooking is not necessary. During surgery, it is more likely that the surgeon will encounter hemorrhage. The use of topical epinephrine (or other decongestant) is helpful. To reduce the risk of scleral melting, it is better to minimize the use of cautery as much as possible. A combination of cautery, mitomycin use, and damage from previous surgery will increase the risk of this complication.

How Should One Use Mitomycin C in Recurrent Pterygium Surgery?

There is general consensus that intraoperative mitomycin CPterygium excisionrecurrentmitomycin C should be used in all recurrent cases [4, 5]. One typically has to use a higher concentration (0.04% instead of 0.02%) and/or longer duration (4–5 min instead of 1–2 min). Mitomycin C is never applied to the bare sclera, and instead the soaked sponges are placed in the subconjunctival space to treat the unexcised fibrovascular tissue.

What Is the Best Way to Cover the Conjunctival Defect?

Covering the conjunctival defect can be challenging in recurrent cases. Smaller defects are best covered with aPterygium excisionrecurrentconjunctival defect coverage conjunctival autograft which provides the lowest rate of recurrence. However, when conjunctiva is not available or insufficient, Amniotic membrane grafting pterygium excision amniotic membrane must be used. One option is to combine AM with conjunctival graft. In such cases, the conjunctival strip will be attached near limbus and the AM is used to cover the gap area between the graft and remaining conjunctival rim [6]. While some studies suggest there may be lower recurrence rate with the use of conjunctivolimbal autograft [7, 8], the evidence is not very strong, while there is greater risk of inducing partial stem cell deficiency at the donor site. We do not usually Pterygium excision recurrent conjunctival defect coverage include any limbal tissue in the graft.

The surgery for this patient was done under general anesthesia. After placing a limbal traction suture with 6-0 Vicryl, 1% lidocaine with epinephrine was injected subconjunctivally. We started to dissect the conjunctiva near the limbus at the superior border of pterygium and extended the dissection to the inferior border. After hooking of medial rectus, dissection of the fibrotic tissue over the muscle was carried out. No cautery was performed and 3-min mitomycin C 0.04% applied under the conjunctival rim. A conjunctival graft was harvested from superotemporal site and fixed with fibrin glue. At the end of

surgery, a bandage contact lens was placed and subconjunctival long-acting betamethasone was injected.

Postoperatively, chloramphenicol drops were used for 1 week and betamethasone drops for 1 month were prescribed. Thereafter, loteprednol was slowly tapered off by 3 months with careful monitoring of intraocular pressure. At 15-month follow-up, the patient had a BCVA of 20/20 after correcting residual with-the-rule astigmatism of 1.5 diopters.

Case 3: Impending Recurrence

A 35-year-old male underwent bare sclera pterygium excision with mitomycin C application. Figures 20.1 and 20.2 show the eye at 1 and 6 months after surgery, respectively Figure 20.3a and 20.3b.

One-month postoperative appearance of the eye demonstrating an avascular area corresponding to the mitomycin treatment (a) and 6 months later demonstrating an impending recurrence of the pterygium inferior to the excision site (b).

What Does This Clinical Picture Represent and How Should It Be Managed?

Outcome of Pterygium excision impending recurrence classification pterygium surgery has been classified into four grades: grade 1, the conjunctiva having no signs of recurrence; grade 2, only fine abnormal episcleral vessels being present at the surgical site; grade 3, fibrovascular tissue accompanying abnormal vessels in the excised area without involving cornea; and grade 4, fibrovascular tissue invading the cornea (true recurrence). Grade 3 lesion is considered an "impending recurrent pterygium" due to the possibility of progression to true recurrence [9].

The first step in these cases is to increase the frequency of steroid drops or, better yet, to inject the active Pterygium excision impending classification fibrovascular area with steroids (e.g., triamcinolone). There are some studies describing the use of bevacizumab for management of impending recurrence [10, 11]. Prabhasawat et al. studied the effect of 5-fluorouracil and triamcinolone injection for inhibiting pterygium recurrence [12]. The results showed that both 5-fluorouracil and triamcinolone injection decrease the chance of corneal involvement in cases with impending recurrencePterygium excisionimpending recurrencetreatment. Dua et al. showed effective suppression of recurrence (93%) by 5-fluorouracil injections [13]. Two main factors in this study were early time of treatment (within 1 month after surgery) and necessity of multiple injections. Mitomycin C injection has been used 1 month before pterygium surgery instead of intraoperative mitomycin C application. There is no study about postoperative mitomycin C injection for preventing recurrence.

Triamcinolone injection prevented further progression of the fibrovascular tissue onto the cornea in this patient.

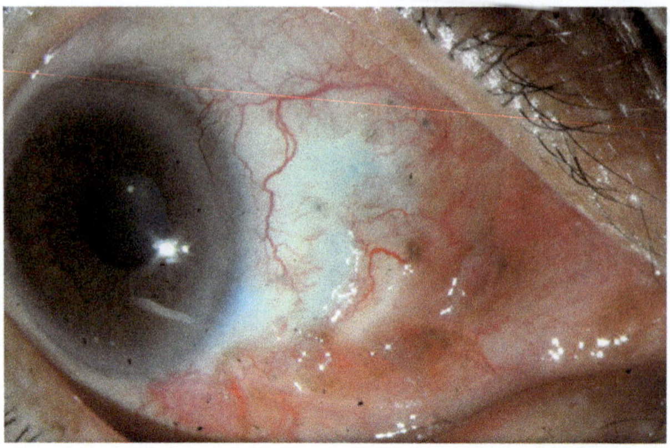

Fig. 20.3 One year after pterygium excision with amniotic membrane grafting. There is a relatively avascular area surrounded by injected fibrovascular tissue nasal and inferior to the graft site

Case 4: Poor Cosmesis

A 47-year-old patient underwent pterygium surgery nearly 1 year ago. The surgery consisted of excision, mitomycin C application, and amniotic membrane transplantation. He had good compliance for postoperative medications and follow-up. The patient is not satisfied with the appearance. The exam demonstrates a prominent area of whitening and avascularization surrounded by conjunctival irregularity and redness inferiorly and nasally (Fig. 20.3).

How Important Is Cosmesis in the Outcome of Pterygium Surgery?

It is well known that most patients choose to undergo pterygium surgery mainly to improve their cosmesis. The surgeons should consider postoperative cosmetic appearance to be just as important as pterygium recurrence. The goal is to have the pterygium excision site look just like the other side of the conjunctiva. The common complaints about cosmesis after surgery are excessive whitening of conjunctiva, bulky/red conjunctiva, conjunctival excess, scar line, and corneal scar/whitening.

What Are Some Strategies to Maximize the Cosmetic Outcome of Pterygium Surgery?

Conjunctival whitening is particularly common after mitomycin C application, especially in bare sclera or amniotic membrane transplantation techniques (Fig. 20.4). Extensive cauterization of episcleral vessels can also be a contributing factor. A conjunctival autograft (especially a thin graft with minimal Tenon's tissue) provides the most natural-looking appearance. A meta-analysis study found better cosmetic result with conjunctival autograft compared to AM transplantation [14].

Another complaint is having a thick and red conjunctiva surrounding the excision site. This is typically because there is excessive Tenon's tissue left behind. It is very important to dissect and excise all of the Tenon's in the subconjunctival space (especially inferiorly and nasally which are more visible) and leave a thin remaining conjunctival rim. Likewise, nasally the pterygium should not be excised too close to the limbus, and typically we recommend the excision site to be around 4 mm from the limbus. Finally, the use of sutures can induce inflammation and therefore fibrin glue is preferred.

Conjunctival excess can also create folds which become inflamed due to recurrent trauma with blinking. It may develop after a large and overlapping conjunctival graft or from epithelialization of the amniotic membrane under the conjunctival rim, especially in preexisting conjunctivochalasis. The surgeon sometimes overestimates the size of conjunctival defect because of excessive traction of globe in abduction which expands the defect size.

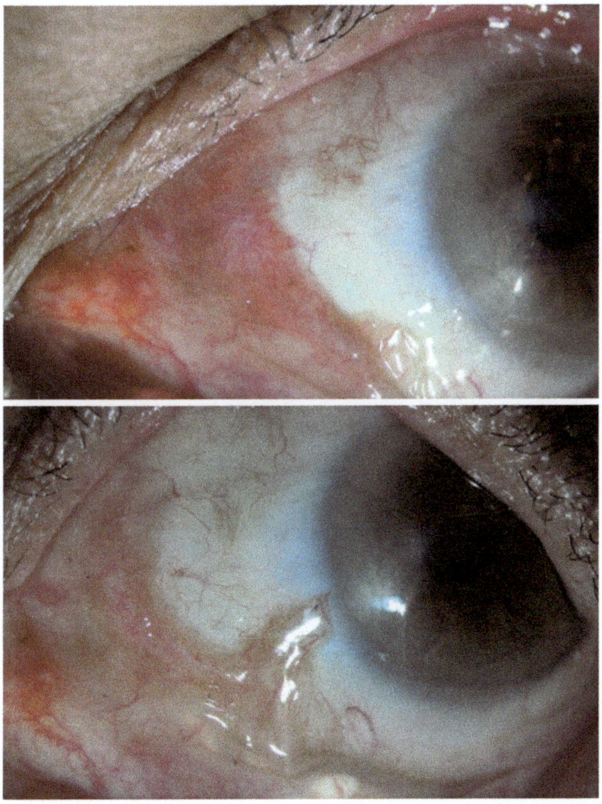

Fig. 20.4 One-month postoperative appearance of the eye demonstrating an avascular area corresponding to the mitomycin treatment (*top*) and 6 months later demonstrating an impending recurrence of the pterygium inferior to the excision site (*bottom*)

Finally, there can be a visible scar line. This can be avoided by close apposition of the conjunctival rim and the graft. Judicious use of steroids (topical/subconjunctival) can likewise decrease inflammation and scar formation.

Corneal haze and opacity can persist after surgery especially in patients with long-lasting pterygium. It is best to avoid trying to remove the stroma haze given the risk of stromal thinning and inducing astigmatism. The management of corneal haziness and scarring in the optical zone should be postponed for future surgery based on visual outcomes.

What Is a Suitable Plan for this Patient?

The surgeon can consider some steps to deal with patients' dissatisfaction in regard to cosmesis. First, the appearance of the surgical site usually improves with time. So, waiting for a few more months is usually advisable for mildly affected patients. Steroid drops or injection and sometimes 5-FU injections are useful to suppress inflammation, vascularization, and scar formation. We do not have any method to treat avascularization and whitening other than a conjunctiva graft or flap used only rarely for just cosmetic issue, but it is the effective treatment for severe scleral avascularization and impending scleral melting. For conjunctival redundancy and tags, especially those that move with lid movement, similar to conjunctivochalasis, excision may be necessary.

This patient did not want to undergo any further surgery and instead underwent an injection of steroids in the fibrovascular area which partially reduced the injection.

References

1. Prabhasawat P, Barton K, Burkett G, Tseng SC. Comparison of conjunctival autografts, amniotic membrane grafts, and primary closure for pterygium excision. Ophthalmology. 1997;104(6):974–85.
2. Küçükerdönmez C, Akova YA, Altinörs DD. Comparison of conjunctival autograft with amniotic membrane transplantation for pterygium surgery: surgical and cosmetic outcome. Cornea. 2007;26(4):407–13.
3. Ti SE, Chee SP, Dear KB, Tan DT. Analysis of variation in success rates in conjunctival autografting for primary and recurrent pterygium. Br J Ophthalmol. 2000;84(4):385–9.
4. Shehadeh-Mashor R, Srinivasan S, Boimer C, Lee K, Tomkins O, Slomovic AR. Management of recurrent pterygium with intraoperative mitomycin C and conjunctival autograft with fibrin glue. Am J Ophthalmol. 2011;152(5):730–2.
5. Narsani AK, Nagdev PR, Memon MN. Outcome of recurrent pterygium with intraoperative 0.02% mitomycin C and free flap limbal conjunctival autograft. J Coll Physicians Surg Pak. 2013;23(3):199–202.

6. Barbosa JB, De Farias CC, Hirai FE, Pereira Gomes JÁ. Amniotic membrane transplantation with narrow-strip conjunctival autograft vs conjunctival autograft for recurrent pterygia. Eur J Ophthalmol. 2016;12:0.
7. Al Fayez MF. Limbal versus conjunctival autograft transplantation for advanced and recurrent pterygium. Ophthalmology. 2002;109(9):1752–5.
8. Mutlu FM, Sobaci G, Tatar T, Yildirim E. A comparative study of recurrent pterygium surgery: limbal conjunctival autograft transplantation versus mitomycin C with conjunctival flap. Ophthalmology. 1999;106(4):817–21.
9. Prabhasawat P1, Barton K, Burkett G, Tseng SC. Comparison of conjunctival autografts, amniotic membrane grafts, and primary closure for pterygium excision. Ophthalmology. 1997 Jun;104(6):974–85.
10. Lekhanont K, Patarakittam T, Thongphiew P, Suwan-apichon O, Hanutsaha P. Randomized controlled trial of subconjunctival bevacizumab injection in impending recurrent pterygium: a pilot study. Cornea. 2012;31(2):155–61.
11. Fallah MR, Khosravi K, Hashemian MN, Beheshtnezhad AH, Rajabi MT, Gohari M. Efficacy of topical bevacizumab for inhibiting growth of impending recurrent pterygium. Curr Eye Res. 2010;35(1):17–22.
12. Prabhasawat P, Tesavibul N, Leelapatranura K, Phonjan T. Efficacy of subconjunctival 5-fluorouracil and triamcinolone injection in impending recurrent pterygium. Ophthalmology. 2006;113(7):1102–9.
13. Pherwani A, Vakil V, Eatamadi H, Singh R, Dua HS. Postoperative subconjunctival 5-fluorouracil in the management of recurring pterygium. Br J Ophthalmol. 2007;91(3):398–9.
14. Li M, Zhu M, Yu Y, Gong L, Zhao N, Robitaille MJ. Comparison of conjunctival autograft transplantation and amniotic membrane transplantation for pterygium: a meta-analysis. Graefes Arch Clin Exp Ophthalmol. 2012;250(3):375–81.

Chapter 21
Evaluation and Management of Acute Stevens-Johnson Syndrome

Jessica B. Ciralsky, Kimberly C. Sippel, and Darren G. Gregory

Case 1

A 5-year-old male was admitted with a 6-day history of high fevers and blistering on his lips and oral mucosa, which had limited his ability to eat and drink. One day prior to admission, conjunctivitis and a blistering rash on the hands and feet had also developed. He was intubated due to poor oxygen saturation and labored breathing. Although the skin involvement was limited to a few blisters on the hands and feet, the patient was diagnosed with SJS due to the coexistent significant mucous membrane involvement.

When and How Should the Eyes Be Evaluated in Acute SJS/TEN?

Studies have shown that the severity of ocular involvement in acute SJS/TEN does not always correlate with the severity or extent of skin involvement and systemic illness [16–18]. Therefore, an ophthalmologic evaluation of the lids and ocular surface should be part of the initial admission process for all cases of SJS/TEN,

J.B. Ciralsky, MD • K.C. Sippel, MD
Weill Cornell Medical College, New York, NY, USA

D.G. Gregory, MD (✉)
University of Colorado School of Medicine,
1675 Aurora Ct., Mailstop f.731, Aurora, CO 80238, USA
e-mail: darren.gregory@ucdenver.edu

A.R. Djalilian (ed.), *Ocular Surface Disease*,
https://doi.org/10.1007/978-3-319-15823-5_21

regardless of the severity of skin involvement. The goal of the initial ophthalmic examination is primarily to assess the extent of sloughing of the epithelium of the cornea, conjunctiva, and lid margins. Following the application of topical anesthetic drops, the eyes and eyelids should be rinsed with sterile saline to remove mucus. Fluorescein dye should then be applied to the surface of the eyes. Using fluorescein strips, rather than drops, gives a more controlled application of the dye. The extent of fluorescein staining can be easily assessed with the cobalt blue light available on penlights or direct ophthalmoscopes. It is crucial that the lids be retracted and if possible even everted, so the entire palpebral conjunctiva (in particular the portion covering the tarsus) can be inspected for staining. Studies have shown that tarsal scarring from SJS/TEN is a major source of long-term visual disability [19]. The condition of the eyes can change rapidly in the acute phase, so daily exams should be performed until it is clear that the areas of sloughing are healing.

Initial ophthalmologic exam showed 8 mm epithelial defects on both corneas with mild conjunctival injection but minimal staining of the bulbar and palpebral conjunctiva. There was staining along the lid margins of all four eyelids with whitening of the skin at the mucocutaneous junction (Fig. 21.1).

An exam under anesthesia was performed in the operating room on Day 2 of hospitalization. The whitened areas on the lid margins were grasped with toothed forceps and with gentle traction of the entire epithelium on the lid margins, and palpebral conjunctiva is peeled off. AMT was immediately performed on all four eyelids, and a 15 mm Prokera was placed on each eye.

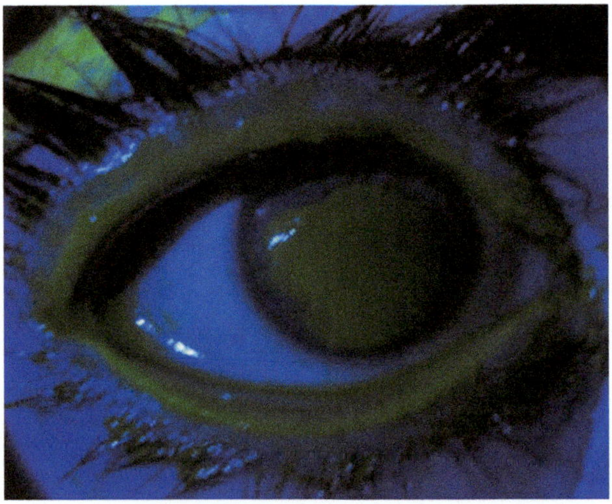

Fig. 21.1 Case 1: Fluorescein stain showing quiet bulbar conjunctiva but extensive sloughing of epithelium on the lid margins, tarsal conjunctiva, and cornea

How Do You Decide What Type of Amniotic Membrane to Use and How It Should Be Applied?

The decision to use amniotic membrane is based on the extent and location of epithelial sloughing as highlighted by fluorescein staining (Table 21.1). Small areas of conjunctival sloughing (less than 1 cm in longest dimension) will generally heal without significant scarring if they are not expanding, and there are not multiple such areas adjacent to one another. If enough normal mucosa is retained, it can heal in the small areas of sloughing with normal mucosa. If the areas of staining are extensive, however, the sloughed areas tend to heal in with scar tissue rather than normal mucosa.

Any sloughing of the *corneal* epithelium is concerning, as it increases the risk for corneal infection and ulceration. Additionally, intense inflammation and sloughing of the limbal areas may lead to limbal stem cell deficiency in the long term and an inability to maintain a normal corneal epithelium.

Staining of the lid margins is also concerning as it may lead to damage of the meibomian gland orifices and eyelash follicles. In addition to misdirected lashes, there may also be distichiasis in areas that have had severe inflammation along the lid margins. Even if lid margin staining is limited, whitening of the lid margins is concerning. The lid margins may not stain if the dead skin has not yet sloughed off, but whitening suggests that significant necrosis and inflammation are occurring in this area.

Table 21.1 Classification of severity of acute SJS/TEN ocular involvement with treatment recommendations

Severity	Description	Treatment recommendations
Mild	Conjunctival hyperemia with no conjunctival, corneal, or lid margin staining	Medical, with close monitoring
Moderate	– Small area of conjunctival staining (<1 cm diameter) – Minimal lid margin staining – No corneal epithelial defect	Medical, with close monitoring
Severe	– Extensive lid margin staining (>1/3 of length) – Larger, more diffuse conjunctival staining (>1 cm diameter) – Any corneal epithelial defect	Urgent AMT to lid margins, palpebral conjunctiva, and ocular surface. May use Prokera on the ocular surface if not multiple areas of bulbar conjunctival stain but must still always cover the lid margins and palpebral conjunctiva with sutured AMT
Extremely severe	– Same as severe but multiple areas involved [multiple areas of severe involvement on lid margin, conjunctiva (bulbar and palpebral), and cornea]	Same as for severe but more likely to need sutured AMT to ocular surface, rather than just a Prokera. Also more likely to have prolonged inflammation that will need repeat AMT 1 week after the initial AMT

Cryopreserved amniotic membrane is the only form of the membrane that has been described in the treatment of acute SJS/TEN [1–4, 6, 7, 9–13, 15]. We begin the AMT procedure by trimming all the eyelashes as close to the skin as possible so that the membranes will be in close contact with the inflamed lid margins. We also debride any necrotic tissue from the lids and conjunctiva. Amniotic membrane is then applied to the lid margins and palpebral conjunctiva. A 3.5 cm square of amniotic membrane (AmnioGraft, Bio-Tissue, Miami, FL) is cut in half and each half is used to treat one eyelid. The membrane is fixated to the external eyelid skin 1–2 mm peripheral to the lash line using an 8–0 nylon running suture. The membrane is oriented with the stromal surface in contact with the epidermal surfaces being treated. Using muscle hooks, the remainder of the amniotic membrane sheet is then tucked over the eyelid margin onto the palpebral conjunctiva and into the fornix. This portion of the membrane is fixated to the posterior lid surface using a double-armed 6–0 polypropylene suture with both ends passed full thickness through the membrane, palpebral conjunctiva, and the eyelid, then tied over bolsters on the external eyelid skin. Generally two separate sets of full-thickness sutures and bolsters are required per eyelid, and all four eyelids are treated in this fashion.

Attention is then turned to the surface of the globe. If the staining involves only a limited area of the bulbar conjunctiva, then a Prokera (Bio-Tissue, Miami, FL) may be used to treat this portion of the eye. A Prokera is a 15 mm diameter symblepharon ring with amniotic membrane stretched across the lumen of the ring. The device is applied in a manner similar to a bandage contact lens (Fig. 21.2). A Prokera only covers the cornea and perilimbal conjunctiva with amniotic membrane, however. If there is extensive staining of the bulbar conjunctiva, it is better to apply a sheet of amniotic membrane that covers the bulk of the ocular surface. A full 3.5 cm square of AmnioGraft is a good size for this step. We prefer to attach the membrane to the bulbar conjunctiva with nylon sutures rather than using fibrin glue. We place a 10–0 nylon running suture circumferentially around the cornea approximately 1–2 mm peripheral to the limbus. We then place a single interrupted suture in each

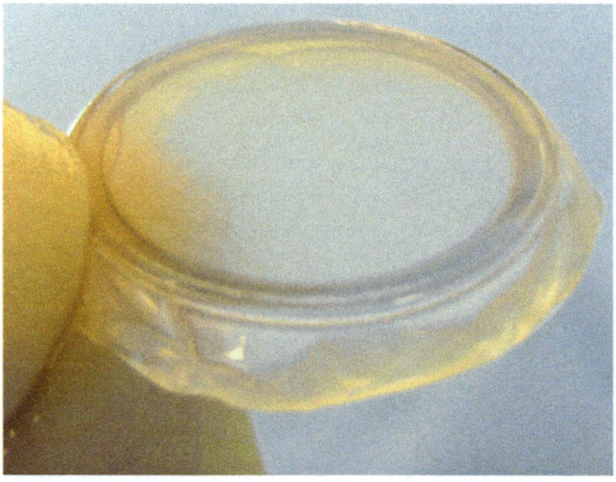

Fig. 21.2 Prokera device. Cryopreserved amniotic membrane stretched across the lumen of a symblepharon ring. Amniotic membrane covers only the cornea and perilimbal conjunctiva. In cases with limited bulbar conjunctival sloughing, a Prokera may be used in combination with amniotic membrane sutured to the lids and palpebral conjunctiva but is not an adequate treatment by itself

oblique quadrant and at the medial and lateral canthi. Leaving the suture tails long allows them to lie flat and also facilitates finding the sutures for later removal. This suturing may require a trip to the operating room, but we find it is more reliable in this situation than fibrin glue. Fibrin glue will not reliably attach the membrane if there are areas of intact epithelium interspersed among the areas of sloughing. If the ocular surface is treated with sutured AMT rather than a Prokera, we place a separate symblepharon ring on the eye once the membranes have been fixated in place.

It needs to be stressed that a Prokera alone, while easy to apply, does not constitute adequate treatment for acute SJS. It is imperative that the tarsal conjunctiva and lid margins be treated with AMT as well. Patients treated with Prokera alone have a higher risk of long-term problems from tarsal and lid margin scarring.

Twelve days after the initial AMT, another exam under anesthesia was performed. The lid sutures and Prokeras were removed. The corneal and conjunctival epithelial defects had resolved, with minimal ongoing inflammation. No further AMT was performed. The patient was discharged after 29 days of hospitalization.

What Is the Follow-Up and Treatment Regimen Following Discharge from the Hospital?

If stable without corneal epithelial defects, patients may be rechecked after 1–2 weeks. We generally continue a topical steroid drop such as fluorometholone 0.1% two to four times per day, cyclosporine 0.05% drops two times per day (Restasis, Allergan, Irvine, CA), and tobramycin 0.3%/dexamethasone 0.1% ointment to the lid margins for 1–2 months depending on the patient's symptoms and intraocular pressure.

After 9 months of follow-up, the patient had no dry eye symptoms and BCVA was 20/20 in each eye. There was mild scarring of the inferior tarsal conjunctiva in each eye without keratinization (Fig. 21.3). No other ocular surface sequelae had occurred.

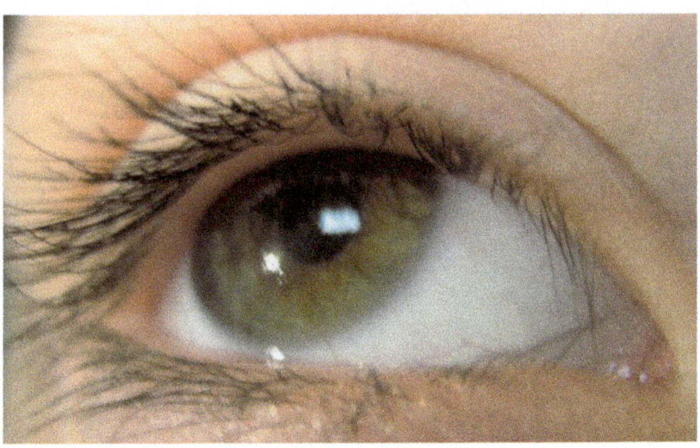

Fig. 21.3 Case 1 outcome 6 months after amniotic membrane transplantation for acute Stevens-Johnson syndrome. Minimal scarring and no dry eye problems

Case 2

A 70-year-old woman with a past medical history of gout had recently been started on allopurinol treatment. She presented to the emergency room with a 1-day history of bilateral eye pain, epiphora, conjunctival injection, and oral mucosal sloughing and was admitted for suspected SJS.

What Is Your Treatment Approach to This Patient?

In patients with acute SJS, ophthalmic involvement can be severe and devastating. Damage wrought to the ocular surface in the acute phase of disease can lead to permanent ocular sequelae, including blindness and debilitating eye pain. Furthermore, ocular involvement can rapidly evolve. Therefore, these patients should be thoroughly examined and followed closely, as described in the previous case. Many reports have shown that aggressively treating inflammation during the acute phase limits long-term damage and ocular sequelae. Treatment with intensive topical anti-inflammatory medications (corticosteroids and possibly cyclosporine) and prophylactic antibiotic drops (especially in the presence of a corneal epithelial defect) may be initiated, and consideration should be given to AMT, depending on the extent of epithelial sloughing on the ocular surface and eyelids (Table 21.1). Additionally, daily eye examinations should be performed to assess for any worsening.

The patient was started on hourly topical fluorometholone ointment (FML 0.1 %, Allergan, Irvine, CA) and a broad-spectrum topical antibiotic drop four times a day. Daily eye examinations were performed and included thorough inspection of her eyelids, conjunctivae (bulbar and palpebral), and corneas for fluorescein staining.

Over the next 48 hours, the patient worsened from both an ophthalmic and systemic standpoint, eventually requiring intubation for respiratory distress. Her ophthalmic findings included worsening injection and the development of conjunctival epithelial defects involving both the bulbar conjunctiva and eyelid margins of both eyes.

How Would Your Management Change at This Stage?

In the acute stage of Stevens-Johnson syndrome, progression can occur quickly. Initiating therapy with medical treatments alone is often the first step for patients with similar ophthalmic presentations. Every 24 hours, the patient should be reevaluated to assess the amount of ophthalmic involvement and the response to medical therapy. In this patient, when the ophthalmic picture worsened despite aggressive topical medical treatment, surgical intervention with amniotic membrane was considered.

After a long discussion with the family about the proposed treatment with amniotic membrane, including the risks, benefits, and alternatives, it was decided to initially treat only the left eye with amniotic membrane. Both eyes continued to receive aggressive topical medical therapy.

What Surgical Technique Should Be Used? Where Should the Procedure Be Performed?

The surgical technique for amniotic membrane application in acute SJS/TEN should ensure that all denuded and inflamed surfaces are completely covered with amniotic membrane. We used the technique described by Gregory and covered the lid margins, all conjunctival surfaces (palpebral, forniceal, and bulbar), and the cornea with amniotic membrane [5, 8] For this particular patient, surgery was performed at the bedside based on the recommendation of the primary team. If possible, our preference is to perform surgery in the operating room as this allows for the use of the ophthalmic microscope. However, if the patient is deemed too unstable for transport to the operating room, surgery can safely be performed at the bedside. As is usually the case with the bedside technique, Prokeras were used to cover the cornea and perilimbal bulbar conjunctiva (the bulbar conjunctiva beyond the perilimbal region would require a sheet of sutured amniotic membrane, and suturing to the bulbar surface is difficult without an operating microscope). Four sheets of amniotic membrane were used to cover the lid margins and palpebral conjunctiva of the four eyelids; this can readily be performed without an operating microscope.

Daily examinations were continued. The surgically treated left eye stabilized. The right eye, however, developed pseudomembranes and early symblepharon on Day 6 after disease onset.

How Would You Proceed at This Stage?

Given the deterioration in the right eye and the successful halting of progression in the left eye, application of amniotic membrane to the right eye should be strongly considered.

Amniotic membrane was applied to the right eye using a similar surgical approach on Day 6. Both eyes stabilized in the ensuing weeks and the patient was eventually discharged.

Follow-up examinations revealed significant differences in the clinical outcome of the two eyes. The patient had much more significant complaints of irritation and fluctuating vision in the right eye. Furthermore, the right eye

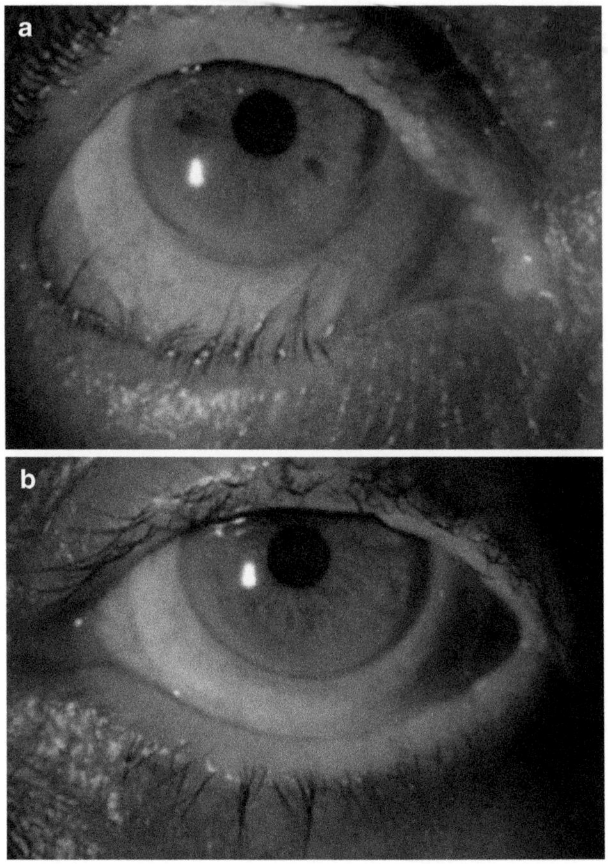

Fig. 21.4 Case 2 outcome at 4 months showing a significant difference between the right and left eye. (**a**) The top eye, treated 6 days into the illness, showed cicatricial entropion, trichiasis, and conjunctival injection. A fluid-filled scleral contact lens (PROSE) is in place. (**b**) The bottom eye, treated 2 days into the illness showed normal lid position with no entropion or trichiasis. A PROSE device is also in place (Reprinted with permission from Dove Medical Press Ltd) [14]. *PROSE* prosthetic replacement of the ocular surface ecosystem.

revealed a lower lid cicatricial entropion, palpebral conjunctival cicatrix, trichiasis, and resultant breakdown of the cornea epithelium. The left eye had a normal eyelid contour and appearance (Fig. 21.4).

What Is the Proper Timing of Amniotic Membrane Application?

Many reports have touted the benefits of amniotic membrane in acute SJS/TEN, but the exact timing of application is not clearly defined. After a diagnosis of SJS/TEN, if the initial sloughing is not severe, it is acceptable to allow a day or two to determine the amount of ophthalmic involvement and the response to medical therapy alone. If the ophthalmic surface is severely affected or worsens with medical therapy alone, amniotic membrane application should be performed urgently. In this particular patient, the left eye was treated in the hyperacute phase (<72 h after disease onset), whereas the right eye was treated within the first week (Day 6). The left eye had a clearly superior result. The earliest possible intervention with amniotic membrane, when indicated for severe acute ophthalmic involvement, is recommended for better outcomes in patients with SJS/TEN.

What Is the Role of Systemic Steroids in Acute SJS/TEN?

There is strong evidence from the groups in Kyoto, Japan, that IV pulse steroids (methylprednisolone 500–1000 mg per day for 3–4 days) given within the first few days of the onset of disease can significantly reduce the cytokine storm that develops in SJS/TEN and significantly improve the outcome of the ocular disease [21]. The main downside of this treatment may be an increased risk of infection, and thus many burn centers in the USA tend to be reluctant in instituting this therapy. Nonetheless, it has clearly been shown to be beneficial and is a good choice to consider in patients where the etiology of the SJS/TEN is known to be drug-related. Intravenous immunoglobulin (IVIG) has likewise been used in steroid-resistant cases.

Case 3

A 44-year-old male was transferred to the burn intensive care unit (ICU) with a blistering rash involving 60% of his body surface area. The rash began 7 days ago (4 days after beginning oral sulfamethoxazole and trimethoprim for treatment of a urinary tract infection). The patient had notified his doctor's office when the rash began but was told to continue the antibiotics. Over the next 4 days on the antibiotics, he developed progressive mouth, throat, and eye pain, prompting hospital admission and cessation of the antibiotics. He was hospitalized at the other facility for 3 days prior to the transfer being completed.

What Should the Initial Management Include?

The first management step in acute SJS/TEN is to stop any potential trigger for the illness. Medications are frequently a cause, with sulfa antibiotics being one of the most common. Recognition of a new medication as a possible culprit is crucial because continuing the medication can further worsen the adverse reaction.

Transfer to a burn ICU is another important initial step. Studies have shown that patient outcomes in acute SJS and TEN are improved if patients receive the specialized care and support available in a burn ICU [20]. It is important that they will be transferred early in the course if there is progressive skin, airway, or eye involvement. In addition to the systemic support provided, a burn ICU is more likely to be

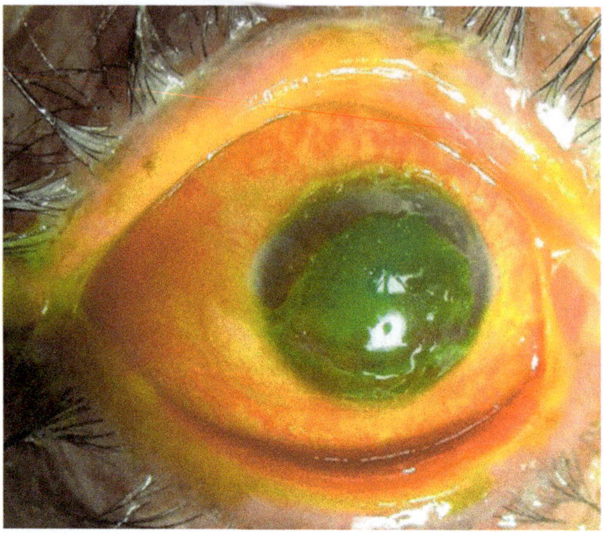

Fig. 21.5 Case 3: Extremely severe eye involvement in acute Stevens-Johnson syndrome, with extensive sloughing of the ocular surface, palpebral conjunctiva, and lid margins. For such cases it is important to remove the necrotic tissues and to cover the denuded surfaces with sutured amniotic membrane

aware of the eye issues and the possible need for AMT. An ophthalmology consult should be part of the initial evaluation of any patient suspected of having SJS/TEN, and the ophthalmologist must be aware that urgent AMT may be necessary in cases with significant ocular surface sloughing. If AMT is not an option at the initial admitting facility, the ophthalmologist may have to push for transfer to a facility where AMT can be performed. There needs to be an urgency to this process as the effectiveness of AMT decreases significantly after the first week of the illness.

On initial exam, both eyes were found to have extensive sloughing of the corneas, bulbar conjunctiva, palpebral conjunctiva, and lid margins (Fig. 21.5).

What Ophthalmologic Treatment Would You Initiate Based on These Findings? If AMT Is Planned, How Would You Apply It?

Urgent AMT is indicated in this case. Considering that the inflammation has been going on already for 7 days, AMT should be treated as an emergency and done as soon as feasible. Although they can be overnight shipped when needed, having cryopreserved amniotic membrane and Prokeras in stock and available is crucial in hospitals where SJS and TEN are managed with any frequency.

It is important that sutured AMT be applied to the lid margins and palpebral conjunctiva in *all* cases where AMT is used. If there is limited bulbar conjunctival sloughing, a Prokera may be used for the cornea/perilimbal bulbar conjunctival treatment, but it must always be in combination with separate sutured AMT to the palpebral conjunctiva and lid margins. In a case like this with extensive bulbar conjunctival sloughing, however, a Prokera is not sufficient for treatment of the bulbar conjunctiva. A sheet of cryopreserved amniotic membrane must be applied to the entire surface of the globe. As described earlier, a combination of interrupted and running sutures can fixate the membrane effectively [5, 8]. A symblepharon ring should be placed on the eye once the AMT is sutured into place. The suturing of the amniotic membrane to the bulbar conjunctiva generally requires an operating microscope in an operating room. It is rare for the patient to be too unstable to go to the operating room, but if that is the case, the lid and palpebral conjunctival AMT may be performed at the bedside using sedation, local anesthesia, and loupes. A Prokera may be substituted for the bulbar surface AMT, but again it is not optimal if there is extensive bulbar conjunctival sloughing.

On the day of admission, the patient was taken to the operating room. Necrotic epithelium was excised, and sutured AMT was applied to the lid margins, palpebral conjunctiva, and the entire bulbar surface of both eyes. Symblepharon rings were placed on both eyes following the AMT.

What Should the Management Be Following AMT?

We start these patients on fluoroquinolone antibiotic drops four times per day, topical steroids 2–4 times per day, and cyclosporine 0.05% drops (Restasis, Allergan, Irvine, CA) two times per day. Combination of tobramycin 0.3% and dexamethasone 0.1% ointment (Tobradex, Alcon, Fort Worth, TX) is also applied to the lid margins four times per day. It is important to keep the AMT on the lid margins moist with ointment or the membranes will desiccate and no longer be effective. Instructing the nurses on the proper application of the drops and ointment is crucial for success.

Following the placement of AMT, a daily ophthalmologic exam is performed to make sure the membranes remain intact and that there are no corneal infiltrates developing. It is important to rinse any serosanguinous debris off the eyes with sterile saline. If there are whitish areas over the cornea, the AMT can be moved with a cotton-tipped swab to see if the whitish area is on the membrane or on the cornea underneath. Usually it is just an irregularity on the membrane, but if it appears to be on the cornea, the membrane may need to be removed in that area for better inspection. Any suspected corneal infection should be cultured for bacterial and fungal pathogens. Patients in the ICU on antibiotic and steroid drops are at a higher risk for infections with rare or multidrug-resistant pathogens. Cultures play an important role in deciding what treatment is most likely to be effective.

At 10 days post AMT, the membranes were beginning to degrade (Fig. 21.6). The patient's skin involvement was beginning to heal.

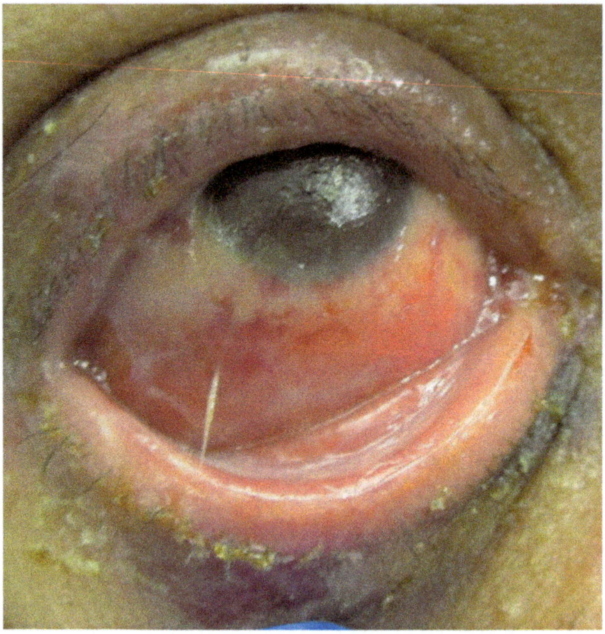

Fig. 21.6 Case 3: Ten days after the initial application of amniotic membrane. Repeat amniotic membrane transplantation was performed due to the persistent inflammation on the ocular surface and eyelids

What Should the Management Be at This Point?

Figure 21.6 shows significant inflammation of the lid margins and ocular surface. Repeat AMT should be considered. In many cases the eyes are quiet and appear to be healing after 10–14 days. In cases with extremely severe initial sloughing, however, the inflammation may persist longer. Repeat AMT can decrease the level of inflammation and tendency for scarring in these cases. Membranes that are not tightly adherent to the underlying surfaces should be removed and replaced. The lids require sutured AMT. Depending on the intensity of inflammation and sloughing, however, a Prokera may be considered in place of sutured AMT for the bulbar surface.

Repeat AMT was undertaken 11 days after the initial procedure. Amniotic membrane sheets were reapplied to the lid margins and palpebral conjunctiva of all four lids. Prokeras were placed on the surface of both eyes. The Prokeras and eyelid sutures were removed 12 days later. The eyes were quieter and no further AMT was applied. At 2 months post AMT, the patient had best corrected visual acuity of 20/25 in each eye with moderate dry eye symptoms and photophobia. There was mild to moderate scarring of the tarsal conjunctiva and significant meibomian gland dysfunction.

Why Did the Patient Develop Sequelae Even Though AMT Was Used Twice?

Despite two rounds of AMT, the patient still had some significant sequelae. Multiple factors contributed to this. First, the initial application of AMT was performed 7 days after the onset of eye symptoms. Earlier intervention is more likely to effectively suppress the destructive inflammation and subsequent scarring. Additionally, the degree of inflammation and sloughing in this case was extremely severe. In such cases, AMT still helps to prevent the devastating sequelae of SJS, but it may not prevent all sequelae. The sequelae that do occur, however, tend to be less debilitating. Patients treated with AMT are much less likely to develop the corneal blindness or severe eyelid and tarsal scarring that lead to a need for complex surgical reconstructive procedures.

Summary

The eye involvement in acute SJS and TEN can lead to permanently painful and potentially blinding ocular surface and eyelid damage. If performed early in the initial phase of the disease, AMT effectively prevents the more severe sequelae. The extent of epithelial sloughing on the mucosal surfaces of the lids and eyes is crucial in determining the severity of eye involvement. Ophthalmologists must be aware of the fact that AMT is an effective treatment for acute SJS and TEN and also be aware that the effectiveness of these treatments diminishes rapidly after the first week of the illness. There must be a sense of urgency in the evaluation and treatment of the disease and a recognition of the need to transfer severe cases to a facility where AMT can be performed.

References

1. John T, Foulks GN, John ME, et al. Amniotic membrane in the surgical management of acute toxic epidermal necrolysis. Ophthalmology. 2002;109:351–60.
2. Kobayashi A, Yoshita T, Sugiyama K, et al. Amniotic membrane transplantation in acute phase of toxic epidermal necrolysis with severe corneal involvement. Ophthalmology. 2006;113:126–32.
3. Muquit M, Ellingham R, Daniel C. Technique of amniotic membrane transplant dressing in the management of acute Stevens-Johnson syndrome. Br J Ophthalmol. 2007;91:1536.
4. Tandon A, Cackett P, Mulvihill A, et al. Amniotic membrane grafting for conjunctival and lid surface disease in the acute phase of toxic epidermal necrolysis. J AAPOS. 2007;11:612–3.
5. Gregory DG. The ophthalmologic management of acute Stevens-Johnson syndrome. Ocul Surf. 2008;2:87–93.

6. Shay E, Kheirkhah A, Liang L, et al. Amniotic membrane transplantation as a new therapy for the acute ocular manifestations of Stevens-Johnson syndrome and toxic epidermal necrolysis. Surv Ophthalmol. 2009;54:686–96.
7. Shammas MC, Lai EC, Sarkar JS, et al. Management of acute Stevens-Johnson syndrome and toxic epidermal necrolysis utilizing amniotic membrane and topical corticosteroids. Am J Ophthalmol. 2010;149:203–13.
8. Gregory DG. Treatment of acute Stevens-Johnson syndrome and toxic epidermal necrolysis using amniotic membrane: a review of 10 consecutive cases. Ophthalmology. 2011;118:908–14.
9. Kolomeyer AM, Do BK, Tu Y, et al. Placement of ProKera in the management of ocular manifestations of acute Stevens-Johnson syndrome in an outpatient. Eye Contact Lens. 2012;0:1–5.
10. Hsu M, Jayaram A, Verner R, et al. Indications and outcomes of amniotic membrane transplantation in the management of acute Stevens-Johnson syndrome and toxic epidermal necrolysis: a case-control study. Cornea. 2012;31:1394–402.
11. Hess TM, Chew HF. Successful treatment of acute ocular involvement in Stevens-Johnson syndrome with amniotic membrane transplantation: a case report. Can J Ophthalmol. 2012;47:e44–6.
12. Barua A, McKee HD, Barbara R, et al. Toxic epidermal necrolysis in a 15-month-old girl successfully treated with amniotic membrane transplantation. J AAPOS. 2012;16:478–80.
13. Tomlins PJ, Parulekar MV, Rauz S. "Triple-TEN" in the treatment of acute ocular complications from toxic epidermal necrolysis. Cornea. 2013;32:365–9.
14. Ciralsky JB, Sippel KC. Prompt versus delayed amniotic membrane application in a patient with acute Stevens-Johnson syndrome. Clin Ophthalmol. 2013;7:1031–4.
15. Sharma N, Thenarasun SA, Kaur M, et al. Adjuvant role of amniotic membrane transplantation in acute ocular Stevens-Johnson syndrome: a randomized control trial. Ophthalmology. 2016;123:484–91.
16. Lopez-Garcia JS, Jara LR, Garcia-Lozano CI, et al. Ocular features and histopathologic changes during follow-up of toxic epidermal necrolysis. Ophthalmology. 2011;118:265–71.
17. Gueudry J, Roujeau JC, Binaghi M, et al. Risk factors for the development of ocular complications of Stevens-Johnson syndrome and toxic epidermal necrolysis. Arch Dermatol. 2009;145:157–62.
18. Morales ME, Purdue GF, Verity SM, et al. Ophthalmic manifestations of Stevens-Johnson syndrome and toxic epidermolysis and relation to SCORTEN. Am J Ophthalmol. 2010;150:505–10.
19. Di Pascuale MA, Espana EM, Liu DT, et al. Correlation of corneal complications with eyelid cicatricial pathologies in patients with Stevens-Johnson syndrome and toxic epidermal necrolysis syndrome. Ophthalmology. 2005;112:904–12.
20. McGee T, Munster A. Toxic epidermal necrolysis; mortality rate reduced with early referral to a regional burn center. Plast Reconstr Surg. 1998;102:1018–22.
21. Araki Y, Sotozono C, Inatomi T, et al. Successful Treatment of Stevens-Johnson Syndrome with Steroid Pulse Therapy at Disease Onset. Am J Ophthalmol. 2009;147(6):1004–11.e1.

Chapter 22
The Use of Boston Keratoprosthesis in Severe Ocular Surface Disease

Kimberly M. Hsu and M. Soledad Cortina

Case 1

S.M. is a 35-year-old female with aniridia who came to us with gradually decreasing vision in the last 10 years. She reported 20/80 vision in childhood but had been counting fingers for the last 6 years. She had no history of glaucoma. On examination, her vision was hand motions in the right eye and counting fingers at 6 in. in the left eye. She had advanced aniridic keratopathy and cortical cataracts in both eyes (Fig. 22.1). Intraocular pressure was 11 in the right eye and 8 in the left eye. It was felt that the major cause of decreased vision in this patient was her keratopathy.

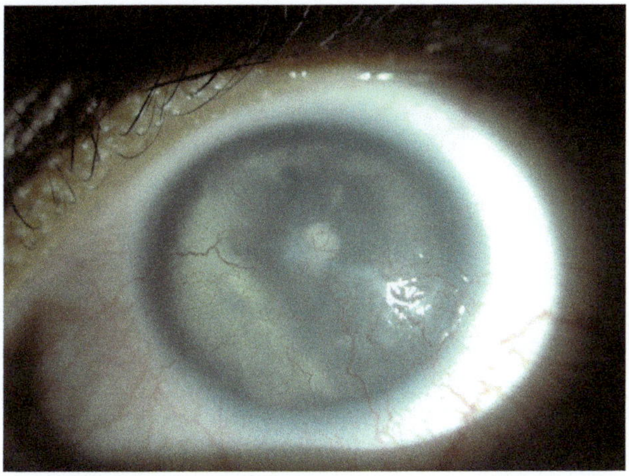

Fig. 22.1 Advanced aniridic keratopathy with conjunctivalization of the entire corneal surface. A cortical cataract is also seen

K.M. Hsu, MD • M. Soledad Cortina, MD (✉)
Illinois Eye and Ear Infirmary, University of Illinois Chicago,
1855 W Taylor St, Chicago, IL 60612, USA
e-mail: mcortina@uic.edu

A.R. Djalilian (ed.), *Ocular Surface Disease*,
https://doi.org/10.1007/978-3-319-15823-5_22

What Treatment Options Would You Recommend?

Aniridic keratopathy develops from limbal stem cell deficiency. Early epitheliopathy and conjunctivalization of the corneal surface starts peripherally and advances centrally with development of subepithelial fibrosis and stromal scarring in later stages. Before the development of significant corneal opacity, keratolimbal allograft or other limbal transplantation procedures can be attempted alone without a penetrating procedure to reverse the keratopathy. However, if the patient has advanced aniridic keratopathy as in our case, a penetrating procedure will be required. In this patient, there are two options: limbal stem cell transplantation followed by corneal transplantation or keratoprosthesis placement.

What Are the Considerations for These Options?

Holland et al. evaluated the success of keratolimbal allograft (KLAL) in aniridia and found that 74.2% of eyes achieved a stable ocular surface and 70% of subsequent penetrating keratoplasties (PKP) remained clear during the study period (mean follow-up 35 months). Long-term immunosuppression was required to improve the odds of maintaining a stable ocular surface [1]. The most likely cause of late failure is graft rejection which argues in favor of continuing immunosuppression beyond the first 2 years. Systemic immunosuppression with a combination of medications, often with cyclosporine/tacrolimus, azathioprine/mycophenolate, and oral prednisone, is required to reduce the risk of limbal graft rejection. Patients taking these medications should be monitored for toxicity, as discussed elsewhere in this book.

In recent years, the Boston keratoprosthesis has become an increasingly accepted option with the advantage of avoiding systemic immunosuppression and faster visual rehabilitation. Studies reporting outcomes of Boston KPro implantation in aniridics with follow-up of 17–28 months on average report visual improvement in 65–94% of patients. However, these patients need to be monitored for unique complications that can be seen after KPro implantation, including retroprosthetic membrane (RPM) formation, melting, worsening glaucoma, infectious keratitis, and device extrusion [2–4]. Although in traditional cases KPro implantation was considered after failure of prior grafts, in these patients KPro placement may be considered as the primary penetrating procedure in advanced keratopathy with or without prior failed KLAL.

Our approach to aniridic patients with limbal stem cell deficiency is as follows: In cases where the disease is limited to the epithelium and there is minimal to no stromal or endothelial disease, limbal transplantation, which is a non-penetrating procedure, is considered first-line treatment (assuming the patient is a good candidate for immunosuppression). Otherwise, when there is coexisting endothelial disease and/or history of previous graft failure, then

KPro may be a preferred option given that the success rate with limbal transplant may be lower. If performing cataract surgery at the time of KPro in aniridic patients, we typically prefer to leave the patient aphakic and use an aphakic KPro given that these patients have a higher likelihood of having zonular instability.

After discussion with the patient, it was decided to proceed with Boston type 1 keratoprosthesis placement in the right eye. Her cataract was removed at the time of surgery and an aphakic KPro was placed. Postoperatively, she was treated with topical antibiotics (gatifloxacin) which was maintained at TID for prophylaxis. A 16.0 mm Kontur bandage contact lens was also placed (changed every 2 months). At postop week 2, she had 20/80 vision but at month 1 had started to develop an RPM with decrease in vision to 20/100 (Fig. 22.2). A YAG membranectomy was performed approximately 5 months postoperatively. The vision improved, but approximately 2 months later, the patient was noted to have circumferential melting around the KPro optic. It was noted that the holes of the KPro backplate were filled with RPM tissue although the optic remained clear.

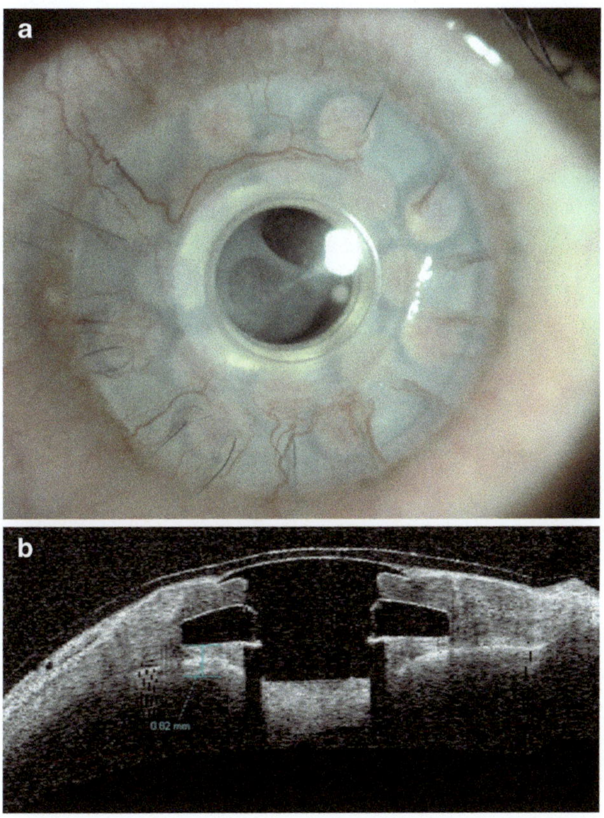

Fig. 22.2 (**a**) RPM formation after Boston type 1 KPro placement, with membrane behind the optic as well as filling the backplate holes. (**b**) Anterior segment OCT image showing the thickness of the RPM behind the optic and backplate

What Risk Factors Did This Patient Have for Corneal Melting?

It has been demonstrated that retro-backplate membranes may be a risk factor for corneal melting, possibly secondary to the impedance of aqueous providing nutritional support to the cornea. In a retrospective study, 100% of eyes that melted had evidence of retro-backplate membrane vs. 34% of eyes that did not melt. In addition, the retro-backplate membrane was thicker in the group that melted [5]. To compound this, patients with aniridia are likely to have an unstable ocular surface that may exacerbate the problem. Although this patient did not have any conjunctival disease, patients with conjunctival deficiency (Stevens-Johnson syndrome and mucous membrane pemphigoid) also appear to have a significantly greater risk of developing a melt after KPro [6].

In our patient, the backplate was noted to be exposed in some areas, although there was no Seidel-positive leak, possibly due to the presence of a dense RPM. Due to this, it was decided to proceed with KPro replacement.

The patient recovered well postoperatively but was noted to develop recurrent RPM which required YAG membranectomy approximately 4 months later. She began to develop increased intraocular pressures and was referred to the glaucoma service. Ultimately her IOP was uncontrolled with drops and oral medication, and she had a pars plana Baerveldt shunt placement approximately 10 months following the KPro replacement. Throughout her clinical course, she had episodes of persistent inflammation postoperatively and intermittent episodes of episcleritis related to her Baerveldt plate (Fig. 22.3), which at times required frequent topical prednisolone or oral steroids. Approximately 2.5 years after KPro replacement, she was found to have recurrent melting around the KPro optic again associated with a very thick retro-backplate RPM.

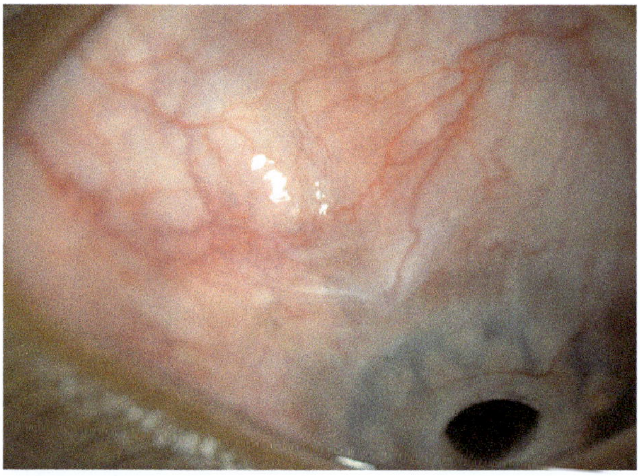

Fig. 22.3 Episcleritis associated with Baerveldt plate

What Options Can Be Considered at This Time?

This patient has recurrent RPM formation, ocular surface inflammation, and most problematic, recurrent corneal melting likely stemming from these issues. Aniridia has been found to be an independent risk factor for RPM formation, although whether this is due to chronic inflammation or another mechanism remains unclear [7]. To our knowledge there is no literature regarding systemic immunosuppression in KPro patients; however, due to this patient's propensity to developing RPM and episodes of ocular inflammation, it was felt that decreasing inflammation could stabilize her ocular surface and perhaps prevent RPM formation. There is some data suggesting that systemic immunosuppression is useful and well tolerated in patients with multiple traditional grafts [8–10]. In addition, a replacement KPro was needed given the amount of melting around the KPro optic.

She was placed on oral mycophenolate (1000 mg bid), and the KPro was replaced. At last follow-up 21 months after her second KPro replacement, she was doing well with 20/70 vision and clear optic.

Patients with aniridia should be monitored carefully after KPro placement, and complications managed promptly. Although melting and device extrusion increases morbidity, prompt treatment including replacement of KPro if necessary usually results in return to baseline vision.

Case 2

E.H. is a 41-year-old male who presented approximately 1 month after a chemical burn. He had sustained a workplace accident of anhydrous ammonia to both eyes, right greater than left. His eyes were flushed immediately afterward. While the left eye had mostly recovered, the right eye continued to have decreased vision, pain, and light sensitivity. On examination, he was counting fingers at 3–4 feet in the right eye and 20/25 in the left eye. He was noted to have superior and temporal ischemia, an epithelial defect covering most of the cornea as well as surrounding conjunctiva, edematous cornea, and cataract (Fig. 22.4). The left eye appeared normal. On presentation he was on ciprofloxacin four times a day, atropine once a day, and prednisolone acetate 1% every 2 h, all in the right eye. Over the next 9 months, he was managed with topical corticosteroids, oral corticosteroids, oral vitamin C, punctal plugs, amniotic membrane, and bandage contact lenses. Scleral lenses were attempted but with poor fit. He continued to have a persistent epithelial defect with decrease in vision to light perception. In addition, his intraocular pressure increased 4 months after

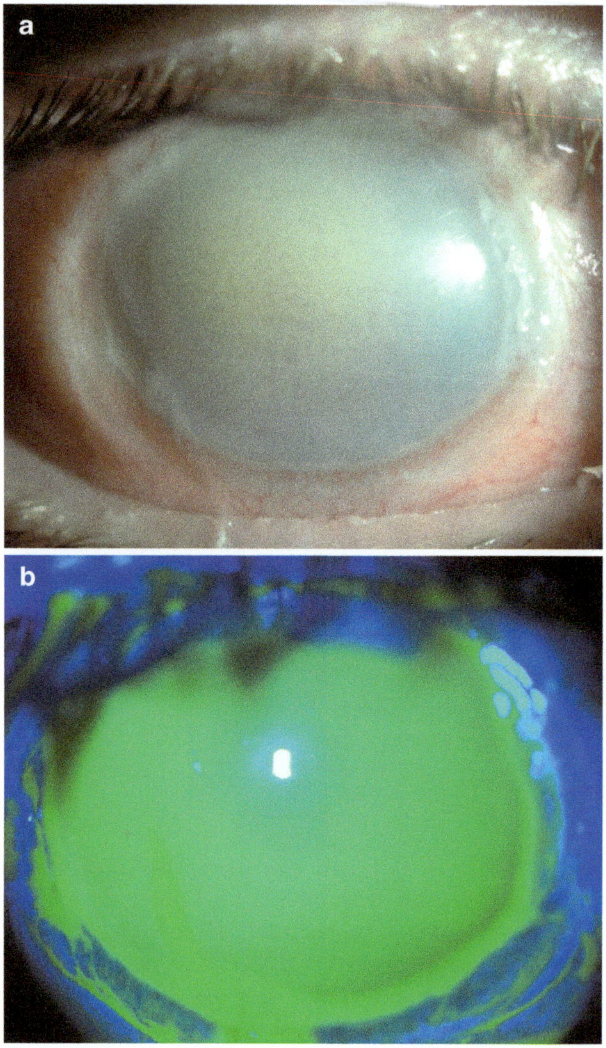

Fig. 22.4 (**a**) Chemical injury with limbal ischemia, diffuse corneal opacification and edema, cataract, and (**b**) limbus-to-limbus epithelial defect highlighted with fluorescein

presentation, necessitating maximal medical therapy and diode cyclophotocoagulation to achieve IOP control. Nine months following presentation, the patient had still a nearly complete epithelial defect of his cornea despite multiple treatment strategies attempted.

What Are Management Options for the Patient at This Point?

This patient has severe limbal stem cell deficiency from his chemical injury and is unable to heal his corneal surface 10 months after injury despite intensive therapy. At this point a strategy for stabilization of the ocular surface and visual rehabilitation should be considered. Severe limbal/corneal injuries usually result in irreversible corneal opacity that requires limbal transplantation with subsequent penetrating keratoplasty. Patients with less severe ocular surface injury may do well after these procedures; however, patients with severe injuries are prone to failure even after these measures are taken with a reported 50–60% or less of patients maintaining a clear cornea [11, 12].

KPro placement for chemical injuries has been reported to be a viable option. Most patients experienced significant improvements in vision, although complications included epithelial defects with sterile melting, likely related to an unstable ocular surface with limbal stem cell deficiency [13, 14]. Efforts to stabilize the ocular surface prior to KPro implantation should be undertaken as much as possible. One study showed that patients with chemical burn had relatively good visual outcome compared to other indications for KPro placement [15]. In addition, in our series of patients who received a primary KPro, that is, without a prior penetrating corneal procedure, we report good outcomes with 100% retention of the KPro in patients whose indication was chemical injury [16].

Keratolimbal allograft vs. keratoprosthesis placement was discussed with the patient, and given the unilateral nature of the disease, it was decided to proceed with Boston type 1 keratoprosthesis placement, lensectomy, amniotic membrane, and permanent lateral tarsorrhaphy. The patient's vision improved to counting fingers following surgery. Postoperatively, he was maintained on vancomycin 15 mg/mL bid. However, he was still noted to have a persistent epithelial defect; therefore, conjunctival flaps over the corneal portion of the graft, amniotic membrane, and a more aggressive tarsorrhaphy were performed 2 months after the initial surgery. Unfortunately, the conjunctiva retracted and the patient's epithelial defect persisted.

A recent study found that in patients with the Boston type 1 keratoprosthesis who required mucosal rehabilitation, free grafting and simple advancement flaps resulted in graft retraction in all cases, whereas vascularized pedicles and bucket handle flaps were stable 50% of the time [17]. Therefore, although these techniques may be effective in patients with cicatrizing conjunctivitis or chemical injury, after keratoprosthesis placement, the ocular environment may not be conducive to survival of these grafts.

In this patient, there was subsequently noted an area of instability at the graft-host junction temporally, and a temporary central tarsorrhaphy was performed in an effort to promote healing. This stabilized the graft-host junction and enabled the healing of the epithelial defect superiorly. After a month the tarsorrhaphy suture broke spontaneously, and the patient was returned to just using Kontur contact lenses; however, he had difficulty with keeping the contact lens in and frequently lost lenses.

What Other Options Are Available to Help Stabilize the Ocular Surface?

This patient has had some success with tarsorrhaphy although with only partial healing of his epithelial defect and with eventual loss of the temporary tarsorrhaphy suture. He frequently loses his contact lens. Conjunctival flaps and amniotic membrane grafts have not helped him. He requires a better solution to maintain coverage of his ocular surface at all times. While a permanent tarsorrhaphy could be an option, this would likely require a large tarsorrhaphy blocking any useful vision. Another option is a vaulted contact lens. Vaulted contact lenses such as scleral lenses or hybrid lenses are often good options for patients with ocular surface disease, providing ocular stability, comfort, and improved vision [18, 19]. There is little literature on the use of scleral or hybrid lenses in patients with an implanted KPro; however, in patients such as these who have persistent epithelial defects with or without melting despite a Kontur lens, these vaulted lenses provide a reservoir of fluid that often promotes healing. In addition, the suction effect between the rigid part of the hybrid lens and the KPro optic gives this lens an excellent retention compared to Kontur lenses, and we have found them very useful in patients with frequent lens loss.

He was referred to the contact lens service and fitted with a SynergEyes A hybrid lens (14.5 mm). This lens stayed in well and was effective in healing his persistent epithelial defect. After 3 months with the hybrid lens the epithelial defect had completely healed (Fig. 22.5).

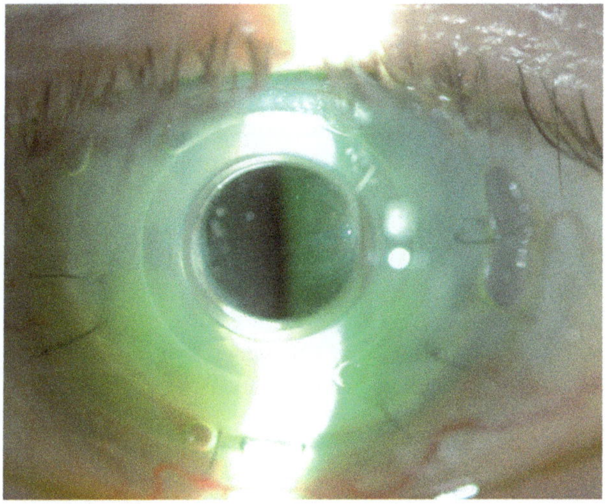

Fig. 22.5 Boston type 1 KPro with hybrid lens, which has healed the chronic epithelial defect

What Other Ocular Comorbidities Should Be Considered and Monitored in This Patient?

1. Cystoid macular edema (CME)
   Patients with chemical injury and chronic inflammation, as well as many other patients who have complex ocular histories leading to KPro placement, are prone to CME. Many patients likely have preexisting CME prior to KPro placement, but for most of these patients, fundus examination is difficult preoperatively. In addition, KPro placement may incite chronic inflammation that can lead to chronic CME. Fundus examination and macular OCT in the early postoperative period should be considered. Chronic CME in these patients can be difficult to treat and require multiple intravitreal injections.
2. Glaucoma
   Secondary glaucoma is not uncommon in patients with chemical injury. IOP pre-operatively can be monitored, but good optic nerve assessment and visual field testing may be difficult. glaucoma management such as the placement of a pars

plana glaucoma shunt at the time of KPro placement should be considered for patients who may be at risk for developing worsened iop control. Postoperatively, glaucoma testing should be performed on a regular basis and treated as necessary.

Shortly after KPro placement, since the visual acuity was only limited to count fingers, an OCT was performed which demonstrated significant cystoid macular edema (CME). This was treated with topical steroids without benefit. He then received intravitreal injections of triamcinolone and subsequently an Ozurdex implant which resolved his CME for a period of time. He had a waxing and waning course and received a total of three Ozurdex implants. His vision improved to 20/150 when his CME was under control. The patient also developed an RPM and this was treated with YAG membranectomy.

Patients with chemical injury often develop secondary glaucoma, and in this case, this was likely exacerbated with chronic steroids used for the treatment of CME. Following KPro placement, the patient's intraocular pressure was controlled with medical therapy for nearly 3 years. He then developed uncontrolled pressures, and the decision was made to proceed with placement of a pars plana glaucoma shunt with pars plana vitrectomy.

Case 3

J.B. is a 42-year-old female who has been followed for many years in our cornea clinic with a history of ectrodactyly, ectodermal dysplasia, and clefting syndrome (EEC). She had limbal stem cell deficiency in her left greater than right eye and for many years had relied on her right eye for functional vision. She had a history of corneal thinning and perforations in the left eye. At the time of her KPro evaluation, she was 20/50 in the right eye and counting fingers at 1 foot in the left eye. As characteristic of EEC, she was noted to have absent meibomian glands. In the right eye, the superior cornea was clear, while she had vessels and corneal haze inferiorly. Her left eye showed complete conjunctivalization with superior symblepharon extending onto her cornea. She was seen for a Boston type 1 KPro evaluation for the left eye.

How Can You Make This Patient a Better Candidate for KPro Implantation?

It is important to note and treat significant symblepharon and forniceal foreshortening in patients who are considering KPro placement. A healthy conjunctival fornix is important for ocular surface stability; forniceal foreshortening and symblepharon may restrict movement of the globe leading to decreased protection of the cornea, eyelid malposition with irritation of the ocular surface, and inadequate distribution

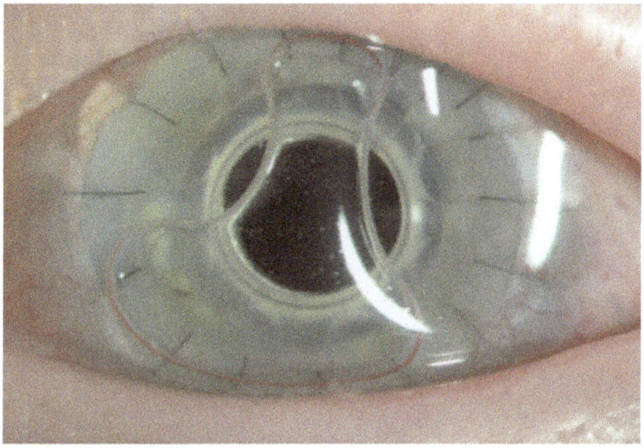

Fig. 22.6 Boston type 1 KPro in a patient with EEC, with absent meibomian glands, inflamed ocular surface, and poorly fitting contact lens

of tears. It may also limit contact lens fitting. Fornix reconstruction has been suggested to be beneficial prior to both limbal stem cell transplant and keratoprosthesis placement [17, 20] and was suggested for this patient. Once the patient is stable from this procedure with open fornices and ocular surface stability, she may then proceed with KPro placement.

The patient underwent fornix reconstruction with amniotic membrane graft on the left eye and subsequently did well with maintenance of a deep fornix postoperatively. Approximately 6 months later, she underwent KPro placement with pars plana tube shunt, and the shunt was able to be placed in the area of her fornix reconstruction (Fig. 22.6). Postoperatively, she was maintained on vancomycin 15 mg/mL bid which was later switched to polymyxin/trimethoprim for prophylaxis. Her vision improved postoperatively and was 20/40 at postoperative month 1; however, she was noted to develop an RPM within the first month. She experienced transient hypotony with choroidals as her tube opened. After about 3 months, she had a YAG membranectomy and vision improved to 20/25. In the next few months, she experienced decreased vision to 20/50 and was found to have CME. This was treated with topical prednisolone and ketorolac with improvement. However, after 2 months she returned to clinic after her contact lens had fallen out and was found to have mild stromal melting around the KPro optic.

What Issues May Have Led to Her Stromal Melting and What Would You Do Next?

Although the patient's ability to maintain a stable ocular surface was improved with forniceal reconstruction prior to KPro placement, she may still be prone to ocular surface instability due to her underlying condition, EEC. In addition, the topical steroid and NSAID that she required for CME treatment may have contributed to poor

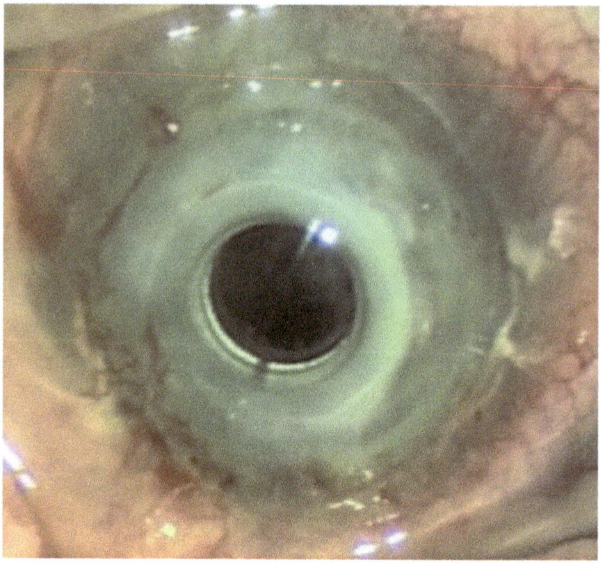

Fig. 22.7 KPro with melt and exposure of backplate temporally

healing of an epithelial defect and subsequent stromal melting. This is often a difficult balance to make; the treatment of CME can be at odds with ocular surface stability. Compounding this is the loss of the contact lens to protect the corneal surface. At this point, her CME is improved, and it would be reasonable to decrease or stop the steroid and NSAID and replace her contact lens as a first step with close follow-up.

Her prednisolone was decreased and ketorolac was stopped, and the bandage contact lens was replaced. Her epithelial defect healed with these measures; however, she experienced recurrent CME. She was placed back on prednisolone and ketorolac four times a day, and her corneal surface remained stable for 7 months when she returned with decreased vision and tearing. She was found to have a large area of melting with KPro extrusion and was hypotonous but Seidel negative at the slit lamp (Fig. 22.7). The decision was made to replace the KPro, and this was done the following day. She did well postoperatively and her vision returned to 20/25 at week one. However, 3 months later she presented with a new epithelial defect covering approximately 50% of the corneal surface with thinning. She also had intraocular inflammation related to the epithelial defect.

What Can Be Done to Help Stabilize Her Ocular Surface at This Point?

In the last case, a vaulted lens was used to heal a chronic epithelial defect. These lenses can also be used in an acute phase of an epithelial defect in this patient who has demonstrated the propensity for melting with a Kontur lens. In addition, if the patient does well with this, they should be kept in a vaulted lens for the long term to protect the ocular surface.

It was decided to place a scleral lens, and she was seen on a daily basis for removal and reinsertion of the scleral lens. After 5 days, the epithelial defect had mostly healed, and she was switched back to a Kontur lens while being fitted for a SynergEyes Duette hybrid lens (14.5 mm). Her surface stabilized, but she continued to have decreased vision and was 20/60 at last follow-up with macular ERM and CME. She is continued on topical prednisolone, and we have chosen to avoid topical NSAIDs given her propensity for corneal melting.

Conclusion

The Boston type 1 keratoprosthesis is a reasonable option in patients with ocular surface disease such as aniridia, chemical injuries, or limbal stem cell deficiency from any etiology. These patients are considered higher risk than patients who undergo KPro placement for indications such as multiple failed grafts because of inherent ocular surface instability and inflammation. They may also have other concurrent ocular morbidities such as glaucoma or retinal issues. However, patients can do very well and maintain large gains in vision postoperatively with close follow-up and prompt treatment of any complications. A multidisciplinary approach involving cornea, contact lens, oculoplastics, glaucoma, and retina is necessary to maximize the outcome of KPro implantation. Prior to placement of the KPro, the ocular surface should be optimized as much as possible including eyelid and fornix surgery if necessary. Ocular surface reconstruction and limbal transplantation may be considered prior to KPro and may improve the final outcome by providing a more stable surface [21]. Corneal melting can lead to device extrusion and may be exacerbated by thick RPM formation. Persistent epithelial defects can be a difficult problem, and we have had good success with scleral or hybrid lenses for the healing and long-term maintenance of ocular surface stability in these patients. Systemic immunosuppression may play a role in long-term management of patients with severe ocular surface disease and KPro implantation. Fortunately, infectious complications after Boston KPro have become significantly less common with the use of prophylactic antibiotics. Our current regimen, as described in the three cases above, varies depending on the risk. The one group of patients in whom we prefer not to perform KPro implantation unless absolutely necessary is Stevens-Johnson syndrome given their higher propensity to develop complications. When we do, we carefully select patients in the chronic phase with relatively controlled ocular surface inflammation.

Acknowledgments *Financial disclosures*: None.
Conflict of interest: None.

References

1. Holland E, Djalilian A, Schwartz G. Management of aniridic keratopathy with keratolimbal allograft: a limbal stem cell transplantation technique. Ophthalmology. 2003;110:125–30.
2. Akpek EK, Harissi-Dagher M, Petrarca R, Butrus SI, Pineda R, Aquavella JV, Dohlman CH. Outcomes of Boston keratoprosthesis in aniridia: a retrospective multicenter study. Am J Ophthalmol. 2007;144(2):227–31.
3. Rixen JJ, Cohen AW, Kitzmann AS, Wagoner MD, Goins KM. Treatment of aniridia with Boston type I keratoprosthesis. Cornea. 2013;32(7):947–50.
4. Hassanaly SI, Talajic JC, Harissi-Dagher M. Outcomes following Boston type 1 Keratoprosthesis implantation in aniridia patients at the University of Montreal. Am J Ophthalmol. 2014;158(2):270–6.
5. Sivaraman KR, Hou JH, Allemann N, de la Cruz J, Cortina MS. Retroprosthetic membrane and risk of sterile keratolysis in patients with type I Boston Keratoprosthesis. Am J Ophthalmol. 2013;155(5):814–22.
6. Chan CC, Loverde L, Qiang J, Nordlund ML, Holland EJ. Incidence, risk factors and surgical management of Boston type I keratoprosthesis corneal melts, leaks and extrusions. Cornea. 2016;35:1049–56.
7. Rudnisky CJ, Belin MW, Todani A, et al. Risk factors for the development of retroprosthetic membranes with Boston keratoprosthesis type 1: multicenter study results. Ophthalmology. 2012;119(5):951–5.
8. Birnbaum F, Mayweg S, Reis A, Böhringer D, Seitz B, Engelmann K, Messmer EM, Reinhard T. Mycophenolate mofetil (MMF) following penetrating high-risk keratoplasty: long-term results of a prospective, randomised, multicentre study. Eye (Lond). 2009;23(11):2063–70.
9. Birnbaum F, Böhringer D, Sokolovska Y, Sundmacher R, Reinhard T. Immunosuppression with cyclosporine A and mycophenolate mofetil after penetrating high-risk keratoplasty: a retrospective study. Transplantation. 2005;79(8):964–8.
10. Joseph A, Raj D, Shanmuganathan V, Powell RJ, Dua HS. Tacrolimus immunosuppression in high-risk corneal grafts. Br J Ophthalmol. 2007;91(1):51–5.
11. Burcu A, et al. Surgical rehabilitation following ocular chemical injury. Cutan Ocul Toxicol. 2014;33(1):42–8.
12. Chan CC, Biber JM, Holland EJ. The modified Cincinnati procedure: combined conjunctival limbal autografts and keratolimbal allografts for severe unilateral ocular surface failure. Cornea. 2012;31(11):1264–72.
13. Magalhães FP, Hirai FE, de Sousa LB, de Oliveira LA. Boston type 1 keratoprosthesis outcomes in ocular burns. Acta Ophthalmol. 2013;91(6):e432–6.
14. Phillips DL, Hager JL, Goins KM, Kitzmann AS, Greiner MA, Cohen AW, Welder JD, Wagoner MD. Boston type 1 keratoprosthesis for chemical and thermal injury. Cornea. 2014;33(9):905–9.
15. de Rezende Couto Nascimento V, de la Paz MF, Rosandic J, Stoiber J, Seyeddain O, Grabner G, Alvarez de Toledo J, Barraquer RI, Michael R. Influence of primary diagnosis and complications on visual outcome in patients receiving a Boston type 1 keratoprosthesis. Ophthalmic Res. 2014;52(1):9–16.
16. Kang JJ, de la Cruz J, Cortina MS. Visual outcomes of Boston keratoprosthesis implantation as the primary penetrating corneal procedure. Cornea. 2012;31(12):1436–40.
17. Rootman DB, Kim MJ, Aldave AJ, Douglas R, Hwang C, Goldberg R. Ocular surface, fornix, and eyelid rehabilitation in Boston type I keratoprosthesis patients with mucous membrane disease. Ophthal Plast Reconstr Surg. 2015;31(1):43–9.
18. Rosenthal P, Croteau A. Fluid-ventilated, gas-permeable scleral contact lens is an effective option for managing severe ocular surface disease and many corneal disorders that would otherwise require penetrating keratoplasty. Eye Contact Lens. 2005;31(3):130–4.

19. Rosenthal P, Cotter JM, Baum J. Treatment of persistent corneal epithelial defect with extended wear of a fluid-ventilated gas-permeable scleral contact lens. Am J Ophthalmol. 2000;130(1):33–41.
20. DeSousa JL, Daya S, Malhotra R. Adnexal surgery in patients undergoing ocular surface stem cell transplantation. Ophthalmology. 2009;116(2):235–42.
21. Hou JH, De La Cruz J, Djalilian AD. Outcomes of Boston keratoprosthesis implantation for failed keratoplasty after keratolimbal allograft. Cornea. 2012;31(12):1432–5.

Chapter 23
Ocular Surface Reconstruction Using Cultivated Corneal and Oral Mucosal Epithelial Transplantation

Tsutomu Inatomi, Takahiro Nakamura, Noriko Koizumi, Chie Sotozono, and Shigeru Kinoshita

Basic Concept and Indication of Cultivated Epithelial Sheet Transplantation

The cultivated epithelial sheet that we use for successful ocular surface reconstruction consists of several key biological elements [1, 2]. First, the primary cells used for initial culture should contain the appropriate number of progenitor cells in order to maintain the long-term survival and wound healing post transplantation. When properly constructed, the epithelial cell sheet used in the transplantation provides rapid coverage of the ocular surface, thus resulting in reduced inflammation and postoperative complications [3]. The second aspect is sufficient stratification and differentiation prior to the surgery, which is essential for efficient initial attachment onto the ocular surface. In order to obtain good differentiation, amniotic membrane (AM) is used for the substrate to provide for good hemidesmosome formation at the basal side, and the "air lifting" process promotes the terminal differentiation and tight barrier function [4]. The quality of the cell sheet is routinely confirmed at the end of the culture process, and fluorescein staining is performed on the transplanted sheet at the end of surgery. The third aspect is application of autologous non-ocular tissue as a source of the regenerative epithelial

T. Inatomi, MD, PhD (✉) • T. Nakamura, MD, PhD • C. Sotozono, MD, PhD
Department of Ophthalmology, Kyoto Prefectural University of Medicine, Kyoto, Japan
e-mail: tinatomi@koto.kpu-m.ac.jp; tnakamur@koto.kpu-m.ac.jp; csotozon@koto.kpu-m.ac.jp

N. Koizumi, MD, PhD
Department of Biomedical Engineering, Faculty of Life and Medical Sciences, Doshisha University, Kyoto, Japan

Department of Ophthalmology, Kyoto Prefectural University of Medicine, Kyoto, Japan
e-mail: nkoizumi@mail.doshisha.ac.jp

S. Kinoshita, MD, PhD
Department of Frontier Medical Science and Technology for Ophthalmology, Kyoto Prefectural University of Medicine, Kyoto, Japan
e-mail: shigeruk@koto.kpu-m.ac.jp

A.R. Djalilian (ed.), *Ocular Surface Disease*,
https://doi.org/10.1007/978-3-319-15823-5_23

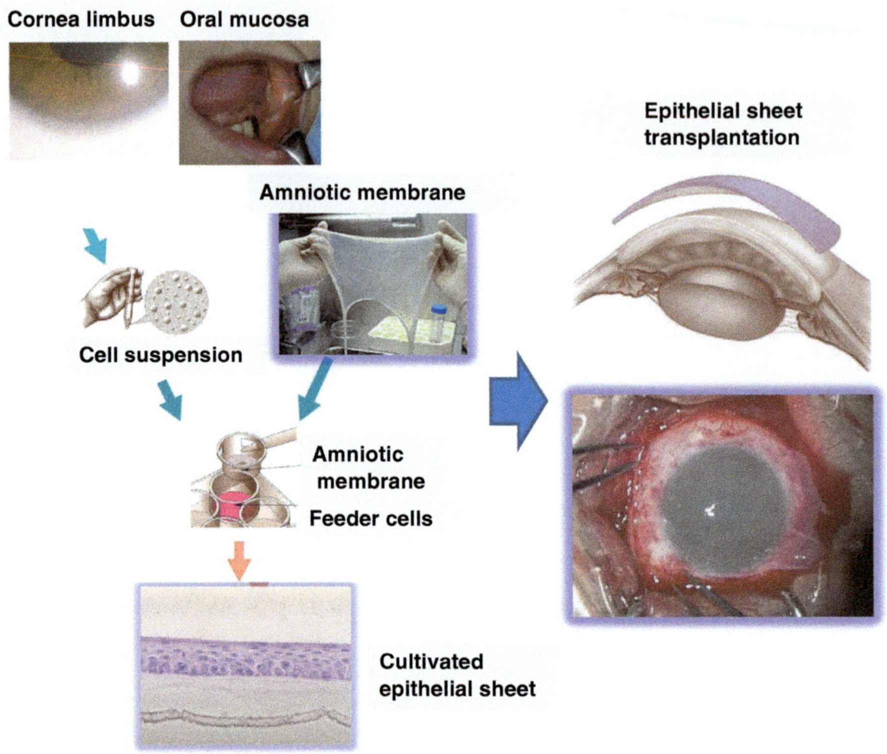

Fig. 23.1 Ocular surface reconstruction using novel regenerative medicine

sheet to eliminate the risk of allogeneic immune response. Our current protocols allow us to select from two different cell sources, corneal epithelium and oral mucosal epithelium. Sufficient understanding of the clinical characteristics of each transplantation technique is necessary in order to determine the proper indications (Fig. 23.1).

Cultivated Limbal Epithelial Transplantation (CLET) for Limbal Stem Cell Deficiency

Case 1: Treatment of Unilateral Stem Cell Deficiency with Auto-CLET

Autologous cultivated limbal epithelial transplantation (i.e., auto-CLET) is an ideal surgical modality used for avoiding the risk of immunological reaction when treating unilateral cases [5]. In such cases, a 2 × 3 mm limbal biopsy is performed, with the biopsy specimen then cultured on AM to obtain the cultivated sheet. The cultured sheet is then transplanted over the corneal surface after the scarred tissue is removed. Systemic steroids are then used for a maximum of 1–3 weeks postoperative for quick reduction of the surgically induced inflammation. Antibiotics and 0.1% betamethasone are used for 1–3 months postoperative and then tapered and switched to 0.1% fluorometholone to maintain the stable reconstructed ocular surface. A medical-use soft contact lens is used for 3–6 months postoperative to promote complete graft attachment and to prevent any physiological damage caused by a scarred lid margin or dry eye. For long-term postoperative maintenance a minimum dose of 0.1% fluorometholone and protective agents such as 0.1% sodium hyaluronate are used to protect the ocular surface.

The case shown in Fig. 23.2 was a 53-year-old male who suffered from unilateral chemical burn. For treatment, he underwent auto-CLET using a healthy limbal biopsy from his fellow eye. His corneal surface was successfully reconstructed via the cultivated

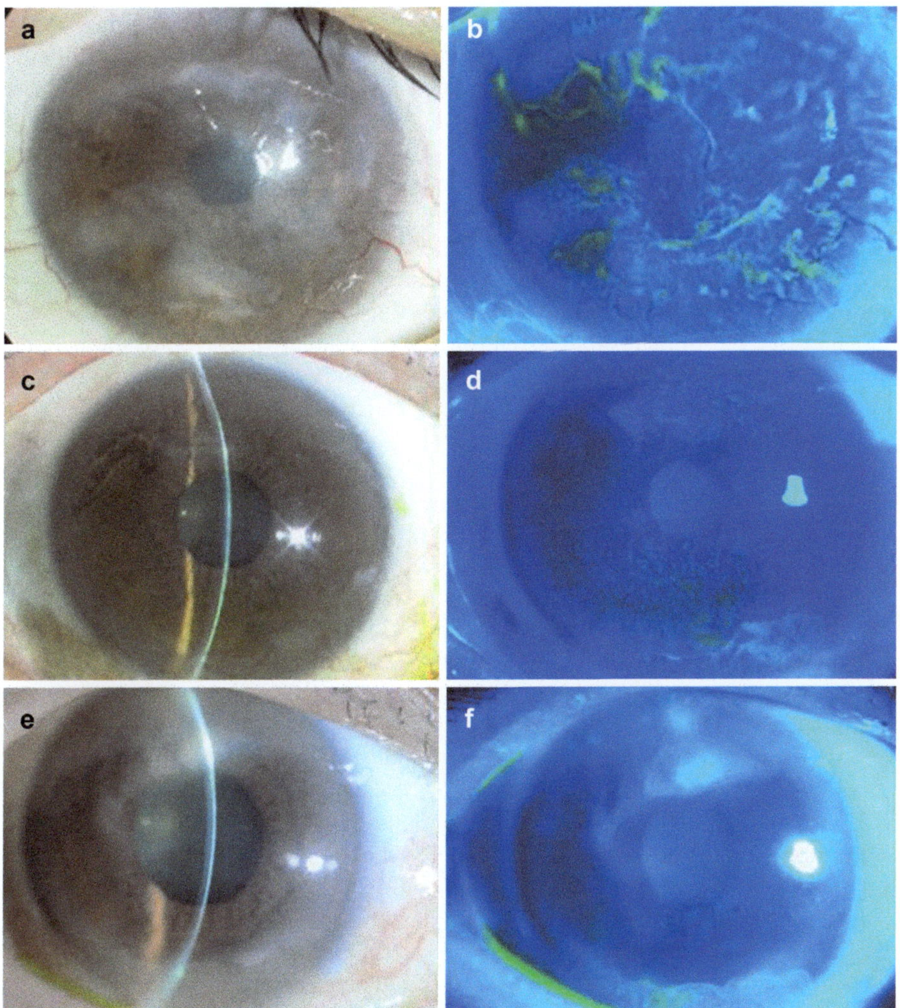

Fig. 23.2 Auto-CLET in a case of unilateral chemical burn. (**a**, **b**) presurgery; (**c**, **d**) 4 years post-CLET; (**e**, **f**) 14 years post-CLET

autologous corneal epithelium, and his visual acuity (VA) recovered to 0.7. Although mild conjunctival invasion was observed at 14-years [5] postoperative, a clear optical zone was maintained in the transplanted corneal epithelium, thus suggesting a long-term supply of regenerative epithelial progenitor cells in the transplanted cell sheet.

Case 2: Allogeneic Cultivated Limbal Epithelial Transplantation (Allo-CLET)

Allo-CLET is an effective procedure that utilizes donor corneal epithelial progenitor cells to enable reconstruction of the diseased host eye without the need of a biopsy [6, 7]. However, long-term intensive immunosuppression post surgery is essential to prevent immunological rejection. Acute-phase corneal-stem-cell depletion, such as in cases of severe chemical burn with persistent corneal epithelial defect that extends over a long period of time and without wound healing, should be considered the indication for allo-CLET [8]. Moreover, allo-CLET. is sometimes indicated in bilateral cases, in which the most intensive treatment is required to obtain visual recovery, as well as unilateral cases, in which preservation of the healthy fellow eye is vital.

General preoperative examination is essential in order to exclude the risk of activation of any possible infections, such as viral hepatitis and obsolete pulmonary tuberculosis, by immunosuppression. Moreover, regular follow-up of the patient's general condition via blood tests is required in order to uncover any drug-related complications such as hepatic and renal toxicity and cytopenia. Monitoring of the drug concentration in plasma is also important in order to adjust the amount of drug needed to maintain an effective level in the blood (Fig. 23.3).

The case of a 58-year-old male who sustained bilateral chemical burns is shown in Fig. 23.4. Prior to surgery, his left eye showed total conjunctival invasion with minimum stromal scarring. No severe cicatrization was observed, and the tear film was well preserved. After undergoing allo-CLET, his VA recovered to 0.8. Following our standard protocol for allo-CLET, intensive immunosuppression was applied both topically and systemically. As a local treatment in such cases, 0.1% betamethasone should be used for as long as possible, except in cases with steroid-associated complications. The additional use of tacrolimus eye drops should be considered for cases with severe inflammation or steroid-induced high intraocular pressure (IOP). After sufficient stabilization, 0.1% betamethasone can be tapered and switched to 0.1% fluorometholone to reduce the risk of complications associated with long-term steroid use. It is vitally important to apply sufficient systemic immunosuppression for at least 1.5-years postoperative to prevent the rejection. For intensive immunosuppression, 125 mg of methylprednisolone is administered intravenously on the day of surgery and at 3-days postoperative. A combination of three immunosuppressive medications (i.e., steroid, cyclosporine, and mycophenolate mofetil) is systemically used. Daily administration of 1–2 mg of betamethasone is initially used for 2-weeks postoperative, and then switched to 5–15 mg prednisolone. Moreover, 2–3 mg/kg of body weight (BW) of cyclosporin is initially used until the ocular

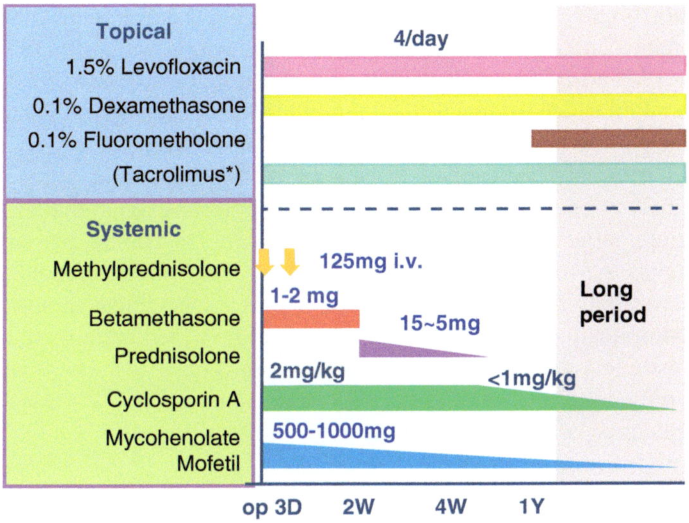

Fig. 23.3 Schema illustrating the standard postoperative treatment protocol for allo-CLET

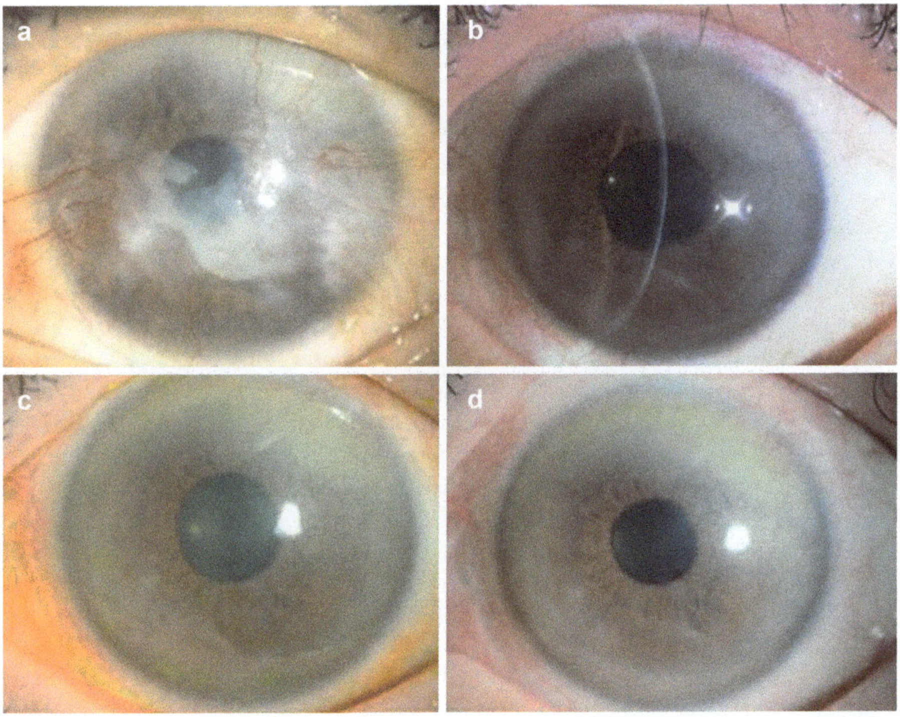

Fig. 23.4 Long-term results post allo-CLET for bilateral chemical burn. (**a**) pre surgery (**b**) 4-years postoperative; (**c**) 12-years postoperative; (**d**) 17-years postoperative

inflammation is sufficiently stabilized. The level of cyclosporin in the plasma should be monitored to prevent excessive absorption. The trough value should be adjusted to between 150 and 200 ng/mL to obtain effective immunosuppression. After reduction of the initial inflammation, 25–50 mg of low-dose cyclosporin is administered to the patient for a long-term immunosuppression of over 1.5 years. Blood tests should be routinely performed to monitor the liver and renal functions. Mycophenolate mofetil is an effective immunosuppressive agent that is suitable for preventing epithelial rejection, and it should be started at 100 mg per day, and then tapered to 500 mg following stabilization of the ocular inflammation. Since allo-CLET requires long-term immunosuppression post surgery, close monitoring of any systemic complications is essential. In the above-described case, the patient's cornea remained clear at over 17-years postoperative (Fig. 23.4). There were no episodes of epithelial rejection, and his VA was maintained at 0.8 via a twice-daily topical application of 0.1% fluorometholone.

Major Complications of Allo-CLET and Associated Solutions

Since allo-CLET requires long-term intensive immunosuppression post surgery, it is important to understand and prepare for any possible major complications that might occur. The primary disease, combined with the immunocompromised condition of the host, is associated with the risk of infection. Close monitoring of the bacterial flora in the conjunctiva is helpful for the selection of the proper antibiotics to successfully treat any growth of bacteria that might occur. Preexisting dry eye is one of the risk factors for epithelia-related problems, and strict adherence to the use of preservative-free artificial tears is crucial for proper maintenance of the epithelium.

Persistent Epithelial Defect

Epithelial defect is the most common problem when performing ocular surface reconstruction, and it has the possibility of developing into severe complications such as corneal ulceration, perforation, and infection. Prompt modification of the local treatment is crucial in order to promote epithelial healing and prevent further progression. To promote epithelial proliferation and migration, it is essential to minimize any possible drug-related toxicity. Switching to preservation-free eye drops and oral medication is a first step in the solution. A sufficient amount of artificial tears without preservatives should be supplied, and punctal plugs or occlusion should be considered. The use of an eye patch and temporal tarsorrhaphy is necessary for severe cases that are not effectively treated by local medications.

Epithelial Rejection

The risk of epithelial rejection is high, similar to when performing conventional limbal transplantation, and ciliary injection and surface-cell infiltration around the epithelial defect are typical clinical signs. Thus, intravenous injection of 125 mg of methylprednisolone is effective for the initial phase, and for increased local and general immunosuppression, systemic steroids (1–2 mg betamethasone for 1–2 weeks and then switched to prednisolone for a long-term use) and 1–3 mg/Kg BW of cyclosporine should be combined.

Infection

Resistant bacteria such as methicillin-resistant *Staphylococcus aureus* (MRSA) or methicillin-resistant coagulase-negative staphylococci (MR-CoNS) and yeast-type fungi such as candida are the most common organisms for infectious keratitis under the immunosuppression. Thus, slit-lamp observation and microbial examination are vital for selection of the optimal medication. During an active infection, local immunosuppressive agents should be tapered or interrupted, and laboratory testing should be conducted in order to select the proper antimicrobial agent. Natamycin ointment should be applied for fungal infection, yet its use should be limited and determined by the diagnosis of each case due to possible excessive toxicity to the epithelium. Performing regular bacterial cultures is important to monitor the growth of resistant bacteria, and is also helpful for the initial selection of the medication. Rotations of different types of antibiotics are effective to prevent the growth of resistant bacteria.

Steroid-Induced Glaucoma

Regular monitoring of the patient's IOP is necessary and is the best solution for steroid-induced glaucoma, especially in cases of severe chemical or thermal burn. Optic nerve examination via optical coherence tomography (OCT) and regular visual field examination should also be performed in order to avoid any possible inaccuracy of the IOP measurement. Topical steroid use should be tapered or interrupted, and an antiglaucoma agent should be applied. Moreover, a topical or systemic immunosuppressive agent such as cyclosporine or FK506 should be added in high-risk cases.

Benzalkonium chloride-free antiglaucoma eye drops in combination with an oral decarboxylase inhibitor should be selected to minimize the epithelial damage. Glaucoma surgery should be considered as the first-line surgical procedure for any uncontrolled cases.

COMET for Severe Bilateral Ocular Surface Disease

Cultivated autologous oral mucosal epithelial transplantation (COMET) is a new and effective surgical option for treating severe bilateral ocular surface diseases, including Stevens-Johnson syndrome (SJS) and ocular cicatricial pemphigoid (OCP) [9, 10]. Advancements in tissue engineering techniques and culture systems have enabled the development of a well-differentiated stratified oral mucosal epithelial sheet on AM that has a cornea-like epithelial structure [11]. COMET can provide a stabilized ocular surface with clinical advantages in comparison to CLET, especially in cases with chronic inflammation and severe dry eye [12–15]. COMET has no risk of immunological rejection, helps to minimize the use of anti-inflammatory medications, and reduces the allo-CLET-associated postoperative complications described above. Although the epithelial morphology appears to be similar with corneal epithelium, our previous study demonstrated that the ectopically survived oral mucosal epithelium maintained its original biological characteristics [16]. Neovascularization is observed in most cases, so it is important to control the postoperative inflammation and maintain the stable ocular surface condition. In severe cases, the apical surface exhibits metaplastic change and thickening of the epithelial layer. These biological changes are not ideal for the VA; however, it has the advantage that the stronger epithelial barrier and surface integrity prevent complications and limbal supported hard contact lens wear.

Postoperative Medication

As opposed to allo-CLET, COMET requires only minimal steroid and immunosuppressive agent usage to control the postoperative inflammation and primary disease. Antibiotics and 0.1% betamethasone eye drops are locally applied. Intravenous injection of 125 mg of methylprednisolone is used on the day of surgery and at 3-days postoperative. An oral dose of 1 mg of betamethasone is used from 14 to 30 days to reduce any surgically induced inflammation. An oral dose of 50–150 mg of cyclosporine is used from 1 to 3 months to reduce inflammation resulting from the primary disease, and it is effective for preventing the recurrence of cicatrization and neovascularization in the COMET graft. Frequent instillation of preservative-free artificial tears should be used to prevent an epithelial defect. A punctal plug and surgical occlusion should be applied if the puncta is open. Continuous wearing of a medical-use soft contact lens is essential to protect the transplanted oral mucosal epithelium and prevent defects.

Case 3: COMET and Limbal Supported Hard Contact Lens for SJS

The following case involved a 25-year-old female with SJS, who developed the disease when she was 4 years old after taking cold medicine for a high fever. As shown in Fig. 23.5, the surface of her right eye was severely cicatrized and keratinized, with no indication for COMET, and her left eye had severe symblepharon and conjunctivalization over the cornea. Although the Schirmer's test result was 2 mm, the presence of a low tear meniscus and wet mucous surface (i.e., not complete keratinaization) is a minimum requirement for the COMET indication. Her preoperative VA was 0.01, and she underwent ocular surface reconstruction via COMET when she was 26 years old. Her preoperative corneal thickness, as measured by OCT, was

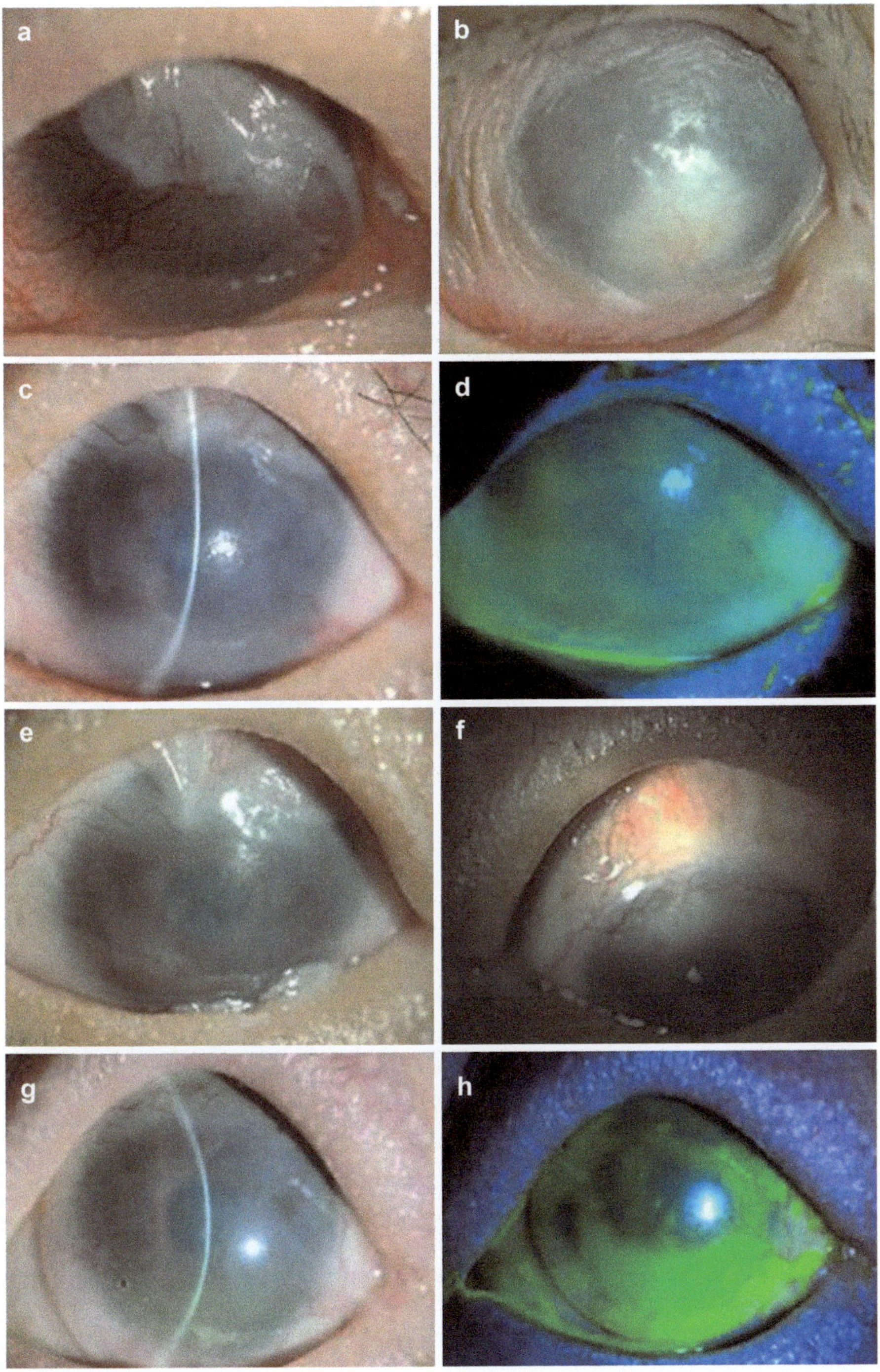

Fig. 23.5 COMET combined with limbal-supported HCL for visual rehabilitation. (**a**) preoperative condition of the patient's right eye; (**b**) the patient's left eye; (**c**) ocular surface reconstructed by COMET; (**e**) recurrence of symblepharon; (**f**) removal of cicatrization by amniotic membrane transplantation (AMT); (**g**, **h**) limbal-supported HCL

490 um, and a preoperative culture examination detected no bacteria. After removal of the scar tissue, intraoperative 0.04% mitomycin C (MMC) was applied to the subconjunctival space for 5 min, followed by AM transplantation (AMT) being performed over the entire ocular surface. She then underwent COMET using a 19-mm-diameter cultivated oral mucosal epithelial sheet. Post-COMET, her VA recovered to 0.4. In addition to the topical treatments, a systemic steroid (1 mg betamethasone per day) and cyclosporine A (50–100 mg per day) were administered for 1 month and 3 months, respectively. After stabilization of the reconstructed ocular surface, the survived oral mucosal epithelium was maintained via a twice-daily administration of topical antibiotics and 0.1% fluorometholone. Preservation-free artificial tears were applied every 30 min to 1 h to maintain moisture and prevent any severe metaplastic changes. At 6-years postoperative, symblepharon at the upper region was removed via a 3-min intraoperative application of 0.04% MMC and AMT so that the patient could wear a limbal-supported HCL (Kyoto-CS™; San Contact Lens, Kyoto, Japan) [17]. Daily wear of the limbal-supported HCL improved her VA to 0.5 and corrected the irregular astigmatism. It also effectively preserved tears in the interface between the corneal surface and the HCL, thus contributing to the clarity and wettability of the transplanted oral mucosal epithelium.

Case 4: Severe Bilateral Chemical Burn Treated with COMET and Delayed Lamellar Keratoplasty

The following case involved a 58-year-old male who was injured in both eyes with an acid burn at age 42. He is a steroid responder who lost vision in his left eye at the end stage of secondary glaucoma after a repeated limbal transplantation and LKP. The preoperative VA in his right eye was 0.02. COMET was selected for treatment in consideration of the fact the he was a steroid responder and the clinical course of his left eye.

Post COMET, his VA recovered to 0.1 and was well maintained with a twice-daily administration of 0.1% fluorometholone. He experienced a slow reduction of visual function following corneal opacification and the progression of cataract. Lamellar keratoplasty (LKP) was performed to remove lipid precipitates and hazy stroma. At 5-months post LKP and suture removal, cataract surgery was performed and his VA improved to 0.5. Step-by-step surgical management was effective for the long-term prognosis (Fig. 23.6) [18].

Fig. 23.6 Long-term surgical managements post-COMET in severe chemical burn. (**a, b**) Pre-COMET (VA: hand motion HM); (**c, d**) 1 year post-COMET (VA: 0.2); (**e**) 3 years post-COMET (VA: 0.08); (**f**) 8 years post-COMET (VA: 0.03); (**g**) post-LKP with cataract (VA:0.08); (**h**) post-phacoemulsification + IOL at 10 years post-COMET (VA: 0.5)

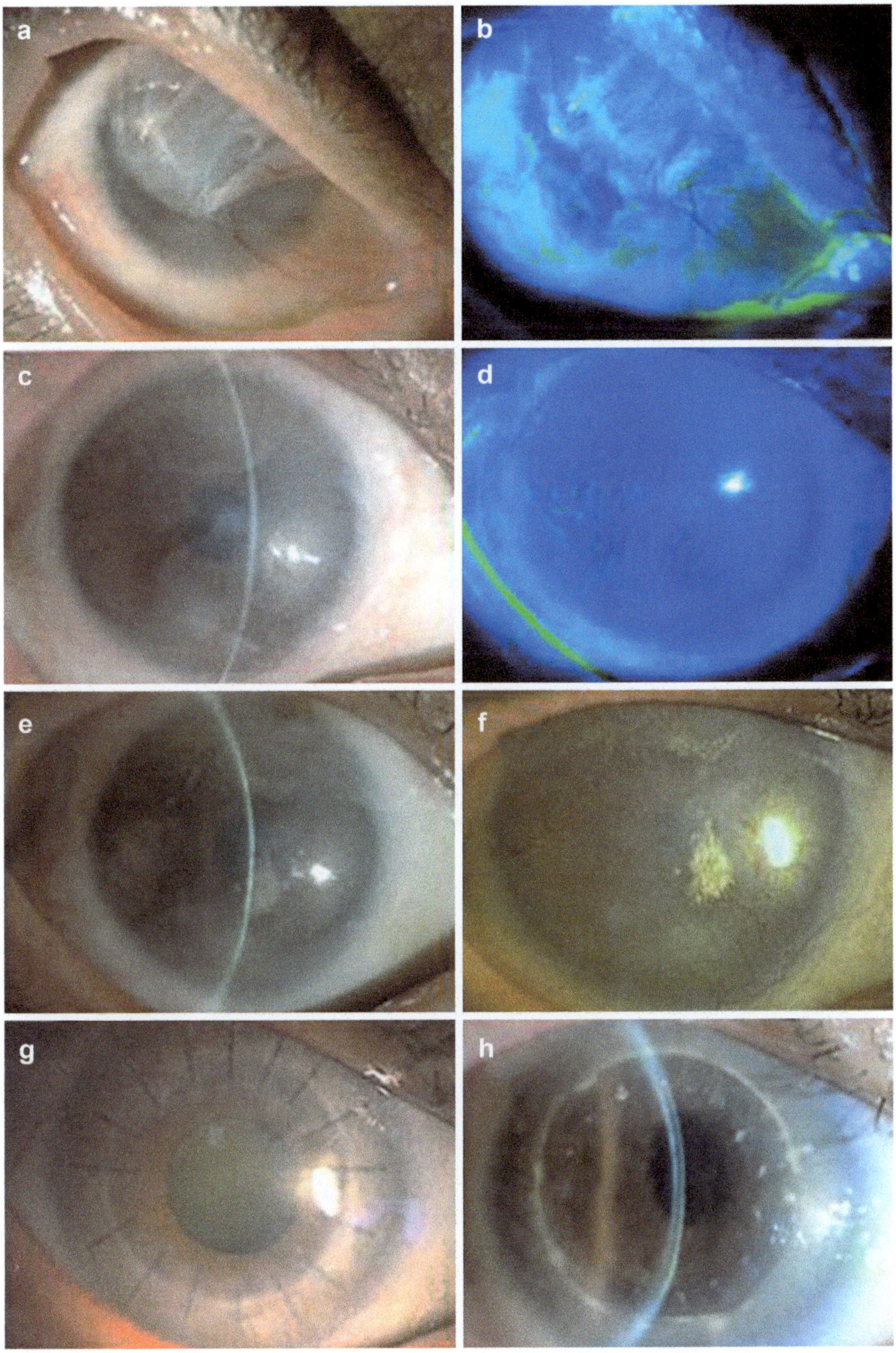
a
b
c
d
e
f
g
h

Summary

Tissue engineering techniques have brought a paradigm shift for ocular surface reconstruction and have provided us with the ability to improve the prognosis of untreatable cases using conventional procedures. The quality of the cultivated epithelial sheet used for transplantation is vital for the initial postoperative success. The choice of autologous non-ocular cells (i.e., oral mucosal epithelium) opens a new pathway for treating inflammation-associated severe bilateral cases without risk of rejection. COMET has been shown to be an extremely effective procedure to eliminate immunosuppression-associated complications and maintain a stabilized ocular surface. However, careful postoperative care and an understanding of the pathogenesis of the primary disease are essential to obtain long-term survival of the transplanted epithelium and a satisfactory prognosis. Current progress has been made to improve the tissue-engineering techniques and quality of epithelial sheet without using exogenic and undefined components for future treatments [19].

References

1. Kinoshita S, Koizumi N, Sotozono C, Yamada J, Nakamura T, Inatomi T. Concept and clinical application of cultivated epithelial transplantation for ocular surface disorders. Ocul Surf. 2004;2(1):21–33.
2. Nakamura T, Inatomi T, Sotozono C, Koizumi N, Kinoshita S. Ocular surface reconstruction using stem cell and tissue engineering. Prog Retin Eye Res. 2016;51:187–207.
3. Ang LP, Sotozono C, Koizumi N, Suzuki T, Inatomi T, Kinoshita S. A comparison between cultivated and conventional limbal stem cell transplantation for Stevens-Johnson syndrome. Am J Ophthalmol. 2007;143(1):178–80.
4. Koizumi N, Fullwood NJ, Bairaktaris G, Inatomi T, Kinoshita S, Quantock AJ. Cultivation of corneal epithelial cells on intact and denuded human amniotic membrane. Invest Ophthalmol Vis Sci. 2000;41(9):2506–13.
5. Nakamura T, Inatomi T, Sotozono C, Koizumi N, Kinoshita S. Successful primary culture and autologous transplantation of corneal limbal epithelial cells from minimal biopsy for unilateral severe ocular surface disease. Acta Ophthalmol Scand. 2004;82(4):468–71.
6. Koizumi N, Inatomi T, Suzuki T, Sotozono C, Kinoshita S. Cultivated corneal epithelial stem cell transplantation in ocular surface disorders. Ophthalmology. 2001;108(9):1569–74.
7. Nakamura T, Sotozono C, Bentley AJ, Mano S, Inatomi T, Koizumi N, Fullwood NJ, Kinoshita S. Long-term phenotypic study after allogeneic cultivated corneal limbal epithelial transplantation for severe ocular surface diseases. Ophthalmology. 2010;117(12):2247–54.
8. Koizumi N, Inatomi T, Suzuki T, Sotozono C, Kinoshita S. Cultivated corneal epithelial transplantation for ocular surface reconstruction in acute phase of Stevens-Johnson syndrome. Arch Ophthalmol. 2001;119(2):298–300.
9. Nakamura T, Inatomi T, Sotozono C, Amemiya T, Kanamura N, Kinoshita S. Transplantation of cultivated autologous oral mucosal epithelial cells in patients with severe ocular surface disorders. Br J Ophthalmol. 2004;88:1280–4.
10. Nakamura T, Takeda K, Inatomi T, Sotozono C, Kinoshita S. Long-term results of autologous cultivated oral mucosal epithelial transplantation in the scar phase of severe ocular surface disorders. Br J Ophthalmol. 2010;95(7):942–6.

11. Nakamura T, Endo K, Cooper LJ, Fullwood NJ, Tanifuji N, Tsuzuki M, Koizumi N, Inatomi T, Sano Y, Kinoshita S. The successful culture and autologous transplantation of rabbit oral mucosal epithelial cells on amniotic membrane. Invest Ophthalmol Vis Sci. 2003;44(1):106–16.
12. Inatomi T, Nakamura T, Koizumi N, Sotozono C, Yokoi N, Kinoshita S. Midterm results of ocular surface reconstruction using cultivated autologous oral mucosal epithelial transplantation. Am J Ophthalmol. 2006;141(2):267–75.
13. Takeda K, Nakamura T, Inatomi T, Sotozono C, Watanabe A, Kinoshita S. Ocular surface reconstruction using the combination of autologous cultivated oral mucosal epithelial transplantation and eyelid surgery for severe ocular surface disease. Am J Ophthalmol. 2011;152(2):195–201.
14. Sotozono C, Inatomi T, Nakamura T, Koizumi N, Yokoi N, Ueta M, Matsuyama K, Miyakoda K, Kaneda H, Fukushima M, Kinoshita S. Visual improvement after cultivated oral mucosal epithelial transplantation. Ophthalmology. 2013;120(1):193–200.
15. Sotozono C, Inatomi T, Nakamura T, Koizumi N, Yokoi N, Ueta M, Matsuyama K, Kaneda H, Fukushima M, Kinoshita S. Cultivated oral mucosal epithelial transplantation for persistent epithelial defect in severe ocular surface diseases with acute inflammatory activity. Acta Ophthalmol. 2014;92(6):e447–53.
16. Nakamura T, Inatomi T, Cooper LJ, Rigby H, Fullwood NJ, Kinoshita S. Phenotypic investigation of human eyes with transplanted autologous cultivated oral mucosal epithelial sheets for severe ocular surface diseases. Ophthalmology. 2007;114(6):1080–8.
17. Sotozono C, Yamauchi N, Maeda S, Kinoshita S. Tear exchangeable limbal rigid contact lens for ocular sequelae resulting from Stevens-Johnson syndrome or toxic epidermal necrolysis. Am J Ophthalmol. 2014;158(5):983–93.
18. Inatomi T, Nakamura T, Kojyo M, Koizumi N, Sotozono C, Kinoshita S. Ocular surface reconstruction with combination of cultivated autologous oral mucosal epithelial transplantation and penetrating keratoplasty. Am J Ophthalmol. 2006;142(5):757–64.
19. Nakamura T, Yokoo S, Bentley AJ, Nagata M, Fullwood NJ, Inatomi T, Sotozono C, Yamagami S, Kinoshita S. Development of functional human oral mucosal epithelial stem/progenitor cell sheets using a feeder-free and serum-free culture system for ocular surface reconstruction. Sci Rep. 2016;6:37173.

Index

A.R. Djalilian (ed.), *Ocular Surface Disease*,
https://doi.org/10.1007/978-3-319-15823-5

D

O

P

R

S

T

CPI Antony Rowe
Chippenham, UK
2018-09-04 22:56